AF878872

THE LUNG
Structure, Function and Disease

INTERNATIONAL ACADEMY OF PATHOLOGY

MONOGRAPHS IN PATHOLOGY

SERIES EDITOR, **Murray R. Abell, M.D.**

Professor, Department of Pathology,
University of Michigan Medical School, Ann Arbor, Michigan

No. 1. **The Lymphocyte and Lymphocytic Tissue**
John W. Rebuck *and* Robert E. Stowell, *Editors*
No. 2. **The Adrenal Cortex**
Henry D. Moon *and* Robert E. Stowell, *Editors*
No. 3. **The Ovary**
Hugh G. Grady *and* David E. Smith, *Editors*
No. 4. **The Peripheral Blood Vessels**
J. Lowell Orbison *and* David E. Smith, *Editors*
No. 5. **The Thyroid**
J. Beach Hazard *and* David E. Smith, *Editors*
No. 6. **The Kidney**
F. K. Mostofi *and* David E. Smith, *Editors*
No. 7. **The Connective Tissue**
Bernard M. Wagner *and* David E. Smith, *Editors*
No. 8. **The Lung**
Averill A. Liebow *and* David E. Smith, *Editors*
No. 9. **The Brain**
Orville T. Bailey *and* David E. Smith, *Editors*
No. 10. **The Skin**
Elson B. Helwig *and* F. K. Mostofi, *Editors*
No. 11. **The Platelet**
K. M. Brinkhous, R. W. Shermer, *and* F. K. Mostofi, *Editors*
No. 12. **The Striated Muscle**
Carl M. Pearson *and* F. K. Mostofi, *Editors*
No. 13. **The Liver**
Edward A. Gall *and* F. K. Mostofi, *Editors*
No. 14. **The Uterus**
Henry J. Norris, Arthur T. Hertig *and* Murray R. Abell, *Editors*
No. 15. **The Heart**
Jesse E. Edwards, Maurice Lev, *and* Murray R. Abell, *Editors*
No. 16. **The Reticuloendothelial System**
John W. Rebuck, Costan W. Berard, *and* Murray R. Abell, *Editors*
No. 17. **Bones and Joints**
Lauren V. Ackerman, Harlan J. Spjut, *and* Murray R. Abell, *Editors*
No. 18. **The Gastrointestinal Tract**
John H. Yardley, Basil. C. Morson, *and* Murray R. Abell, *Editors*
No. 19. **The Lung**
Structure, Function and Disease
William M. Thurlbeck *and* Murray R. Abell, *Editors*
Succeeding Volumes to Be Announced

INTERNATIONAL ACADEMY OF PATHOLOGY MONOGRAPH

THE LUNG

Structure, Function and Disease

by 23 authors

EDITED BY **WILLIAM M. THURLBECK,**
M.B., Ch.B., F.R.C.P.(C), M.R.C. Path., F.C.C.P.

Professor and Head of Pathology
University of Manitoba,
Winnipeg, Manitoba, Canada

AND MURRAY R. ABELL, M.D., Ph.D.

Department of Pathology
University of Michigan Medical School, Ann Arbor, Michigan

SANS TACHE

THE WILLIAMS & WILKINS COMPANY
BALTIMORE, 1978

C11T 2/23/79 $34.00 JB

Copyright ©, 1978
The United States—Canadian Division of
THE INTERNATIONAL ACADEMY OF PATHOLOGY

All rights reserved. This book is protected by copyright. No part of this book may be reproduced in any form or by any means, including photocopying, or utilized by any information storage and retrieval system without written permission from the copyright owner.

Made in the United States of America

Library of Congress Cataloging in Publication Data
Main entry under title:

The Lung: structure, function, and disease.

(Monographs in pathology; no. 19)
Includes bibliographies and index.
1. Lungs—Diseases. 2. Lungs. I. Thurlbeck, William M. II. Abell, Murray R. III. Series: International Academy of Pathology. Monographs in pathology; no. 19.
RC756.L84 616.2'4 77-16655
ISBN 0-683-08274-4

COMPOSED AND PRINTED AT
WAVERLY PRESS, INC.
Mt. Royal and Guilford Aves.
Baltimore, MD. 21202, U.S.A.

Contents

Contributing Authors

JERROLD L. ABRAHAM, B.S., M.D.
Department of Pathology, University of California, San Diego, La Jolla, California.

CHARLES B. CARRINGTON, M.D.,
Associate Professor of Pathology, Stanford University School of Medicine, Stanford, California.

SOLON COLE, M.D.
Department of Pathology, Hartford Hospital, Hartford, Connecticut

MANUEL G. COSIO, M.D.
Assistant Professor of Medicine, University of Minnesota Medical School, Director, Pulmonary Functions Laboratories, Veterans Administration Hospital, Minneapolis, Minn.

JESSIE E. EDWARDS, B.S., M.D.
Department of Pathology, United Hospitals, St. Paul, Minnesota

DAVID FAGAN, M.D.
Department of Pathology, The Hospital for Sick Children, Toronto, Canada.

GORDON T. FORD, M.D.
Department of Medicine, University of Manitoba, Winnipeg, Manitoba, Canada.

EDWARD A. GAENSLER, M.D.
Professor of Surgery & Physiology, Boston University, Boston, Massachusetts.

DENNIS G. GILLETT, M.D.
Department of Pathology, University of Manitoba, Winnipeg, Manitoba, Canada.

J. C. HOGG, M.D., M.Sc., Ph.D., F.R.C.P.(C),
Professor of Pathology, McGill University, Montreal, Quebec, Canada.

KEITH HORSFIELD, PH.D., M.D., F.R.C.P.
Senior Investigator, Midhurst Medical Research Institute, Midhurst, West Sussex, England.

HARRY L. IOACHIM, M.D.
Clinical Professor of Pathology, College of Physicians & Surgeons of Columbia University, New York, New York, Attending Pathologist, Lenox Hill Hospital, New York, New York.

CHARLES KUHN, III, M.D.
Professor of Pathology, Washington University, St. Louis, Missouri.

CLAIRE LANGSTON, B.A., M.D.
Department of Pathology, University of Manitoba, Winnipeg, Manitoba, Canada.

RICHARD L. NAEYE, A. B., M.D.
Professor & Chairman of Pathology, Milton S. Hershey Medical Center, Hershey, Pennsylvania.

DENNIS E. NIEWOEHNER, M.D.
Associate Professor of Medicine, University of Minnesota Medical School, Chief, Pulmonary Section Veterans Administration Hospital, Minneapolis, Minnesota.

GIUSEPPE PIETRA, M.D.
Professor of Pathology and Director, Division of Pathologic Anatomy, Hospital of the University of Pennsylvania, Philadelphia, Pennsylvania.

PHILIP C. PRATT, A.B., M.D.
Professor of Pathology, Duke University Medical Center, Durham, North Carolina.

LYNNE M. REID, M.D., M.R.C.P., F.R.C.Path., F.R.A.C.P.
S. Burt Wolback Professor of Pathology, Harvard Medical Center, Boston, Massachusetts, Chairman of Pathology, Children's Hospital Medical Center, Boston, Massachusetts.

ROBERT M. SENIOR, M.D.
Associate Professor of Medicine, Washington University School of Medicine and Co-director, Pulmonary Disease and Respiratory Care Division, Department of Medicine, The Jewish Hospital of St. Louis, St. Louis, Missouri.

WILLIAM M. THURLBECK, M.B., Ch.B., F.R.C.P.(C), M.R.C.Path., F.C.C.P.
Professor and Head of Pathology, University of Manitoba, Winnipeg, Manitoba, Canada.

PETER A. WARD, M.D.
Professor and Chairman of Pathology, University of Connecticut Health Center, Farmington, Connecticut.

Foreword

This monograph, *The Lung*, is the 19th in the series of *Monographs in Pathology* initiated by the International Academy of Pathology in 1959. The various chapters are based on lectures and illustrative materials that comprised the Academy's Long Course, "Recent Advances in Pumonary Pathology", given at the 66th Annual Meeting of the United States-Canadian Division of the Academy in Atlanta, Georgia, in March, 1977. It is the second monograph that the Academy has published on diseases of the lung, the first being compiled and edited by Dr. Averill A. Liebow in 1968. It contains and reflects the tremendously expanded knowledge of pulmonary structure, function and disease that has accumulated in the interval.

The Long Courses of the Academy, and their offspring the Monographs in Pathology, comprise one of the major facets of the educational program of the Academy and contribute greatly to its educational goals for its members and fellow pathologists in many countries.

Dr. William M. Thurlbeck, Professor and Head of the Department of Pathology, The University of Manitoba, gathered an impressive faculty of scientists and clinicians for the Long Course, "Recent Advances in Pulmonary Pathology". Their presentations in this monograph are an invaluable compilation of information and a permanent reference for all who are interested in and seek further understanding of the Pulmonary Diseases. The wealth of basic and clinical information within these chapters stands as a testimony to the authors' industry and accomplishments in further elucidating the riddles of pulmonary disease.

The Academy expresses its sincere appreciation to Dr. Thurlbeck and to his distinguished faculty who have contributed of their knowledge and effort to this monograph, and to the publishers, The Williams and Wilkins Company, for their valuable support.

Ann Arbor, Michigan

M. R. Abell, M. D., Ph.D.
Series Editor

This Monograph is dedicated to the memory of PROFESSOR AVERILL A. LIEBOW *and to* PROFESSOR JETHRO GOUGH *in recognition of their many contributions to the understanding of pulmonary disease.*

Preface

The lung was last a topic of the annual IAP Long Course in 1966. The course was directed by Averill Liebow, who also edited the IAP monograph, *The Lung*, edited by A.A. Liebow and D. E. Smith, The Williams & Wilkins Company, Baltimore, 1968. It is interesting to read that volume and the present one and it immediately becomes apparent how much the knowledge of the lung has advanced since then. The major advances have been in cell biology and biochemistry and we were perhaps remiss in not including a presentation on the metabolic functions of the lung. The discovery of surfactant provoked profound interest in biochemistry; no longer was it appropriate to consider the lung a metabolically inactive bellows. It is now clear that the lung is an actively secreting endocrine and exocrine organ. In 1966 the ultrastructure of the lung was poorly studied, and only a few physicians were familiar with such information as was available. Today the ultrastructure of the lung is much better understood, many additional cell types are known (depending on the ground rules, there may be at least 40 different cell types in the lung) and most medical students, pathologists, and chest physicians are reasonably well informed concerning lung ultrastructure.

Three of today's participants took part in the 1966 Long Course—Lynne Reid, Richard Naeye, and Charles Carrington. Lynne Reid spoke on mucus secretion at the last course also; her current presentation underlines the considerable advances in cell biologic phenomena made by her in the intervening time. Richard Naeye discussed the pathology of the pulmonary vasculature and it was his experience and interest in the pulmonary vascular changes in hypoxemia that were in part responsible for his insight into the pathogenesis of the Sudden Infant Death Syndrome, which has created so much excitement and interest recently. Charles Carrington, who had just joined the faculty at Yale, read a paper describing techniques in investigating the lung but was also intimately concerned with Dr. Liebow's contribution "New Concepts in Pulmonary Disease." Items discussed that Dr. Carrington has helped elucidate include the eosinophilic pneumonias and the limited form of Wegener's granuloma. The chapter also included an early account of the classification of the interstitial pneumonias, a topic that is covered particularly in this monograph by Drs. Carrington and Gaensler.

Two other items of interest emerge from perusing the last monograph. Four chapters were primarily concerned with clinical respiratory physiology: little mention is made of pulmonary physiology in this volume and this represents the fact that pulmonary physiology is no longer the cutting edge of research in the lung. The main thrusts today are cellular biology and experimental pathology and a great opportunity exists for pathologists to play a dominant role in lung research. Pulmonary pathology is recognized as an important subject by pulmonary physicians and pathologists alike and there are great opportunities for pathologists to specialize and do research in pulmonary disease, using methods with which they are naturally familiar. The second noteworthy item in the previous monograph comes from reading the chapter "Genetics and Pulmonary Disease." In that excellent review, the problem of familial emphysema was reviewed; two recent reports were discussed and a quotation from a well known textbook was included stating "that available evidence does not support the role of heredity in chronic obstructive pulmonary emphysema." Since then the genetics of the proteinase inhibitor system have been worked out, the biochemistry of $alpha_1$ antitrypsin extensively studied and the significance of $alpha_1$ antitrypsin in relation to emphysema described at great length.

The last volume was an excellent source book. It, of necessity, was not a textbook, nor can this one be a textbook. The participants of this course were chosen because they were recognized authorities in their own field of interest and because these fields are of importance to pathologists and chest physicians at this time. I have taken the liberty of writing a closing chapter which attempts to provide an explanation for the choice of topics and a link between them. It also will fill in a few gaps in recent advances of current knowledge and thus it should provide a broader perspective to the general readership. It also became apparent that the important topic of Drug-Induced Lung Injury had not been covered at the time of the symposium. I thus asked Dr. Dennis Gillett, a fellow in pulmonary pathology at the University of Manitoba, and Dr. Gordon Ford, research fellow in the Department of Medicine, to write a chapter on this topic, although they were not participants at the symposium in Toronto.

This monograph is dedicated to Averill Liebow and Jethro Gough, the founding fathers of modern pulmonary pathology. Coming from different continents, it is also appropriate that their contributions were to a large extent complementary. Professor Gough and the Head of the Department of Pathology at the Welsh National Medical School in Cardiff, Wales. He was primarily interested in medical lung disease and lungs derived from necropsy studies. His major technical contribution was the development of the paper-mounted whole-lung sections which were then used in this department to unravel the complex problems of pulmonary emphysema and coal workers' pneumoconiosis. Dr. Averill Liebow, first at Yale and then as the founding professor of Pathology at the New Medical School in La Jolla, was also responsible for a major technical advance, that of making casting of the pulmonary vasculature and the airways feasible. He made notable advances using this technique in experimental situations and medical conditions. However, Dr. Averill Liebow is perhaps best known for his contributions to the unraveling and understanding of diseases in living patients from tissue obtained by surgical biopsy. The dedication of this volume indicates our debt to them.

Winnipeg, Manitoba

WILLIAM M. THURLBECK
Monograph Editor

Chapter 1

Ultrastructure and Cellular Function in the Distal Lung*

CHARLES KUHN, III

Many of the structures of the normal alveolar wall are near or below the limits of resolution of the light microscope. Consequently, the early application of electron microscopy to the lung was aimed at defining the basic cell populations and the organization of the alveolar walls. More recent studies have been concerned with the functional aspects of pulmonary ultrastructure and, with the localization and organization of biochemical and physiologic process. This chapter will review some examples of studies of this type. Many of the conclusions which will be offered are still quite speculative, indicating how much we have still to learn about the cell biology of even the normal lung.

THE ALVEOLAR EPITHELIUM

The alveolar surface is covered mainly by two types of lining cells (Fig. 1) which are joined by tight junctions.[28, 61] The larger is the squamous or type I epithelial cell. This simple-appearing cell is actually highly specialized, specialized in shape, or, as Weibel and co-workers[62] have stated, topologically specialized. It sends out extensive thin sheets of cytoplasm which cover large areas potentially available for gas exchange (Fig. 2). These cytoplasmic sheets even penetrate pores of Kohn and cover portions of the surface of neighboring alveoli. When these extensive thin cytoplasmic sheets are taken into account, the total cytoplasmic volume of a type I cell is twice that of a type II cell, and its surface exposed to the alveolar gas is 50 times that of a type II cell.[62] Consequently, it is hardly surprising that the type I cell is more susceptible than the type II cell to damage by many inhaled agents. It has 50-fold the surface exposed to the agent, and much of its cytoplasm is far removed from the nucleus where many reparative processes probably begin.

The type II alveolar cell, or granular pneumonocyte, is the secretory alveolar epithelial cell. Type II cells are established as the source of the surface active phospholipids in the alveolar lining.[1] Whatever doubts still lingered were dispelled by the demonstration of active biosynthesis of the phospholipids characteristic of surfactant by isolated cell populations consisting almost entirely of type II cells.[24, 40]

* Supported by Research Grant HL-12650 from the United States Public Health Service.

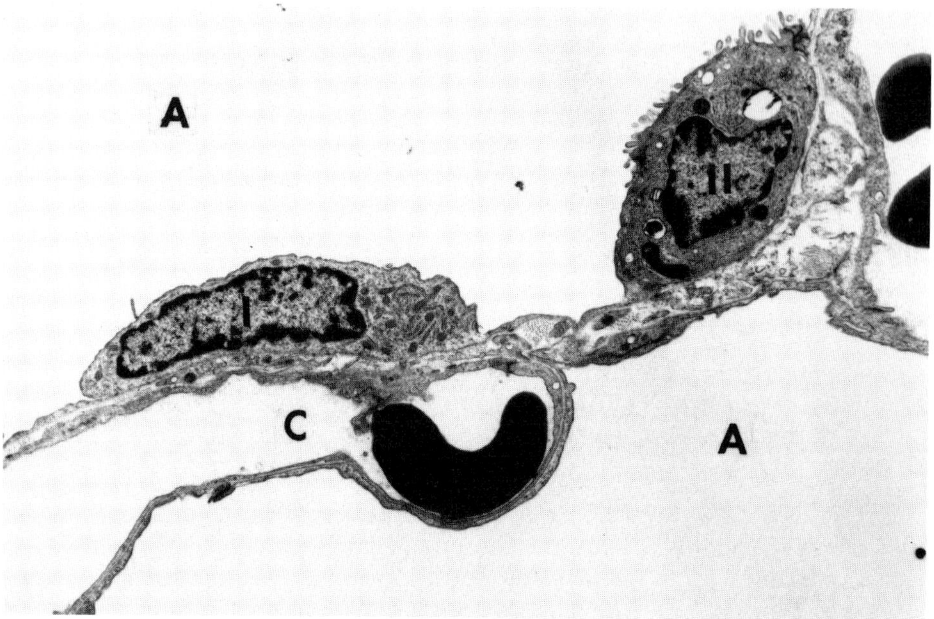

FIG. 1. Alveolar septum of a rat lung showing type I and type II alveolar epithelial cells. *A,* alveolar space; *C,* capillary. × 4,000.

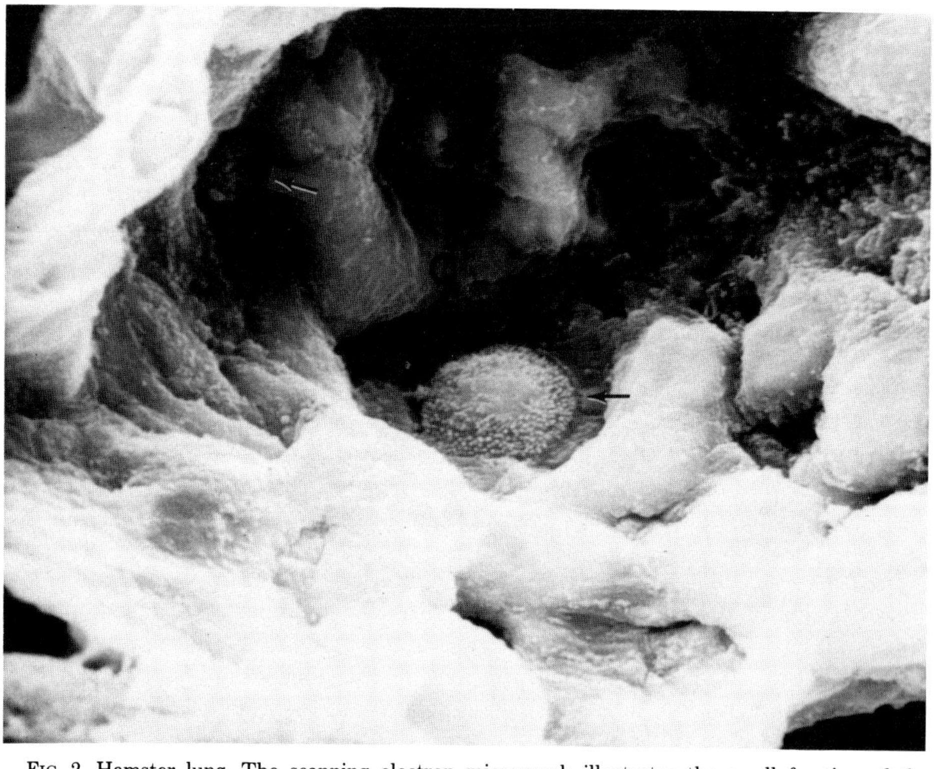

FIG. 2. Hamster lung. The scanning electron micrograph illustrates the small fraction of the alveolar surface which is occupied by type II cells (*arrows*). The capillaries (*C*) form a network of ridges bulging into the alveoli. × 4,500.

In tissue, the type II cells are roughly cuboidal cells typically found in niches in the alveolar walls at the junctions of alveolar septa. They are identified by their microvilli and by their characteristic lamellar cytoplasmic inclusions (Fig. 3). These inclusions are considered to be the storage form of the surfactant. The lamellar inclusions can now be isolated in a high degree of purity by several methods.[16, 20, 45] They have a very high phospholipid content; the phospholipid:protein ratio of most preparations ranges from 3:1 to 6:1. Analysis of the specific phospholipids found in the inclusions shows the similarity to the phospholipids of surface-active fractions purified from washings of the alveolar spaces (Table 1). Particularly characteristic is the large proportion of saturated phosphatidyl choline and the presence of appreciable amounts of phosphatidyl glycerol, a surface-active phospholipid which is unusual in mammalian cells.[11, 18, 49, 60]

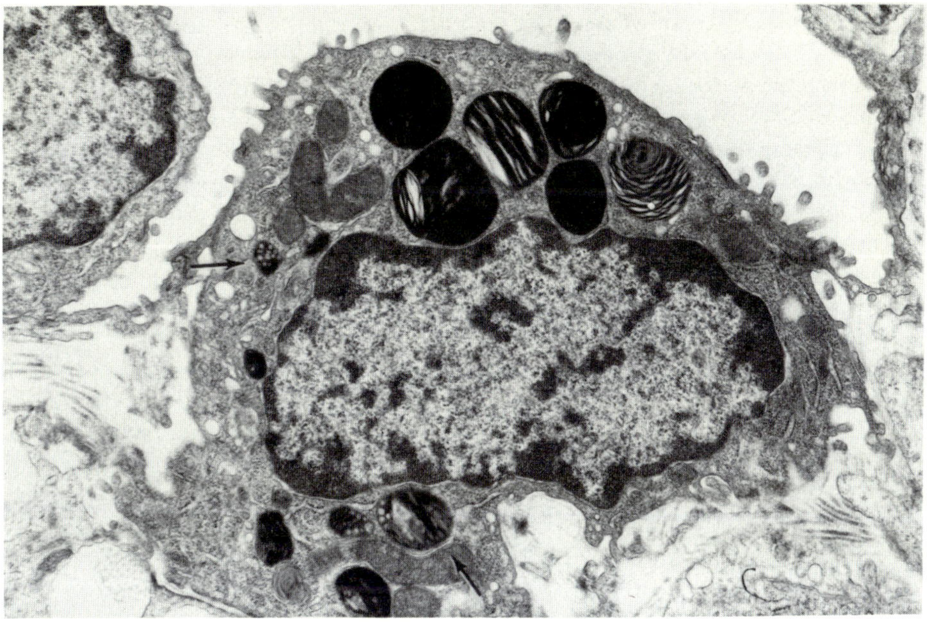

FIG. 3. A type II epithelial cell with typical lamellar inclusions. Several small lamellar inclusions appear to be forming from multivesicular bodies (*arrow*). × 9,000.

TABLE 1. COMPOSITION OF LAMELLAR BODIES AND SURFACTANT*

Components	Lamellar bodies	Surfactant
Phospholipid/Protein (w/w)	3.5–4.7	
Phospholipid	%	
Phosphatidyl choline	71–78	73–88
Phosphatidyl glycerol	8–12	4.9–11
Acidic phospholipids	3–4.9	1.8–4.2
Phosphatidyl ethanolamine	4–7	2–7
Sphyngomyelin	0.7	1.5–1.7
Lecithin fatty acids		
Palmitic	62–86	60–71
Saturated	66–94	63–81

* Based on data in References 11, 16, 18, and 49.

Replicas of freeze-fractured type II cells give additional information about the organization of lamellar bodies. Freeze-fracture replicas are prepared from tissue which has never been exposed to organic solvents, and therefore probably give a more reliable image than routine transmission electron microscopy.

In replicas of freeze-fractured tissue, the lamellae are straight and are stacked with a regular periodicity (Fig. 4), unlike the irregularly spaced wavy lamellae of embedded tissue. The lamellae themselves have smooth surfaces devoid of intramembranous particles.[63] In contrast, the limiting membrane does contain intramembranous particles (Figs. 4 and 5). Thus the limiting membrane, which is cytochemically the site of highest activity of several enzymes,[17,31] has the complex organization of a typical cytoplasmic membrane while the lamellae resemble those of synthetic liposomes. This suggests that a large part of the protein in the lamellar bodies is in the limiting membrane, a conclusion which fits with the high phospholipid:protein ratio of purified surfactant.[25]

The morphologic evolution of the lamellar bodies has been studied extensively. They have many of the cytochemical properties of lysosomes[17, 31] and form multivesicular bodies, a type of lysosome.[31, 57] Whether the lamellar bodies function in the biosynthesis of surfactant, however, is still under active investigation.[60]

Meban[42] has presented cytochemical evidence that one of the enzymes in the biosynthetic pathway to lecithin, phosphatidic acid phosphatase, may be found in the lamellar bodies. The distribution of reaction product was similar to the localization of nonspecific acid phosphatase, however. Most biochemical studies have shown that the enzymes for the biosynthetic reactions leading to phosphatidyl choline are in the microsomes.[60]

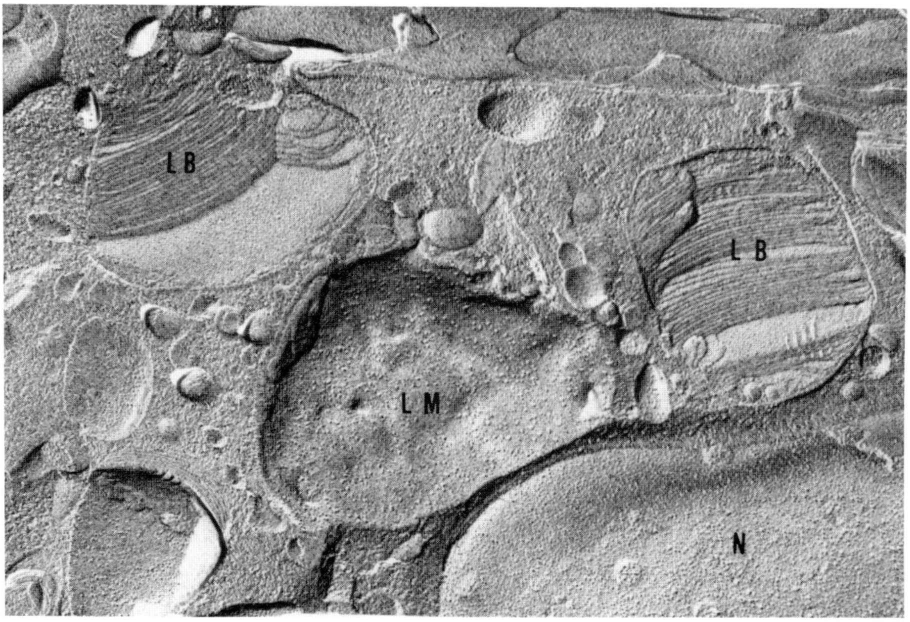

FIG. 4. Replica of a freeze-fractured type II cell. The lamellae in the lamellar bodies (*LB*) are straight and regularly spaced. There are no intramembranous particles on the lamellae. Where the cleavage plane passes through the limiting membrane (*LM*) of a lamellar body numerous intramembranous particles are visible. *N*, nucleus. × 31,000.

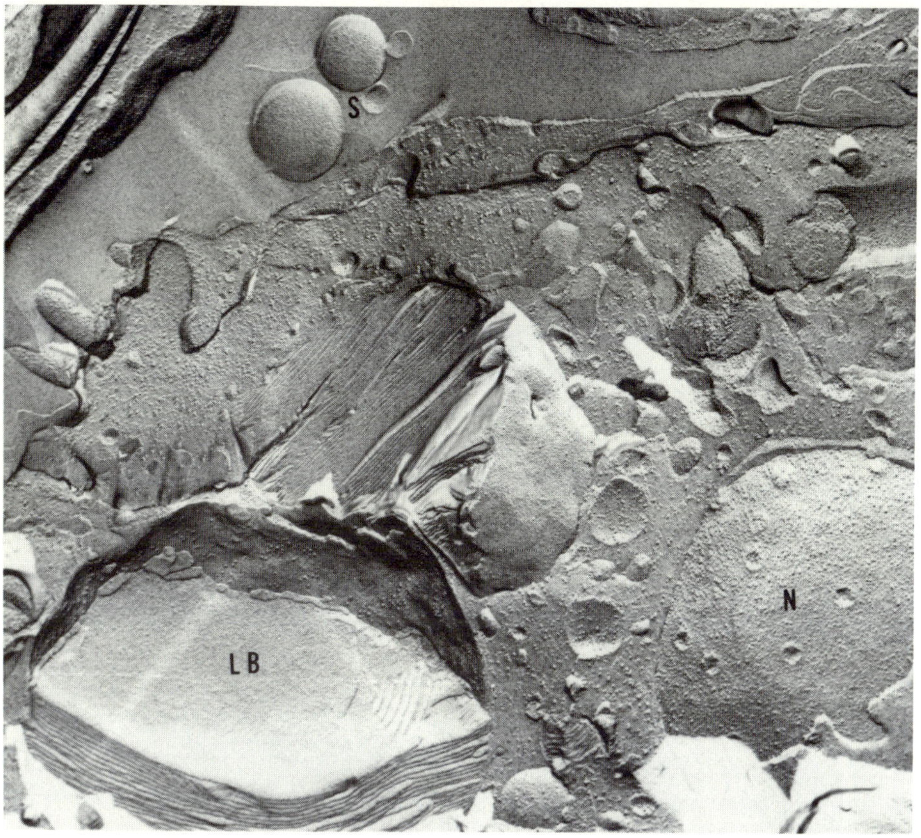

FIG. 5. Freeze-fractured type II cell. Two lamellar bodies (*LB*) with intramembranous particles in their limiting membranes. The lamellae themselves are free of particles. Intraalveolar membranous vesicles of surfactant (*S*) also lack particles. *N*, nucleus. × 29,000.

The phosphatidy choline in surfactant is unusual, however, in that the β position of the lecithin molecule, which is esterified with an unsaturated fatty acid in most tissues, is occupied by palmitic acid in roughly two-thirds of the surfactant lecithin.[25] This could come about in at least two ways. One is through the usual *de novo* pathway of lecithin synthesis (Table 2). This would require either an α-glycerophosphate:acyl CoA transferase with unusual specificity or a substrate pool with little unsaturated fatty acid; in fact, it has been found that the microsomal acyl transferase in lung does not have particular specificity for saturated acyl groups.[59] Another possibility is that a conventional β-unsaturated phospholipid is formed in the endoplasmic reticulum, but is cleaved by a phospholipase A_2 in the lamellar body to 1-acyl-2 lysophosphatidyl choline and reacylated by acyl transferase using palmitoyl CoA (Table 2, reaction 5). Phospholipase A[19] and an acyl transferase with specificity for palmitoyl over oleoyl CoA have recently been identified in lamellar bodies.[11] Currently it seems unlikely that lamellar bodies are primary biosynthetic organelles, but it is likely that some modification of phospholipids can occur within them.

The lamellar bodies are discharged by exocytosis into the alveolar lining fluid.[31] Little is known about the mechanism of secretion. Microtubules may be involved since colchicine and vinblastine inhibit the release of phospholipid from lung slices and isolated type II cells.[8] Furthermore, Beige mice, mice with the Chediak Higashi syndrome, have abnormal intracellular accumulation of lamellar bodies.[5] Mice with this mutation also have evidence of impaired microtubule function.

Morphologic observation on discharging lamellar bodies shows a mesh work of microfilaments associated with the secretory vesicle suggesting involvement of actin in granule release (Fig. 6). As yet the actomyosin system has not been studied biochemically in type II cells, and its involvement in surfactant secretion is unknown.

After the lamellar bodies are released into the alveolar lining fluid, the surfac-

TABLE 2. SOME MAJOR PATHWAYS IN PULMONARY LECITHIN SYNTHESIS

De novo pathway of lecithin synthesis:

1) glycerol-3-phosphate $\xrightarrow[\text{Acyl transferase}]{\text{Acyl-S CoA}}$ 1 acyl-2-lysophosphatidic acid

2) 1-acyl-2-lysophosphatidic acid $\xrightarrow[\text{Acyl transferase}]{\text{Acyl-S CoA}}$ 1,2 Diacylphosphatidic acid

3) 1,2 Diacylphosphatidic acid $\xrightarrow[\text{phosphatase}]{\text{phosphatidic acid}}$ 1,2 Diacylglycerol

4) 1,2 Diacylglycerol + CDP-Choline $\longrightarrow$ Phosphatidyl choline

Deacylation-Reacylation Reaction:

5) Diacylphosphatidyl choline $\xrightarrow{\text{Phospholipase } A_2}$ 1-acyl-2-lysophosphatidyl choline; $\xleftarrow[\text{Acyl transferase}]{\text{Acyl-S CoA}}$

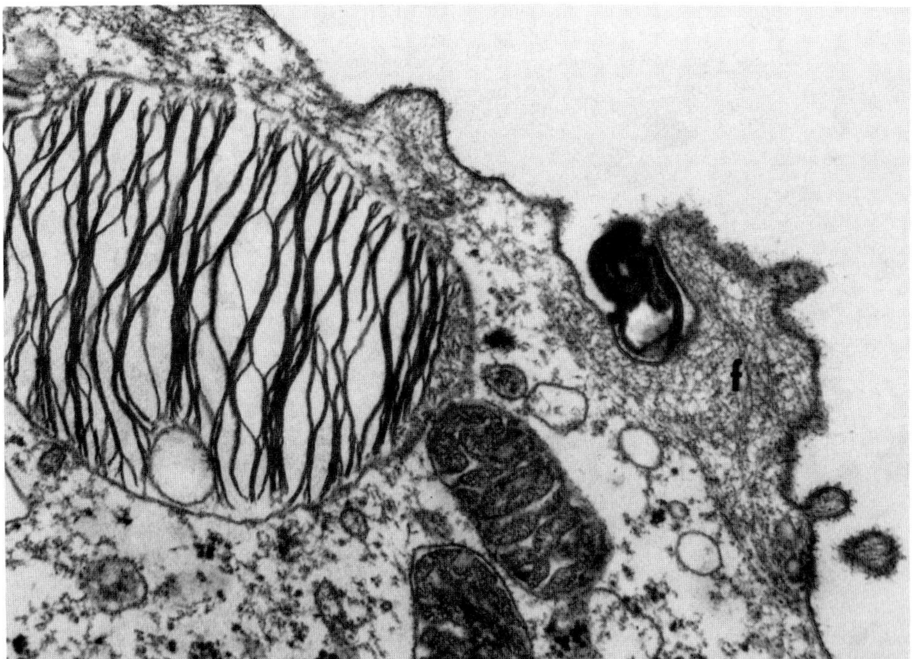

FIG. 6. Exocytosis of a lamellar body. The secretory vacuole which has fused with the plasma membrane is surrounded by a prominent meshwork of microfibrils (*F*).

tant gradually spreads to form a film on the surface of the lining fluid. During the early phase of its dispersion it forms peculiar lattice-like complexes with protein, tubular myelin (Fig. 7).[30, 64] Later it spreads to form a single monomolecular film.[15, 30] The proteins dispersed in the alveolar lining fluid include serum proteins,[4] albumin, IgG, and α_1-antiprotease, as well as specific proteins associated with lamellar inclusions.[26, 46]

THE INTERSTITIAL CELLS

The interstitium of the lung contains cells of several types including smooth muscle, mast cells, rare lymphocytes and monocytes, pericytes, and septal connective tissue cells. These septal cells, which are the most numerous cell in the interstitium, are highly branched and send out cytoplasmic projections of considerable complexity (Fig. 8). Although these cells sometimes resemble fibroblasts, often their cytoplasm appears rather quiescent with few organelles. Characteristically, the cells have one or several lipid droplets and bundles of filaments (Fig. 9). Intuitively one would assume that these cells are active in the maintenance of pulmonary connective tissue. Evidence for this has been obtained from studies

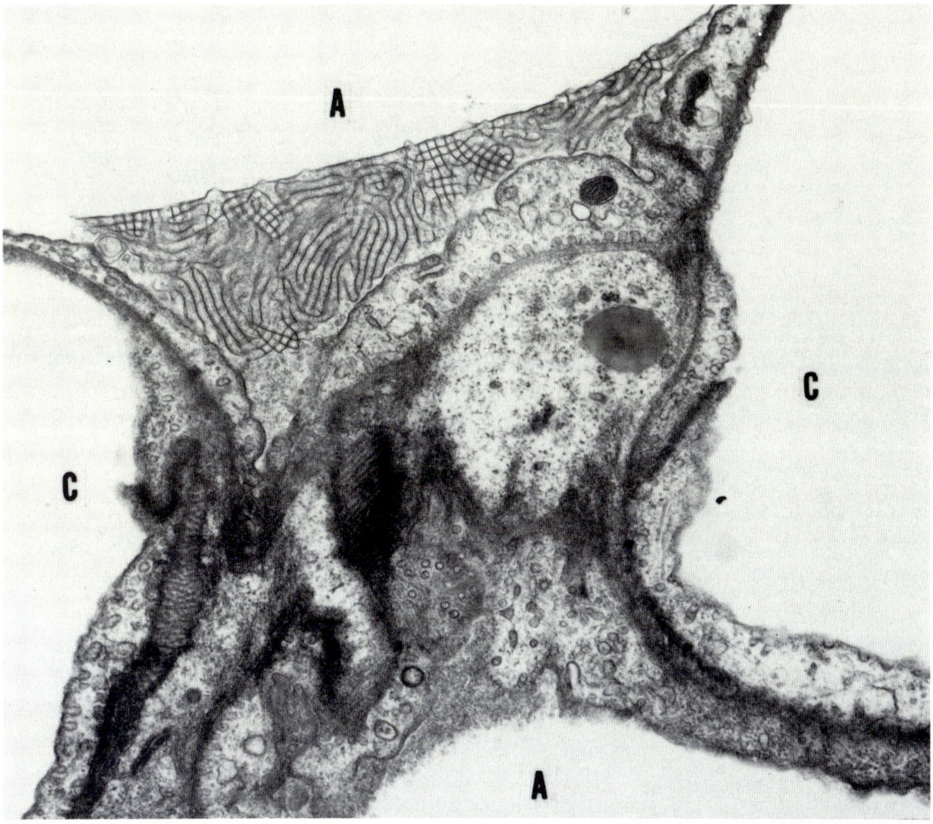

FIG. 7. The alveolar lining layer of a hamster lung fixed by perfusion of the vascular bed. The latice pattern at the alveolar surface is tubular myelin, one morphologic form taken by the surfactant. *A,* alveolus. *C,* capillary. × 23,000.

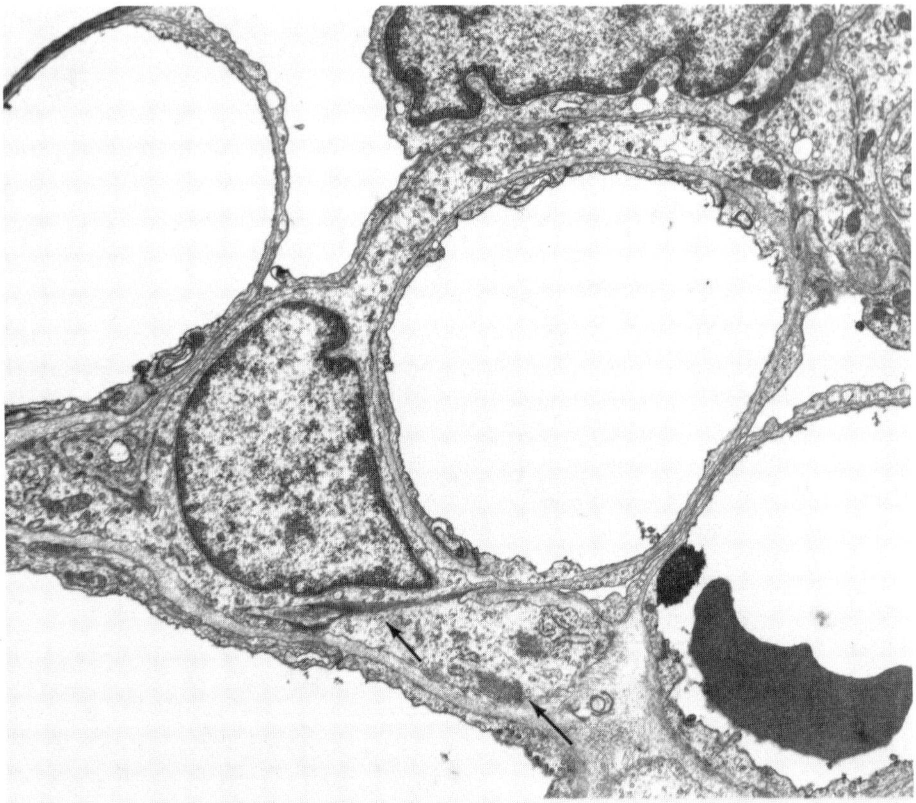

FIG. 8. Interstitial cell in an alveolar septum of a hamster lung. The cell extends processes in the interstitium. There are discrete bundles by myofilaments in the cytoplasm (*arrows*). × 9,600.

of lungs treated with enzymes to produce emphysema.[35] Following the injection of elastase to produce emphysema there is a marked fall in elastin which is followed by rapid resynthesis of elastin. During the period of synthesis, the septal cells are often seen in close contact or partly enveloping tiny, presumably forming, elastic fibers.

A more unexpected function for the septal connective tissue cell was suggested by Kapanci and co-workers.[22, 23] These workers called attention to the presence of bundles of filaments in these cells, identified actin and myosin in the cells by immunofluorescence, and indirectly attempted to study the contractile properties of the cells.[22] Peripheral lung slices from rat lungs do not contain smooth muscle, except in vessels. Therefore they attributed the contractile properties of the parenchymal strips to interstitial cells. These properties differed from those of either vascular smooth muscle from large pulmonary arteries or airway muscle. The lung strips failed to contract in response to serotonin, but specifically contracted in response to hypoxia. Kapanci *et al.*[23] suggested that their contraction in response to hypoxia could decrease capillary perfusion and might play a role in the matching of perfusion to ventilation.

These septal cells with their extensive intermingling of cytoplasmic projections ramifying throughout the alveolar walls appear to form junctions one to another. The junctions have not been critically studied with freeze-fracture or lanthanum tracing, but by routine electron microscopy they appear to be gap junctions which would imply electric coupling of the septal cells such that they would behave as a unit. According to Kapanci's hypothesis, coordinated contraction of these cells in an hypoxic alveolus would decrease alveolar size and presumably ventilation.[23]

This could, in turn, effect perfusion. The air-filled lung presents a smooth contour towards the alveolar space,[34] but in fact, the alveolar walls are extremely plastic and easily deformed by surface forces.[61] They fold inward into the capillary lumen (Figs. 10 and 11) and as lung volume decreases, the depth of these folds increases[2] and may actually interfere with smooth laminar blood flow through the capillaries. Kapanci suggests that hypoxic constriction of the septal connective tissue cells decreases alveolar volume and may thereby cause folds of the alveolar capillary membrane to project into the capillary lumen and impede flow tending to decrease perfusion of poorly oxygenated air spaces.[23] Thus the contractile function of the septal cells may help in the autoregulation of ventilation:perfusion ratios.

THE SEARCH FOR CHEMORECEPTORS

The possible contractile nature of pulmonary interstitial cells does not eliminate the role of the precapillary arterioles, which unquestionably are a major site of hypoxic vasoconstriction.[14] While the arterioles may respond directly to the local PO_2 there has been much interest in attempting to identify a chemoreceptor mechanism. The description of minute chemodectomas surrounding small pulmonary veins[27] suggested that chemoreceptors in that location could sample venous blood and if it were hypoxemic, reflexely decrease perfusion to that area. Unfortunately for this hypothesis, the cellular aggregates of the "chemodectoma" are, in fact, whorls unlike the "zellballen" of paraganglia and by electron micros-

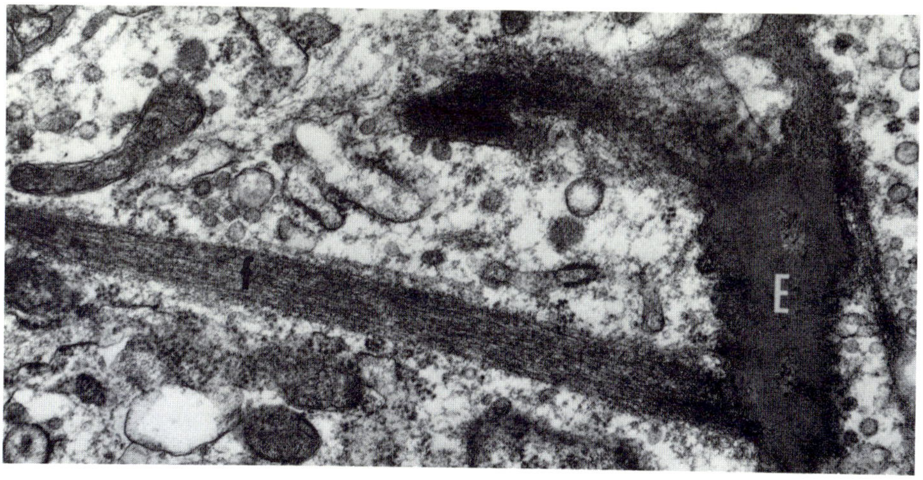

FIG. 9. A bundle of myofilaments (*f*) in an interstitial cell inserts on the cell membrane adjoining an elastic fiber (*E*). × 34,000.

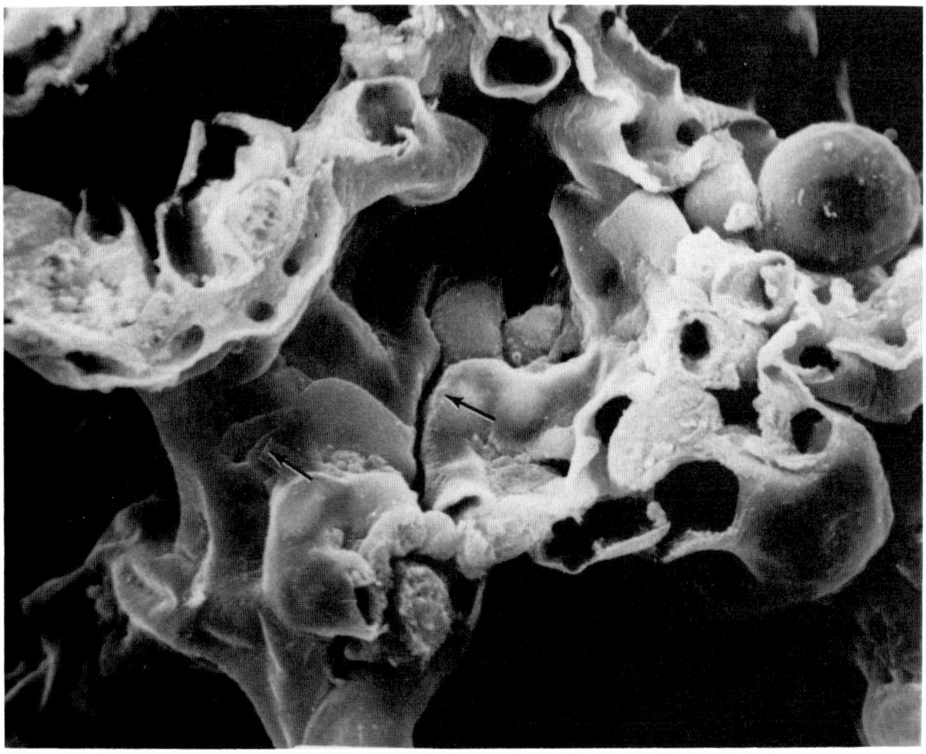

FIG. 10. Scanning electron micrograph of an alveolus fixed near functional residual capacity by perfusion of glutaraldehyde and OsO_4 through the inferior vena cava without opening the thoracic cavity. Notice the numerous infoldings (*arrows*) in the alveolar surface. These are probably not an artifact since the lung did not undergo pneumothorax before fixation. × 2,000.

copy they do not have the features of true paragangliomas such as dense cored granules or basement membrane. Rather they consist of complex interdigitating epithelium which fits together like the pieces of a jigsaw puzzle (Fig. 12).[6, 32] The origin of this lesion is obscure. Its resemblance to meningioma is striking but leads to no rational proposal for its histogenesis. The point to make here is that it does not appear to have the features expected of a chemoreceptor.

Physiologic studies, too, have provided no support for a chemoreceptor in the pulmonary circulation, while there is physiologic evidence that vasoconstriction occurs directly in response to low Po_2 in the inspired air.[13, 14] There is a structure in the airways which does have many of the morphologic features of a chemoreceptor and is appropriately placed to sample the oxygen tension of inspired air. This is the neuroepithelial body, described by Lauweryns, Cokelaere, and Theunynck[37] in airways of various sizes. These bodies are discrete clusters of innervated epithelium, lacking cilia and often producing evagination of the basal lamina (Fig. 13).[21, 36, 37] The epithelial cells are argyrophilic and fluoresce emitting the characteristic spectrum of serotonin.[36] As seen by electron microscopy, they consist of grouped cells with dense-core granules (Fig. 13). In Figure 13, narrow projections of nongranular cytoplasm penetrate the clusters of granule-containing cells like the sustentacular cells of paraganglia. Fenestrated capillaries like those of chemoreceptive paraganglia supply the neuroepithelial bodies.[36, 37] Exposure of animals to hypoxia results in changes in the neuroepithelial bodies suggestive of secretion.[38, 43] Consequently, these structures are currently the leading contenders for the role of pulmonary chemoreceptors.

THE ENDOTHELIUM

The processes discussed so far have been concerned directly or indirectly with the classical gas-exchanging functions of the lung. The endothelium is, of course, one of the three layers of the blood-air barrier. In addition to its passive role in gas exchange, it plays an active part in the metabolic transformation of a variety of materials (Table 3). Since the lung receives the entire cardiac output, it is well situated to detoxify a variety of substances. By the same token it is important that the process be selective, since most hormones must pass through the lung on their way to their target. The localization of several of these metabolic processes has been studied in recent years. Serotonin is taken into cells and metabolized by a monoamine oxidase (MAO). By autoradiography this has been shown to occur extensively in capillary endothelium.[58] In contrast, norepinephrine is taken up and degraded mainly in precapillary arterioles and venules.[44]

A second pattern of metabolism is exemplified by the adenine nucleotides[51] and by the polypeptides angiotensin I and bradykinin.[50] These substances are metabolized almost completely in a single passage through the lung, with quan-

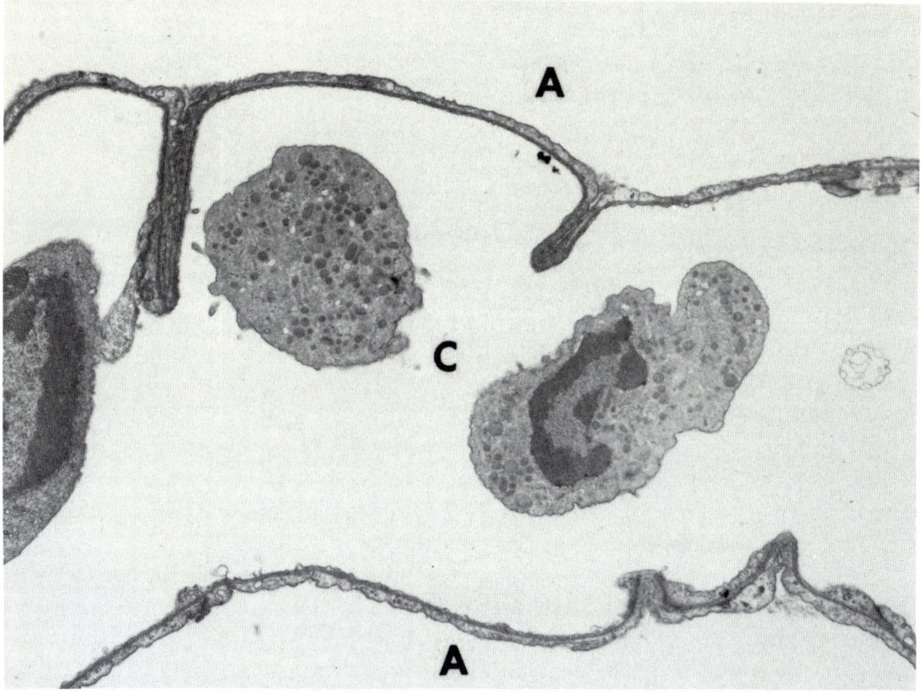

FIG. 11. Transmission electron micrograph of the same lung as in Figure 10. The alveolar-capillary membrane tends to fold into the capillary lumen, forming flaps which could impede laminar flow through the capillary. *A,* alveolus. *C,* capillary. × 6,700.

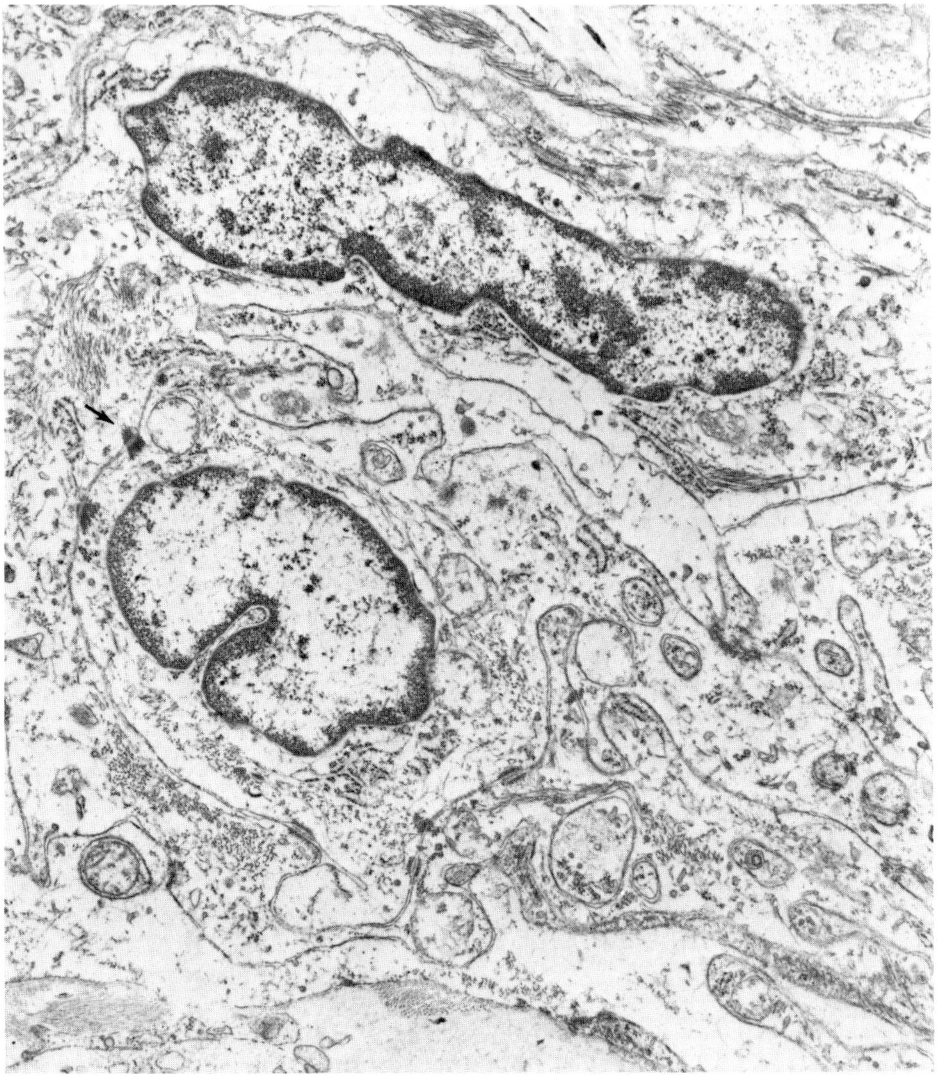

FIG. 12. Minute pulmonary "chemodectoma." The lesion is composed of cells with extensive interdigitating processes joined by occasional desmosomes (*arrow*). There are no secretory granules. × 11,000.

titative recovery of the metabolites in the venous effluent. This suggests that the metabolism occurs at or near the endothelial membrane.

The Ryans and co-workers[54] have suggested that the caveolae in the endothelium are a likely place for such metabolism. The caveolae are covered by a delicate membrane[55] which provides an isolated microenvironment within them (Fig. 14). In freeze-fracture replicas, intramembranous particles are clustered about the caveolae, especially at their necks.[56] Cytochemically, 5′-nucleotidase does appear to be concentrated in the caveolae.[55] The dipeptidyl carboxy peptidase which converts angiotensin I to angiotensin II and inactivates bradykinin has been demonstrated in isolated endothelial membranes.[52, 53] The localization of the enzyme by perioxidase-labeled antibody shows antigen along the entire luminal surface of the endothelium, however.[54] Whether or not the caveolae are

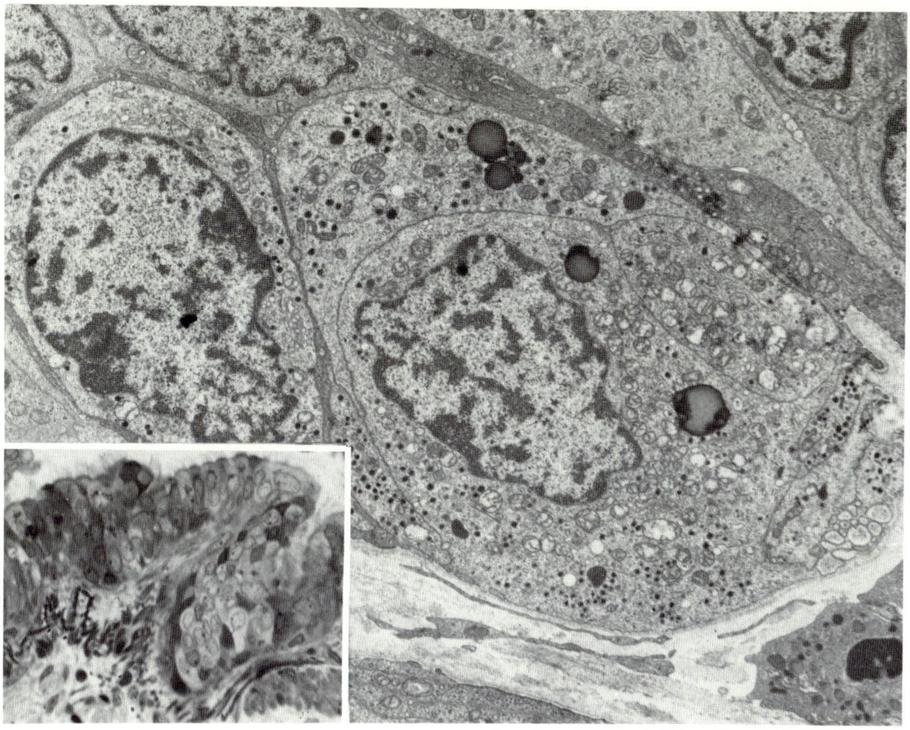

FIG. 13. Human bronchiole. *Inset:* The cluster of epithelial cells to the right with clear cytoplasm is a neuroepithelial body. Epoxy section, toluidine blue-basic fuchsin, × 200. The electron micrograph, taken from an adjacent section, shows that the cells of the cluster contain granules of the neurosecretory type. × 5,000.

TABLE 3. SOME METABOLIC ACTIVITIES OF PULMONARY ENDOTHELIUM*

Class of compound	Metabolized without uptake	Metabolized with uptake	Largely unchanged
Biogenic amines		Serotonin Norepinephrine Acetyl choline	Histamine Epinephrine Dopamine
Adenine nucleotides	AMP ATP		
Peptides	Bradykin Angiotensin I		Angiotensin II Oxytocin Vasopressin VIP
Lipoproteins		VLDL	LDL
Prostaglandins		PGE_1, PGE_2, $PGF_{2\alpha}$	PGA_1 PGA_2

* Based mainly on data from References 12, 41, 44, 47, 48, 50, 51, 53, and 55.

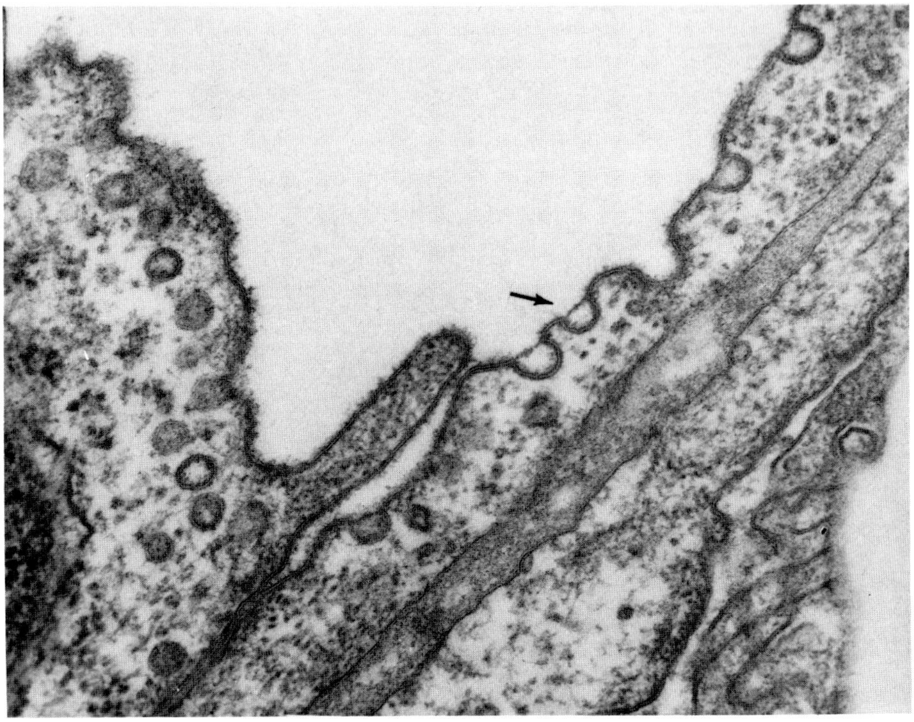

FIG. 14. Endothelial cell of a hamster lung. There are several caveolae, most of which are closed off from the capillary lumen by thin diaphragms (*arrow*) which lack the trilaminar structure of the plasma membrane. × 7,600.

particularly active, these results clearly show that the endothelial membrane is a major site of metabolism of these compounds.

THE BRONCHIOLAR EPITHELIUM

The bronchioles are lined mainly by two types of cells, ciliated cells and Clara cells.[29] Clara cells are tall columnar cells which form domes protruding into the bronchial lumen (Fig. 15). The characteristic feature of Clara cells is the presence, within the dome of the apex, of numerous electron dense granules. The granules are not mucin and are only variably PAS positive.[37, 33] They are insoluble in lipid solvents[7, 33] and stain for basic groups with phosphotungstic acid (Table 4).[33] In the rat they have a crystalline structure with a square or hexagonal lattice with an 80 Å spacing. They appear to consist mainly of protein. The apex of rodent Clara cells has an extensive smooth endoplasmic reticulum in which granules can sometimes form directly, bypassing the Golgi apparatus.[33] The granules appear to be discharged by exocytosis (Fig. 16). The appearance of blebs on the Clara cells, often cited as evidence of decapitation secretion, occurs with equal frequency on ciliated cells and is probably a sign of cell damage or suboptimal fixation.[29]

When the lung is fixed by perfusion through the blood vessels, the cilia can no longer be seen from the lumen, but a continuous film appears to fill the space between protruding Clara cells (Fig. 17).[10] Transmission electron microscopy shows a layer of dense fluid enveloping the cilia (Fig. 18). The film is similar in electron opacity to the matrix of the Clara granules, suggesting that it is derived in part from Clara cell secretions.[33] Ebert and co-workers[9, 10] obtained additional evidence for this. Using a perfusion system to administer labeled amino acids and other precursors for radioautography, they were able to label the apex of Clara cells. After a three-hour or longer chase with unlabeled amino acids, the label left the cells and appeared over the bronchiolar lining.[9]

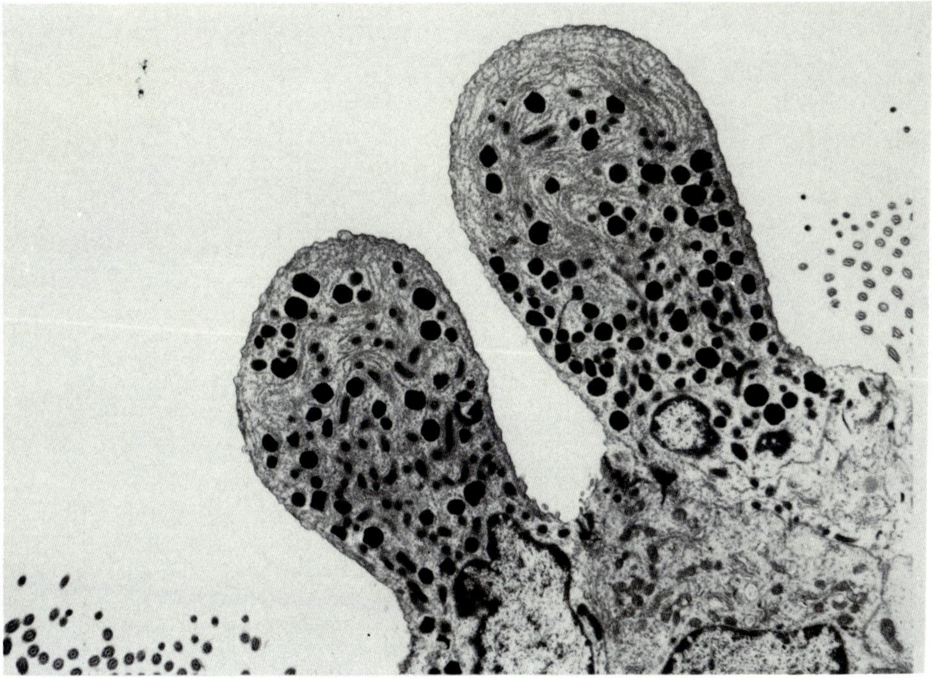

FIG. 15. Clara cells of a rat bronchiole. The prominent bulbous apex of each cell contains secretory granules and extensive smooth endoplasmic reticulum. × 2,700.

TABLE 4. PROPERTIES OF CLARA CELL GRANULES*

LIGHT MICROSCOPIC STAINING	
mucin	negative
PAS	variable
fat	negative
phospholipid	positive
ELECTRON MICROSCOPY	
structure—crystalline	
lipid solvents—insoluble	
pepsin—labile	
phosphotungstic acid—positive	

* Based on data in References 1, 3, 7, and 33.

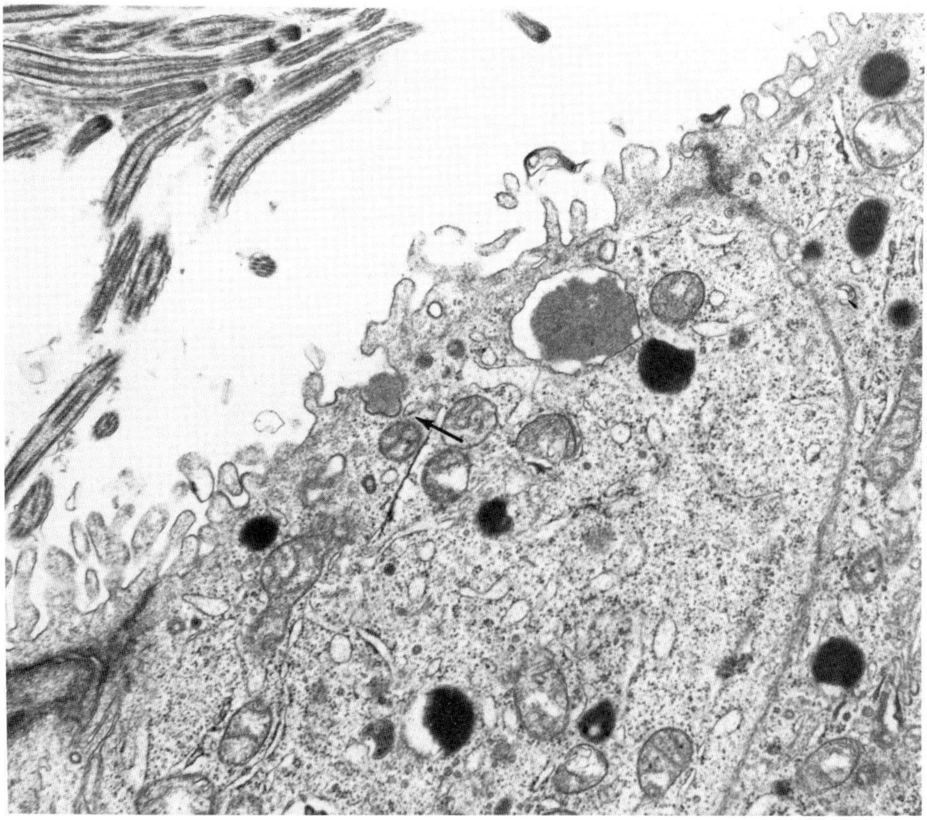

FIG. 16. Human bronchiole. A Clara cell discharging a granule by exocytosis (*arrow*). × 14,000.

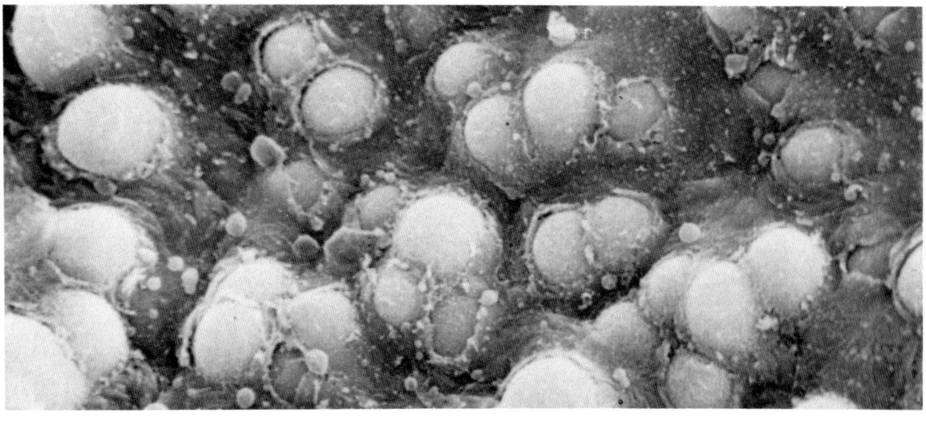

FIG. 17. Scanning electron micrograph of a hamster bronchiole fixed by perfusion through the vascular system. The cilia are not visible as they are covered by a layer of dense fluid. The domes of Clara cells project through the lining layer. × 2,400.

The need for a unique proteinaceous lining in the bronchioles probably stems from the occurrence of bronchiolar closure in late expiration. Reopening requires a lining which is not sticky and has a low surface tension,[39] properties quite different from those of bronchial mucus.

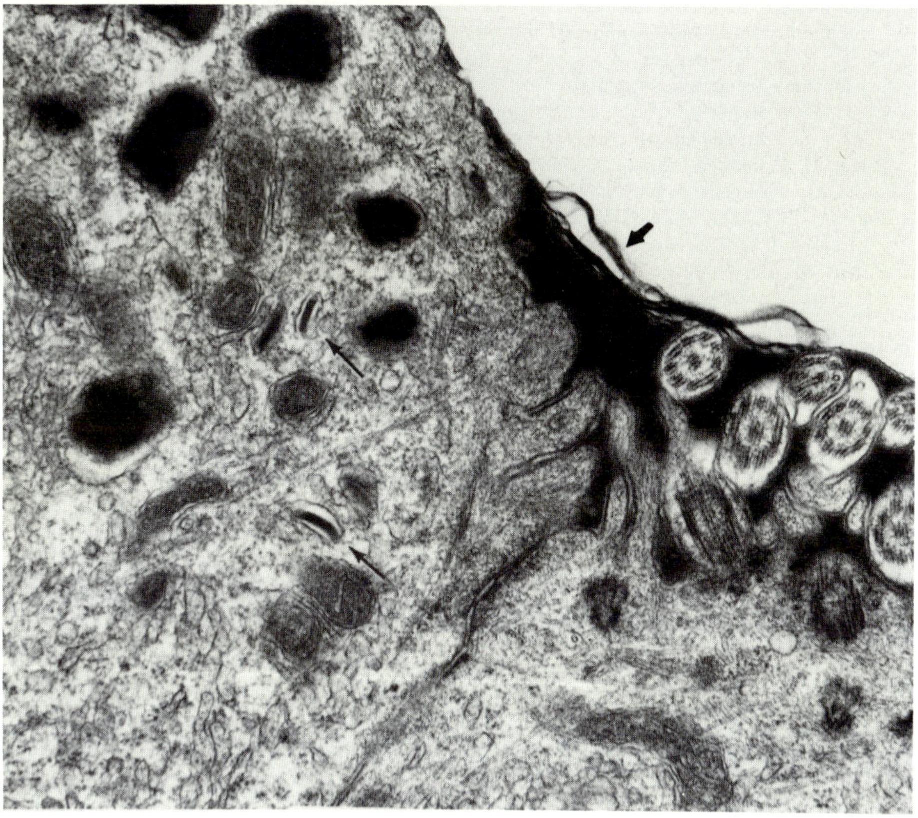

FIG. 18. Transmission electron micrograph of a rat bronchiole after fixation by vascular perfusion. An electron dense lining layer covers the cilia (compare with Fig. 17). A surface film, presumably surfactant, is present on the surface of the lining layer (*thick arrow*). The Clara cell (*left*) has several secretory granules of an electron density similar to the lining layer. Several small granules appear to be forming with dilated cisterns of smooth endoplasmic reticulum (*thin arrows*). × 35,000. (Reproduced by permission, from Crystal, R. G. (ed.): *The Biochemical Basis of Pulmonary Function.* New York, Marcel Dekker, Inc., 1976.)

REFERENCES

1. Askin, F. B., and Kuhn, C.: The cellular origin of pulmonary surfactant. *Lab. Invest. 25:* 260–268, 1971.
2. Assimacopoulos, A., Guggenheim, R., and Kapanci, Y.: Changes in alveolar capillary configuration at different levels of lung inflation in the rat. An ultrastructural and morphometric study. *Lab. Invest. 34:* 10–22, 1976.
3. Azzopardi, A., and Thurlbeck, W. M.: The histochemistry of the nonciliated bronchiolar epithelial cells. *Am. Rev. Resp. Dis. 99:* 516–525, 1969.
4. Bignon, J., Jaurand, M. C., Pinchon, M. C., Sapin, C., and Warnet, J. M.: Immunoelectron microscopic and immunochemical demonstrations of serum proteins in the alveolar lining material of the rat lung. *Am. Rev. Resp. Dis. 113:* 109–120, 1976.
5. Chi, E. Y., Prueitt, J. L., and Lagunoff, D.: Abnormal lamellar bodies in type II pneumocytes and increased lung surface active material in the beige mouse. *J. Histochem. Cytochem. 23:* 863–866, 1975.
6. Churg, A. M., and Warnock, M. W.: So-called "minute pulmonary chemodectoma." A tumor not related to paragangliomas. *Cancer 37:* 1759–1769, 1976.
7. Cutz, E., and Conen, P. E.: Ultrastructure and cytochemistry of Clara cells. *Am. J. Pathol. 62:* 127–142, 1971.

8. Delahunty, T. S., and Johnston, J. M.: The effect of colchicine and vinblastine on the release of pulmonary surface active material. *J. Lipid Res. 17:* 112–116, 1976.
9. Ebert, R. V., Kronenberg, R. S., and Terracio, M. J.: Study of the surface secretion of the bronchiole using radioautography. *Am. Rev. Resp. Dis. 114:* 567–574, 1976.
10. Ebert, R. V., and Terracio, M. J.: Observation of the secretion on the surface of the bronchioles with the scanning electron microscope. *Am. Rev. Resp. Dis. 112:* 491–496, 1975.
11. Engle, M. J., Sanders, R. L., and Longmore, W. J.: Phospholipid composition and acyltransferase activity of lamellar bodies isolated from rat lung. *Arch. Biochem. Biophys. 173:* 586–595, 1976.
12. Ferreira, S. H., and Vane, S. R.: Prostaglandins: Their disappearance from and release into the circulation. *Nature 216:* 868–873, 1967.
13. Fillenz, M., and Widdicombe, D. G.: Receptors of the lungs and airways. In *Handbook of Sensory Physiology: Enteroceptors,* edited by Neil, E., Vol. 3, pt. 1, pp. 81–112. New York, Springer-Verlag, 1972.
14. Fishman, A. P.: Hypoxia on the pulmonary circulation. How and where it acts. *Circ. Res. 38:* 221–231, 1976.
15. Gil, J., and Weibel, E. R.: Improvements in demonstration of lining layer of lung alveoli by electron microscopy. *Resp. Physiol. 8:* 13–36, 1969.
16. Gil, J., and Reiss, O. K.: Isolation and characterization of lamellar bodies and tubular myelin from rat lung homogenates. *J. Cell Biol. 58:* 152–171, 1973.
17. Goldfischer, S., Kikkawa, Y., and Hoffman, L.: The demonstration of acid hydrolase activities in the inclusion bodies of type II alveolar cells and other lysosomes in the rabbit lung. *J. Histochem. Cytochem. 16:* 102–109, 1968.
18. Hallman, M., and Gluck, L.: Phosphatidylglycerol in lung surfactant. II: Subcellular distribution and mechanism of biosynthesis *in vitro. Biochem. Biophys. Acta 409:* 172–191, 1975.
19. Heath, M. F., and Jacobson, W.: Phospholipases A_1 and A_2 in lamellar inclusion bodies of the alveolar epitheluim of rabbit lung. *Biochem. Biophys. Acta 441:* 443–452, 1976.
20. Hoffman, L.: Isolation of inclusion bodies from rabbit lung parenchyma. *J. Cell Physiol. 79:* 65–72, 1972.
21. Hung, K-S, Hertweck, M. S., Hardy, J. D., and Loosli, C. G.: Ultrastructure of nerves and associated cells in bronchiolar epithelium of the mouse lung. *J. Ultrastr. Res. 43:* 426–437, 1973.
22. Kapanci, Y., Assimacopoulos, A., Irle, C., Zwahlen, A., and Gabbiani, G.: "Contractile interstitial cells" in pulmonary alveolar septa: A possible regulator of ventilation-perfusion ratio? Ultrastructural, immunofluorescence and *in vitro* studies. *J. Cell Biol. 60:* 375–392, 1974.
23. Kapanci, Y., Costabella, P. M., and Gabbiani, G.: Location and function of contractile interstitial cells of the lungs. In *Lung Cells in Disease,* edited by Bouhuys, A., pp. 69–82. Amsterdam, Elsevier, North Holland Press, 1976.
24. Kikkawa, Y., Yoneda, K., Smith, F., Packard, B., and Suzuki, K.: The type II epithelial cells of the lung. II: Chemical composition and phospholipid synthesis. *Lab. Invest. 32:* 295–302, 1975.
25. King, R. J.: The surfactant system of the lung. *Fed. Proc. 33 (11):* 2238–2247, 1974.
26. King, R. J., Klass, D. J., Gikas, E. G., and Clements, J. A.: Isolation of apoproteins from canine surface active material. *Am. J. Physiol. 224:* 788–795, 1973.
27. Korn, D., Bensch, K., Liebow, A. A., and Castleman, B.: Multiple minute pulmonary tumors resembling chemodectomas. *Am. J. Pathol. 37:* 641–672, 1960.
28. Kuhn, C.: The cells of the lung and their organelles. In *The Biochemical Basis of Pulmonary Function,* edited by Crystal, R. G., pp. 3–48. New York, Marcel Dekker, 1976.
29. Kuhn, C.: Ciliated cells and Clara cells. In *Lung Cells in Disease,* edited by Bouhuys, A., pp. 91–108. Amsterdam, North Holland Publishing Co., 1976.
30. Kuhn, C.: A comparison of freeze-substitution with other methods for preservation of the pulmonary alveolar lining layer. *Am. J. Anat. 133:* 495–508, 1972.
31. Kuhn, C.: Cytochemistry of pulmonary alveolar epithelial cells. *Am. J. Pathol. 53:* 809–833, 1968.
32. Kuhn, C., and Askin, F. B.: The fine structure of so-called minute pulmonary chemodectomas. *Human Pathol. 6:* 681–691, 1975.
33. Kuhn, C., Callaway, L. A., and Askin, F. B.: The formation of granules in the bronchiolar Clara cells of the rat. 1: Electron microscopy. *J. Ultrastr. Res. 49:* 387–400, 1974.

34. Kuhn, C., and Finke, E. H.: The topography of the pulmonary alveolus: Scanning electron microscopy using different fixations. *J. Ultrastr. Res. 38:* 161–172, 1972.
35. Kuhn, C., Yu, S-Y., Chraplyvy, M., Linder, H. E., and Senior, R. M.: The induction of emphysema with elastase. II: Changes in connective tissue. *Lab. Invest. 34:* 372–380, 1976.
36. Lauweryns, J. M., Cokelaere, M., and Theunynck, P.: Serotonin producing neuroepithelial bodies in rabbit respiratory mucosa. *Science 180:* 410–413, 1973.
37. Lauweryns, J. M., Cokelaere, M., and Theunynck, P.: Neuro-epithelial bodies in the respiratory mucosa of various mammals. A light optical, histochemical, and ultrastructural investigation. *Z. Zellforsch Mikrosk. Anat. 135:* 569–592, 1972.
38. Lauweryns, J. M., and Cokelaere, M.: Hypoxia-sensitive neuro-epithelial bodies. Intrapulmonary secretory neuroreceptors modulated by the CNS. *Z. Zellforsch Mikrosk. Anat. 145:* 521–540, 1973.
39. Macklem, P. T., Proctor, D. F., and Hogg, J. C.: The stability of peripheral airways. *Resp. Physiol. 8:* 191–203, 1970.
40. Mason, R. J.: Phospholipid synthesis in primary cultures of type II alveolar cells. *Am. Rev. Resp. Dis. 115:* (Part 2) 352, 1977 (abstract).
41. Mathé, A. A., Hedqvist, P., Strandberg, K., and Leslie, C. A.: Aspects of prostaglandin function in the lung. *N. Engl. J. Med. 296:* 850–855, 1977.
42. Meban, C.: Localization of phosphatidic acid phosphatase activity in granular pneumonocytes. *J. Cell Biol. 53:* 249–252, 1972.
43. Moosavi, H., Smith, P., and Heath, D.: The Feyrter cell in hypoxia. *Thorax 28:* 729–741, 1973.
44. Nicholas, T. E., Strum, J. M., Angelo, L. S., and Junod, A. F.: Site and mechanism of uptake of ^{3}H-1-norepinephrine by isolated perfused rat lungs. *Circ. Res. 35:* 670–680, 1974.
45. Page-Roberts, B. A.: Preparation and partial characterization of a lamellar body fraction from rat lung. *Biochim. Biophys. Acta 260:* 334–338, 1972.
46. Passero, M. A., Bhattacharyya, S. N., Sahu, S., and Lynn, W. S.: Crosslinking and carbohydrate studies on the hydroxylated glycopeptides which accumulate in alveoli and lamellar bodies. *Chest 67:* 28s–29s, 1975.
47. Pietra, G. G., Spagnoli, L. G., Capuzzi, D. M., Sparks, C. E., Fishman, A. P., and Marsh, J. B.: Metabolism of ^{125}I-labeled lipoproteins by the isolated rat lung. *J. Cell Biol. 70:* 33–46, 1976.
48. Piper, P. J., Vane, J. R., and Wyllie, J. H.: Inactivation of prostaglandins by the lungs. *Nature 225:* 600–604, 1970.
49. Rooney, S. A., Page-Roberts, B. A., and Motoyama, E. K.: Role of lamellar inclusions in surfactant production: Studies on phospholipid composition and biosynthesis in rat and rabbit lung subcellular fractions. *J. Lipid Res. 16:* 418–425, 1975.
50. Ryan, J. W., Niemeyer, R. S., Goodwin, D. W., and Smith, U.: Metabolism of [8-L-(^{14}C) phenylalanine]-Angiotensin I in the pulmonary circulation. *Biochem. J. 125:* 921–923, 1971.
51. Ryan, J. W., and Smith, U.: Metabolism of adenosine 5′-monophosphate during circulation through the lungs. *Trans. Assoc. Am. Physns. 84:* 297–306, 1971.
52. Ryan, J. W., and Smith, U.: A rapid simple method for isolating pinocytotic vesicles and plasma membrane of lung. *Biochim. Biophys. Acta 249:* 177–180, 1971.
53. Ryan, J. W., Smith, U., and Niemeyer, R. S.: Angiotensin I: Metabolism by plasma membrane of lung. *Science 176:* 64–66, 1972.
54. Ryan, U. S., Ryan, J. W., Whitaker, C., and Chiu, A.: Localization of angiotensin converting enzyme (kininase II). II: Immunocytochemistry and immunofluorescence. *Tissue and Cell 8:* 125–145, 1976.
55. Smith, U., and Ryan, J. W.: Substructural features of pulmonary endothelial caveolae. *Tissue and Cell 4:* 49–54, 1972.
56. Smith, U., Ryan, J. W., and Smith, D. S.: Freeze-etch studies of the plasma membrane of pulmonary endothelial cells. *J. Cell Biol. 56:* 492–499, 1973.
57. Sorokin, S. P.: A morphologic and cytochemical study on the great alveolar cell. *J. Histochem. Cytochem. 14:* 884–897, 1966.
58. Strum, J. M., and Junod, A. F.: Radioautographic demonstration of 5-hydroxytryptamine—^{3}H uptake by pulmonary endothelial cells. *J. Cell Biol. 54:* 456–467, 1972.
59. Tansey, F. A., and Frosolono, M. F.: Role of 1-acyl-2-lyso-phosphatidylcholine acyl transferase in the biosynthesis of pulmonary phosphatidylcholine. *Biochem. Biophys. Res. Commun. 67:*

1560–1566, 1975.

60. Van Golde, L. M. G.: Metabolism of phospholipids in the lung. *Am. Rev. Resp. Dis. 114:* 977–1000, 1976.
61. Weibel, E. R.: Morphological basis of alveolar-capillary gas exchange. *Physiol. Rev. 53:* 419–495, 1973.
62. Weibel, E. R., Gehr, P., Haies, D., Gil, J., and Bachhofen, M.: The cell population of the normal lung. In *Lung Cells In Disease,* edited by Bouhuys, A., p. 3. Amsterdam, North Holland Publishing Co., 1976.
63. Weinstein, R. S., Hogg, J. C., Nash, G., and McNutt, N. S.: Proceedings of 1st Annual Conference on Environmental Toxicology, Sept. 9–11, 1970, Fairborn, Ohio. AMRL-TR-70-102, pp. 251–273.
64. Williams, M. C.: Conversion of lamellar body membranes into tubular myelin in alveoli of fetal rat lungs. *J. Cell Biol. 72:* 260–277, 1977.

Chapter 2

Drug-Induced Lung Disease*

D. G. GILLETT AND G. T. FORD

Injury to the lung induced by drugs and chemicals is becoming a common problem facing the clinician and the pathologist. Over the past several years the number of drugs and chemicals recognized to have adverse pulmonary effects has increased rapidly.[17, 32, 95, 123] The variability and nonspecific nature of their presentation makes diagnosis difficult. This discussion is an attempt to describe the toxic effects of oral or parenterally administered drugs or chemicals on the lung. The effects of inhaled substances will not be considered.

The clinical situation often involves the combined effects of multiple agents; *e.g.*, the concurrent administration of several toxic drugs, oxygen in high doses, and viral or bacterial infection. In this setting it may be difficult to distinguish any specific drug-induced morphologic features in the pulmonary lesion even if experimental animal studies suggest that they do exist. Also the earliest and therefore the most specific pulmonary lesion is usually not seen in human disease. For these reasons the most important diagnostic step is a careful consideration of the patient's history. If the histologic features are compatible with drug or chemical exposure, the diagnosis should be considered.

In our approach to this problem, we have attempted to classify drug reactions on the basis of their common clinical presentation (Table 1). Although this approach has limitations, it does provide a framework from which this complex problem may be studied. We hope it will enhance awareness of possible drug reactions when considering the presentation and pathologic changes in lung disease.

DIFFUSE ALVEOLAR DAMAGE - FIBROSING ALVEOLITIS

These two pathologic categories are considered together since there is considerable evidence[16, 28, 65] that interstitial fibrotic lung disease due to drugs, inhalants, and other agents is a response to an initial inflammatory lesion which is often termed diffuse alveolar damage (DAD). This reaction is entirely nonspecific and has been found following shock, severe trauma, multiple fractures, head injury, sepsis, major intra-abdominal surgery, cardiopulmonary bypass, and viral pneumonitis, as well as with a variety of drug or chemically induced injuries. Depend-

* Supported by Grant No. DG-152 from the Medical Research Council. The authors wish to thank Larry Wood, M.D., Ph.D. for his helpful comments and advice given in the preparation of this chapter.

TABLE 1. CLASSIFICATION OF DRUG-INDUCED LUNG DISEASE

I.	Diffuse alveolar damage—fibrosing alveolitis
II.	Pulmonary edema
III.	Hypersensitivity pneumonitis
	a. with eosinophilia
	b. without eosinophilia
IV.	Systemic lupus erythematosus
V.	Pulmonary hypertension
VI.	Bronchospasm
VII.	Respiratory muscle paralysis
VIII.	Pleural disease
IX.	Miscellaneous

ing upon the time course after injury, different stages of a progressive pathologic process are found. This process has been divided into two major steps,[65] the exudative phase and the proliferative phase.

The earliest lesion, the exudative phase, consists of capillary congestion, endothelial edema, inflammatory cell infiltration, and hyaline membrane formation (Fig. 1). The initial sites of injury are the capillary endothelial cells and membranous (type I) pneumocytes. In experimentally induced diffuse alveolar damage, Bowden and Adamson[15] and Adamson, Bowden and Wyatt[2] have shown that hyaline membrane formation is a result of destruction of the membranous pneumocyte. In the normal lung the tight junctions of the epithelial cells form the major barrier to the movement of fluid and protein into the alveolar space. If the pulmonary toxin produces injury to only the endothelial cells, leaving the epithelial layer intact, interstitial edema without hyaline membranes occurs. If the epithelial layer is also destroyed, the air-blood barrier becomes much more permeable resulting in alveolar edema. Hyaline membranes composed of epithelial cell debris, plasma protein, and fibrin then form within the alveolar space.

The proliferative phase is characterized by alveolar lining cell hyperplasia, organization of alveolar fibrin and interstitial fibrosis. Type II pneumocytes proliferate and cover the denuded basement membrane while the interstitium becomes thickened by inflammatory cells, fibroblasts, and collagen. The exact pathophysiologic mechanism leading to interstitial fibrosis is unknown. In fact, biochemical studies have failed to show an increase in the amount of collagen present or an increase in the rate of collagen synthesis.[28] The alveolar interstitium contains two major forms of collagen, termed type I (typical fibrillar collagen found in skin, bone, tendon, vessels, and lung) and type III (reticulin, found in skin, vessels, intestine, and lung). It has been shown that in idiopathic pulmonary fibrosis the relative amount of type III collagen is markedly reduced, while an increased amount of type I collagen is present.[104] Autoimmune reactions to type I collagen, as exhibited by migration-inhibition factor production and lymphocyte-mediated cytotoxicity reactions, also occur.[70]

In drug-induced pulmonary disease, a classic prototype of this type of reaction is produced by chemotherapeutic agents.[94] Bleomycin[1] and cyclophosphamide[49] have been found to induce DAD—fibrosis in experimental animals. Agents implicated in a similar manner in human lung disease are: busulfan,[85] methotrexate,[11, 83] chlorambucil,[98] melphalan,[26] bleomycin,[71, 102] cyclophosphamide.[49, 120]

Busulfan produces the typical chronic pneumonitis, pulmonary fibrosis and dysplastic epithelial changes of all other agents in this category. A possible distinguishing feature is a more prominent intra-alveolar and intraductal fibrosis perhaps resulting from the organization of fibrinous edema and epithelial cell debris[55, 76] (Fig. 2). Although the exact incidence is unknown, the duration of therapy causing lung disease has been reported from 13 days to 120 months with a mean of 49 months, and survival has varied at the time of diagnosis from 1 month or less to 24 months with a mean of 5 months.[85]

Methotrexate causes bilateral diffuse pulmonary infiltrates from 10 days to 5 years after the start of therapy. Again, although the exact incidence is unknown, 39 cases have been reported in the literature.[107] In one study of 92 methotrexate-treated patients, 7 (7.6%) had features compatible with methotrexate-induced lung disease.[107] In addition to the typical histologic changes, poorly defined noncaseating granulomas containing multinucleated giant cells may be present.[25] The illness usually remits with cessation of therapy, and only a few deaths have been reported. It is possible that this agent should be considered in the hypersensitivity category since the presence of granulomas and rapid reversibility suggests an immunologic reaction rather than a direct toxic effect. Figure 3 illustrates the histologic and radiologic features of methotrexate-induced lung disease.

Bleomycin has been reported to cause clinically evident pulmonary disease in 3–6% of patients given the drug. However, pulmonary function studies have shown abnormalities in 33–71%.[57, 126] It has been shown to cause disease after a cumulative dose of 105–165 mg[71] while most investigators have shown a very low incidence until 450–500 mg have been given. In animal studies[1] the initial sites of

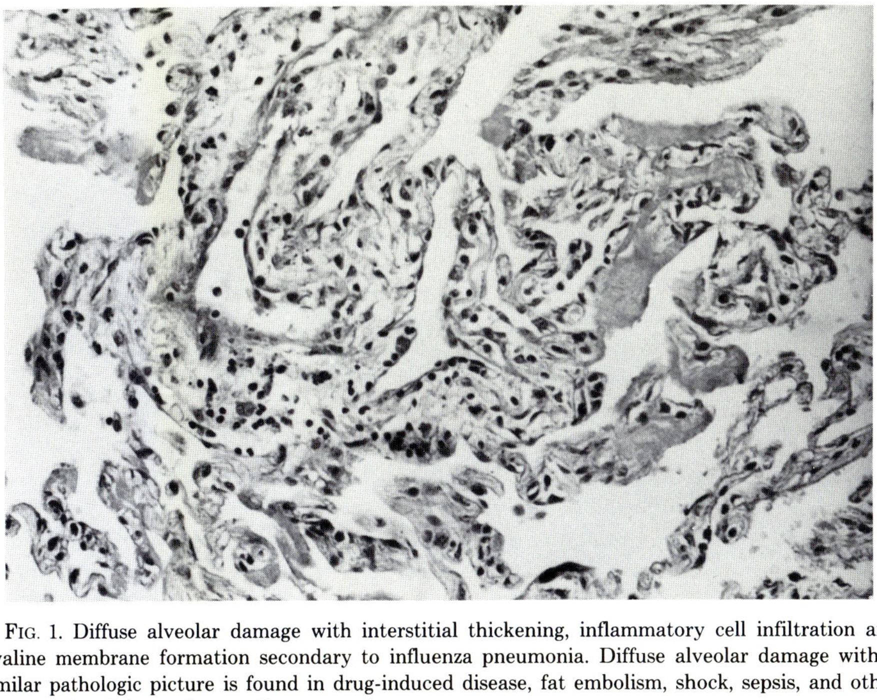

FIG. 1. Diffuse alveolar damage with interstitial thickening, inflammatory cell infiltration and hyaline membrane formation secondary to influenza pneumonia. Diffuse alveolar damage with a similar pathologic picture is found in drug-induced disease, fat embolism, shock, sepsis, and other forms of the adult respiratory distress syndrome.

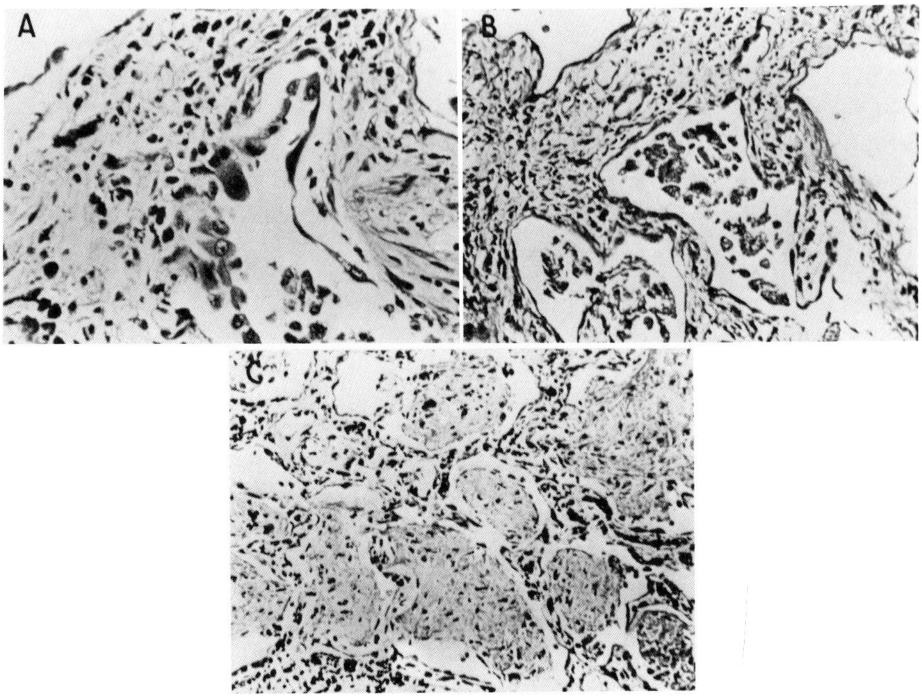

FIG. 2. *A*, Busulfan-Induced epithelial cell dysplasia. (Reproduced by permission, from Podoll, L., Winkler, S: Busulfan lung. *Am. J. Roent. Rad. Ther. Nucl. Med. 120:* 151–156, 1974.) *B*, Interstitial pulmonary fibrosis with intra-alveolar collections of granular pneumocytes. *C*, Early organization of intra-alveolar granular material associated with early interstitial fibrosis. (*B* and *C* reproduced by permission, from Littler, W. A., McKay, J., Hasleton, P. S., and Heath, D.: *Thorax 24:* 639–655, 1969.) 1969.

injury were the endothelial cells of veins and arteries followed by the endothelial cells of the septal capillaries (Fig. 4).

Cyclophosphamide, in addition to causing bronchial hypersecretion, has also been shown to produce the picture of diffuse alveolar damage. Along with the typical hyaline membranes and inflammatory changes, the most conspicuous change was alveolar epithelial cell hyperplasia.[49, 120]

The clinical presentation of diffuse alveolar damage-fibrosing alveolitis due to chemotherapeutic agents usually begins with the onset of cough, fever, and dyspnea associated with diffuse bilateral interstitial and intra-alveolar infiltrates on the chest roentgenogram. Pulmonary function studies show a restrictive pattern, often with severe reduction in carbon monoxide diffusing capacity. Clinical signs are nonspecific and the differential diagnosis usually includes neoplastic infiltration, opportunistic infection, or viral pneumonitis. A lung biopsy is necessary to rule out these possibilities and shows the spectrum of diffuse alveolar damage-interstitial fibrosis previously described. Treatment consists of discontinuation of the drug and a trial of steroids in most cases. Although the value of steroids has not been established, individual case reports have shown some improvement after high dose therapy.

Paraquat, a powerful herbicide, has been shown to produce the typical exudative and proliferative phases of DAD following human and experimental animal ingestion.[119] Classically, pulmonary complications become apparent about a week after ingestion, beginning with diffuse intra-alveolar infiltrates followed by a more reticular pattern on X-ray. Histologically the early phase of injury is characterized by damage to the epithelial cells, in contrast to other agents (*e.g.*, bleomycin). Two distinct forms of subacute fibrotic responses have also been reported.[119] The first is characterized by the formation of microcysts, thought to be due to alveolar wall destruction. The second is the formation of intra-alveolar fibrotic tissue, believed to be due to the organization of protein-rich edema fluid (Fig. 5).

Nitrofurantoin, although better known for the acute syndrome of eosinophilic pneumonia, also produces a fibrosing alveolitis. In the chronic form of nitrofurantoin injury[96] there is usually a lengthy history of exposure (6 months to 6 years). The usual histologic appearance is that of a nonspecific chronic interstitial pneumonitis and fibrosis but desquamative interstitial pneumonia has also been reported[14] (Fig. 6).

Other drugs associated with the development of irreversible fibrosis include

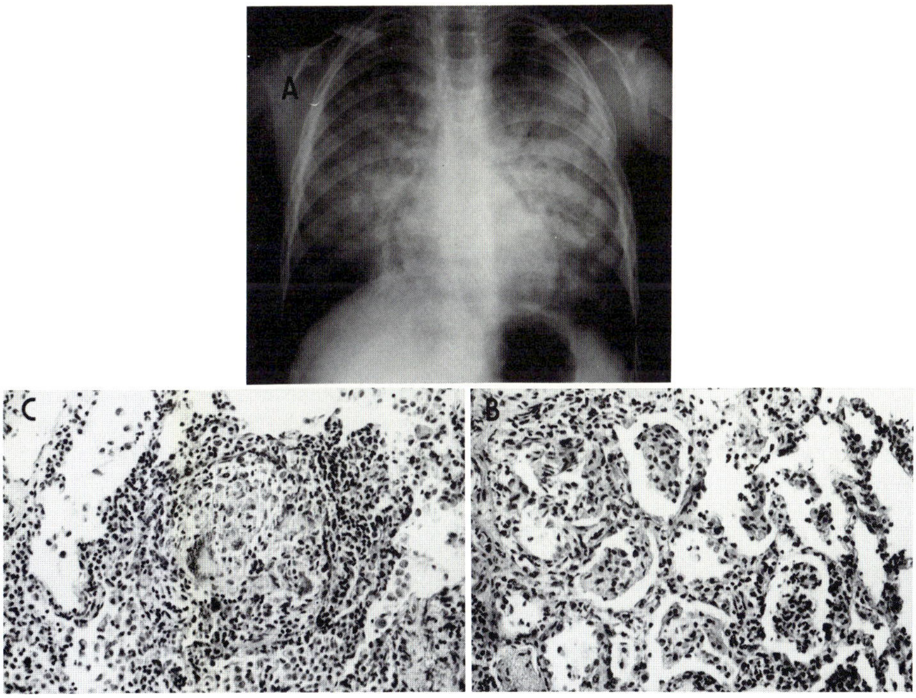

FIG. 3. Four-year-old girl with acute lymphoblastic leukemia treated with methotrexate. Shortly after completing the first course of methotrexate she developed a diffuse reticular nodular infiltrate, seen on the chest roentgenogram (*A*) to involve both lungs. *B*, Lung biopsy showing diffuse alveolar damage, epithelial cell proliferation, and inflammatory cell infiltration extending into intra-alveolar spaces. *C*, Noncaseating granuloma formation with multinucleated giant cells (Courtesy of Dr. Claire Langston).

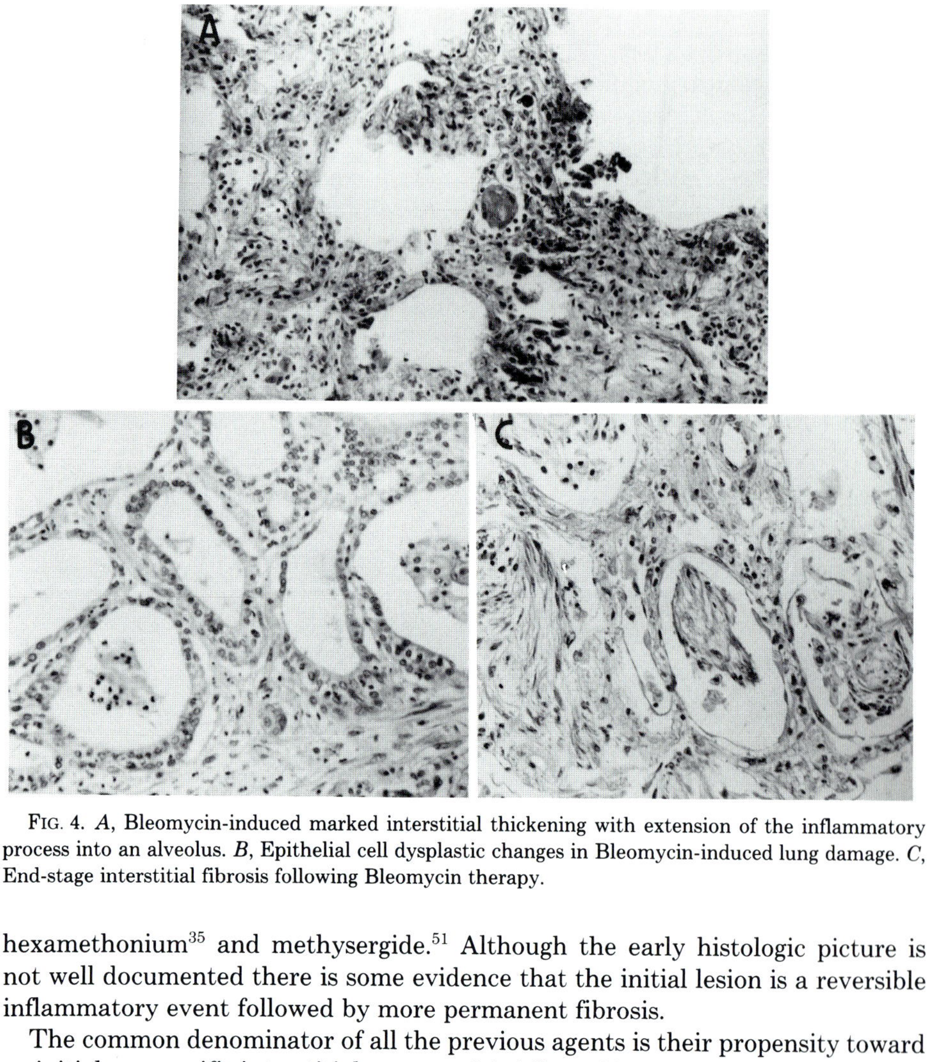

FIG. 4. *A*, Bleomycin-induced marked interstitial thickening with extension of the inflammatory process into an alveolus. *B*, Epithelial cell dysplastic changes in Bleomycin-induced lung damage. *C*, End-stage interstitial fibrosis following Bleomycin therapy.

hexamethonium[35] and methysergide.[51] Although the early histologic picture is not well documented there is some evidence that the initial lesion is a reversible inflammatory event followed by more permanent fibrosis.

The common denominator of all the previous agents is their propensity toward an initial nonspecific interstitial pneumonitis followed by a fairly rapid progression to irreversible pulmonary fibrosis.

PULMONARY EDEMA

Many drugs have been reported to cause pulmonary edema and there are several potential pathophysiologic mechanisms for each (see Chapter 12). In 1896 Starling described a classical approach to fluid movement across endothelium. His equation has recently been modified by Staub[109] who has developed more complex equations describing fluid and solute transport across endothelium, lymphatics, and alveolus. These extend the Starling equation to describe better the physical properties of the membrane separating one compartment from another.

$$Jv = Kf\,[(Pc - Pis) - \sigma(\pi c - \pi is)]$$

Where Jv is the rate of net liquid movement; Kf is the capillary filtration

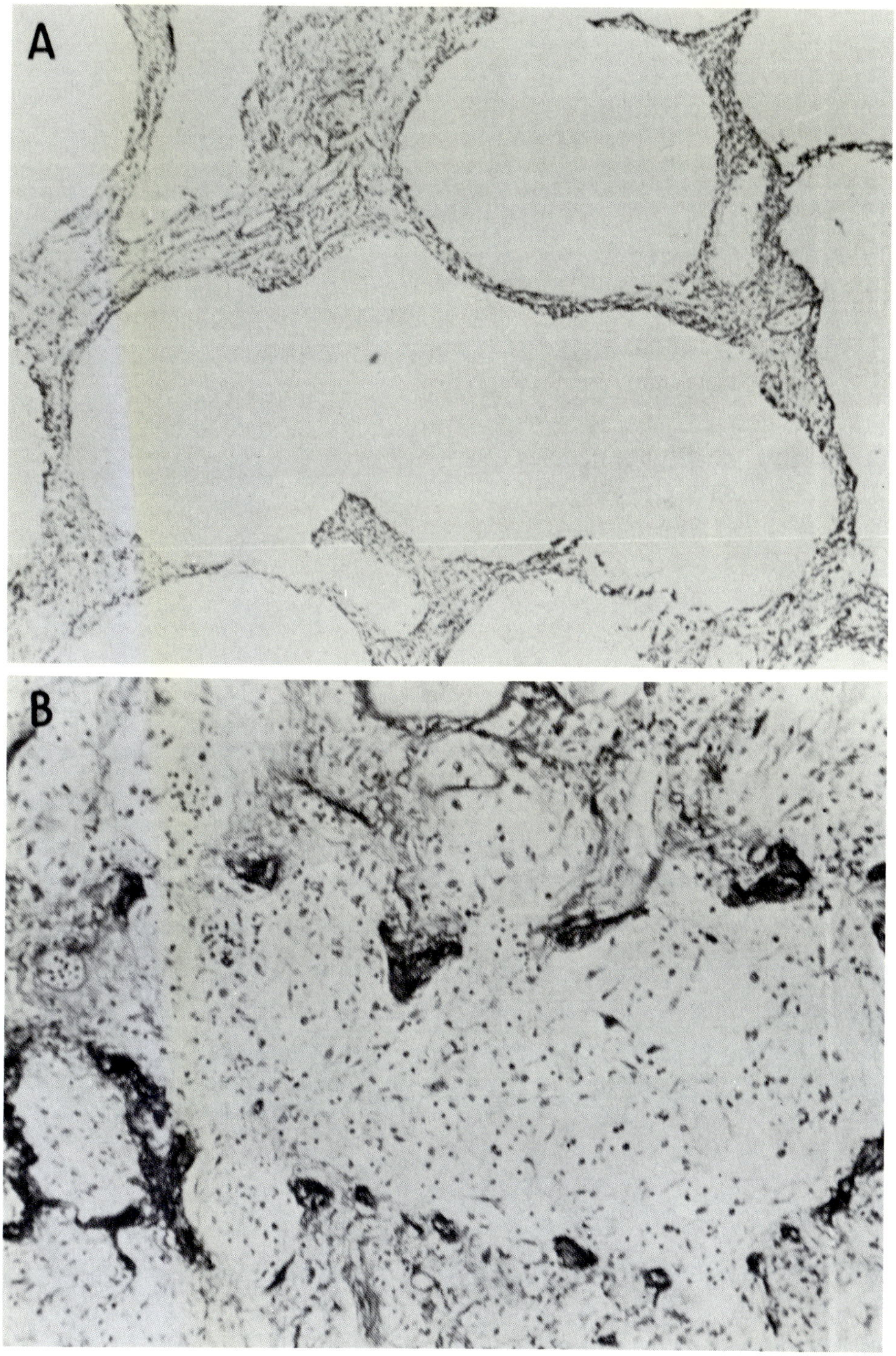

FIG. 5. *A*, Paraquat-induced pulmonary damage resulting in the formation of small cysts separated from each other by fibrous tissue. *B*, Alveolar duct showing loose fibrous tissue filling air spaces. (Reproduced by permission, from Thurlbeck W., and Thurlbeck, S.: Pulmonary effects of paraquat poisoning. *Chest 69 (Suppl.)*: 276–280, 1976.)

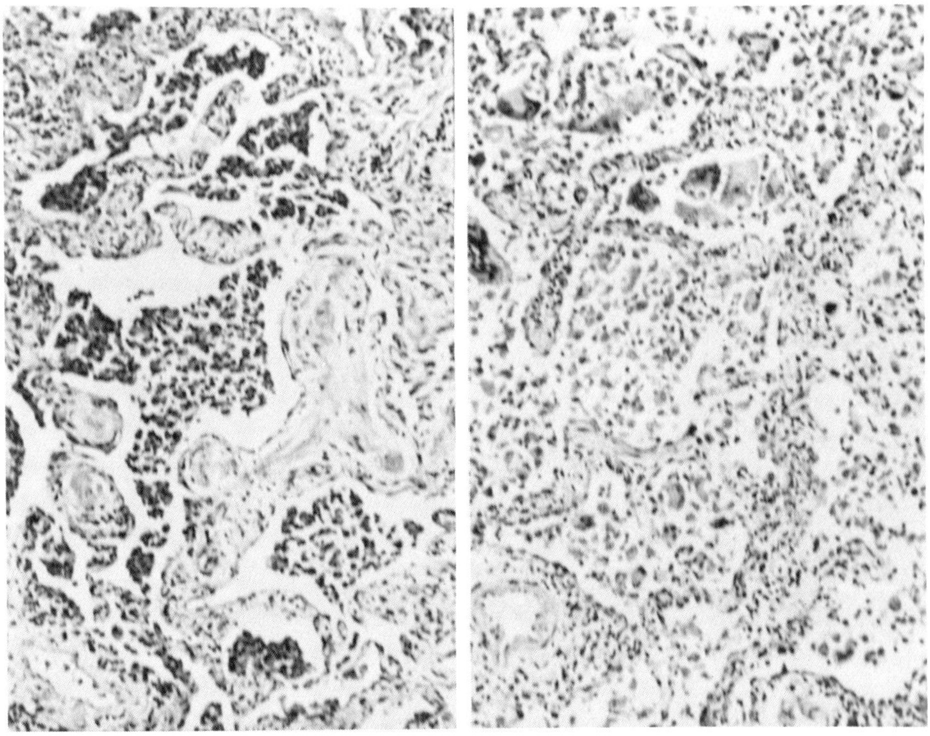

FIG. 6. Desquamative interstitial pneumonia from two cases of chronic nitrofurantoin induced lung disease. (Reproduced by permission, from Bone, R., *et al.*: Desquamative interstitial pneumonia following chronic nitrofurantoin therapy. *Chest 69 (Suppl.)*: 296–297, 1976.)

coefficient (including contribution of capillary permeability and actual microvascular surface area in which exchange occurs); Pc and Pis are the hydrostatic pressures in microvascular and interstitial spaces; πc and πis are the oncotic pressures in the microvascular and interstitial spaces; and σ is the reflection coefficient, which indicates the permeability of the microvascular membrane to plasma proteins.

Because significant alterations in any variable can account for pulmonary edema, the literature on drug-induced pulmonary disease contains many speculations concerning pathophysiology. Interstitial hydrostatic pressure and plasma oncotic pressure are not likely to change abruptly with drug therapy. Accordingly, useful information is provided by reports which include measurements of pulmonary capillary wedge pressure (PCWP). When this estimate of Pc is significantly elevated, pulmonary edema secondary to heart failure, increased plasma volume, or pulmonary venous constriction is suggested. If Pc is normal, pulmonary edema is likely due to the drug effect on the integrity of the microvasculature ($\uparrow$Kf, $\downarrow\sigma$).

Isolated cases in which PCWP was measured and found to be normal are shown in Table 2. It is not known how large a role decreased lymph flow plays in drug-induced pulmonary edema.

Since some drugs affect the microvascular membrane (by altering Kf) it is difficult to distinguish this process from that of the exudative phase of DAD secondary to drugs, and these may share the same mechanism. It is unclear why certain injuries progress to hyaline membrane formation and fibrosis and still others clear spontaneously with aggressive treatment and withdrawal of the inciting agent.

HYPERSENSITIVITY PNEUMONITIS WITH OR WITHOUT EOSINOPHILLA

The agents in this category are thought to produce pulmonary damage via immune or hypersensitivity reactions rather than by exerting a direct toxic effect. As such, their reactions are not dose related and occasionally exhibit immunologically mediated reactions *in vitro*. Nitrofurantoin-induced pulmonary disease has received the most attention and study in the recent literature[8, 14, 47, 60, 80, 108, 118] and may serve as a useful model to characterize hypersensitivity pneumonitis. In acute and subacute reactions, vasculitis, interstitial inflammation, and granulomatous reactions were found.[108] Evidence for an immunologically mediated reaction includes: presence of raised titres of antinuclear antibodies, antibodies to thyroid, renal glomeruli and smooth muscle, raised serum IgG levels, positive lymphocyte-transformation tests, and the production of migration inhibition factor,[47, 108] in response to nitrofurantoin. Albumin - IgG antibody complexes have been associated with nitrofurantoin treatment, and these may cause the vasculitis and interstitial inflammation.[118] Eosinophilia may be indicative of a type III reaction, since eosinophils are attracted to antigen-antibody complexes.[75]

Although agents in this category may eventually produce pulmonary fibrosis, the infiltrates are generally rapidly reversible upon discontinuation of the agent and usually respond well to steroid therapy.

Usually with Eosinophilia

Drugs reported to produce pulmonary infiltrates with peripheral blood eosinophilia are penicillin,[43, 87] sulfonamides,[39] nitrofurantoin (acute reaction),[59] para-

Table 2.

Drug	Pulmonary capillary wedge pressure*
Opiates[41, 86, 111, 127]	Normal
Heroin	Normal
Methadone	Normal
Morphine	Normal
Salicylates[18, 29, 58]	Normal
Pentazocine (Talwin)[7]	
Propoxyphene (Darvon)[12, 114]	Normal
Ethchlorvynol (Placidyl)[45, 46]	Normal
Bromocarbamide[105]	
Dextran[64]	
Propoxur (Baygon)[99]	Normal
Thiazides[110]	
Iodinized Oils[9, 19, 40, 67, 122]	
Sodium diatrizoate (Hypaque)[23, 24, 30]	
Phenylbutazone[84]	

* Normal capillary wedge pressure suggests that the drug affects the capillary membrane coefficient (Kf) to cause pulmonary edema.

aminosalicylic acid,[121] hydralazine,[74] mecamylamine,[74] mephenesin,[93] chlorpropamide,[10] salicylazosulfapyridine,[27, 31, 37, 61] disodium chromoglycate,[20, 78, 88] and imipramine.[124] Although peripheral eosinophilia is not present in every case it is found often enough to warrant consideration as a distinguishing feature.

The clinical presentation is often one of sudden onset of cough, dyspnea, and weight loss with febrile episodes. The chest X-ray shows an increase in linear lung markings often with patchy, wandering, unstable infiltrates more marked at the base. In nitrofurantoin-induced disease there is often an associated pleural effusion.

The histologic picture is one of filling of alveoli with a mixture of mononuclear cells and eosinophils with edema and eosinophilic infiltration of the interstitium. Fibrinous exudates, granulomatous reaction, mucous plugging, and vascular infiltration are also common features.[74]

Usually without Eosinophilia

Agents in this category are generally less easily identified as having an allergic or immunologically mediated mechanism for pulmonary damage. Although peripheral eosinophilia has been reported with some of the agents, it is present in fewer cases than those described above.

For example, intramuscular gold therapy was reported to cause pulmonary reactions with or without associated peripheral eosinophilia.[42, 125] The adverse reactions correlate with a positive lymphocyte transformation test.[34] Procarbazine[62] has also been reported to cause hypersensitivity reactions with or without eosinophilia. Other agents include azathioprine,[77] penicillamine,[36, 113] and colchicine.[56] Among limited histologic data in the above studies, diffuse interstitial infiltration with lymphocytes and plasma cells were reported.

DRUG-INDUCED SYSTEMIC LUPUS ERYTHEMATOSUS (SLE)

A large number of drugs have lupus-inducing or activating potential.[5, 6, 32, 72, 95] Alarcón-Segovia[4–6] has suggested that this group of drugs can be split into two categories on the basis of their mechanism of action.

Drugs that induce SLE because of their peculiar pharmacologic properties. This group includes hydralazine hydrochloride, isonicotinic acid hydrazide (isoniazid), procainamide, chlorpromazine, and many anticonvulsants (*e.g.,* dilantin). Each elicits SLE without evidence of an allergic reaction and appears to react in a dose- or time-related manner. Although the incidence of SLE activation for each agent is not known with certainty, procainamide and hydralazine have the highest potential for activation, in some series up to 30% for procainamide and 10–15% for hydralazine. Anticonvulsants, isoniazid, and chlorpromazine carry a lower risk of activating clinically overt disease. Although the mechanism by which they act is unknown, it is possible that they modify nuclear or cytoplasmic antigens, directly stimulate immunologic phenomenon or even alter the response to a viral infection.

Drugs which elicit allergic reactions leading to the development of lupus. This group of drugs (Table 3)[5] may elicit SLE after brief periods of use, usually associated with allergic reactions, and associated with a low incidence of both antinuclear induction and SLE activation.

TABLE 3. DRUGS REPORTED TO INDUCE OR ACTIVATE SLE (from Reference 5)

Group I (by pharmacologic action)	Group II (by allergic reaction)
Hydralazine	Aminosalicylic acid
Procainamide	Chlorthalidone*
Anticonvulsants	D-Penicillamine
Isoniazid	Griseofulvin
Chlorpromazine	Guanoxan
	Isoguinazepan
	Levodopa
	Methyldopa*
	Methysergide
	Methylthiouracil
	Oral contraceptives
	Oxyphenisatin
	Penicillin
	Phenylbutozone
	Practolol
	Propylthiouracil
	Quinidine
	Reserpine
	Streptomycin
	Sulfonamides
	Tetracycline
	Tolazamide

* May belong to Group I.

Drug-induced SLE and the spontaneously occurring disease differ in at least two ways. First, the clinical manifestations are somewhat different and second, the drug-induced syndrome is usually reversible after discontinuation of the drug. The clinical manifestations of drug-induced SLE are generally milder than those occurring in the natural form. Unlike the naturally occurring disease which predominantes in females with family histories of rheumatic disorders, drug-induced SLE occurs in the more elderly (those who are being treated with antiarrhthymic or antihypertensive medication), with only slight female preponderance. Drug-induced SLE seldom causes renal disease and generally there is a lower incidence of anemia and leukopenia. On the other hand, some drugs (*e.g.*, procainamide), induced a much higher incidence of pleuropulmonary manifestations than the naturally occurring form.[4, 6, 21]

Some drugs are capable of producing immunologic abnormalities, such as positive antinuclear antibody (ANA), without the clinical manifestations of SLE. Twenty percent of tuberculous patients treated with INH have been shown to have positive ANA while only 4% of untreated tuberculous patients have positive ANA.[4] Procainamide therapy after 4 months may lead to the development of ANA in 30–40% with few having symptoms of SLE.[4]

The respiratory manifestations of drug-induced SLE include (1) pleurisy, with or without effusion, usually bilateral and associated with pericarditis and systemic illness; (2) recurrent cough, dyspnea, pleurisy, and fever resembling either pneumonia, interstitial pneumonitis, or pulmonary edema; and (3) dyspnea and tachypnea with alveolar atelectasis. Lung function studies show a restrictive pattern with a decreased diffusing capacity. All manifestations usually respond promptly to corticosteroids.

Histologically, the lung in SLE shows diffuse interstitial lymphocytic infiltrate with lymphoid nodules and organizing bronchiolitis. Often there is a perivascular lymphocytic and plasma cell infiltrate with vasculitis, arteriolar fibrinoid necrosis, and occasionally, fibrocollagenous intimal thickening.

PULMONARY HYPERTENSION

At least two mechanisms for drug-induced pulmonary hypertension exist. One is probably a result of a direct, functional, pharmacologic action on the pulmonary vasculature, and the second is due to an inflammatory reaction causing vascular obstruction.

A group of compounds known as pyrolizidine alkaloids isolated from the seeds of various species of crotalaria and senecio plants have been shown to cause pulmonary arterial hypertension and associated hypertensive pulmonary vascular disease in rats.[66] Although not a major cause of human disease, senecio jacobaen is a plant sold in "health food" stores for a variety of ailments and has been shown to produce pulmonary hypertension in rats. More importantly, it may help explain some of the mechanisms producing epidemics of pulmonary hypertension in Western Europe following the introduction of Aminorex, an appetite-suppressing drug. In Switzerland a sudden 20-fold increase in incidence of primary pulmonary hypertension was reported[52] two years after the introduction of Aminorex. Similar reports followed from other countries where the medication was available, but not in areas where it was not released. Further, the incidence in Switzerland has fallen since the withdrawal of Aminorex. Fatal cases showed plexiform lesions (see Chapter 13) in pulmonary vessels like those occurring in left to right cardiac shunts (Fig. 7). Although convincing epidemiologic evidence exists, no direct proof is available as the response has not been seen in animal studies.[66, 22] It has been postulated that, like the pyrolozidine alkaloids, there is a direct vasoconstriction of the smaller pulmonary arterioles by stimulating α-adrenergic receptors.[81]

The second form of drug-induced pulmonary hypertension is seen in narcotic addicts. The presence of talc and other foreign body granulomas in the lungs of addicts is well known. Pulmonary hypertension has been documented from injection of paragoric plus tripelennamine[117] and methylphenidate (ritalin)[73]. Postmortem examination in these cases has demonstrated the characteristic pulmonary talc granulomatosis and morphologic evidence of severe pulmonary hypertension with cor pulmonale. It has been postulated that the pulmonary hypertension is due to vascular obstruction by granulomas and that the degree is directly related to the amount of talc injected[73] (Fig. 8).

DRUG-INDUCED BRONCHOSPASM

Any drug which is implicated in a type I (IgE mediated) immunologic response may produce some degree of bronchospasm if the lung is involved in the anaphylactic reaction. Bronchospasm may predominate if the lung is the target organ in the reaction. The acute allergic penicillin reaction is the prototype of this response. It is not known whether asthmatics are more prone to this type of drug reaction than the normal population.

Intolerance to acetylsalicylic acid (ASA) with the development of asthma has

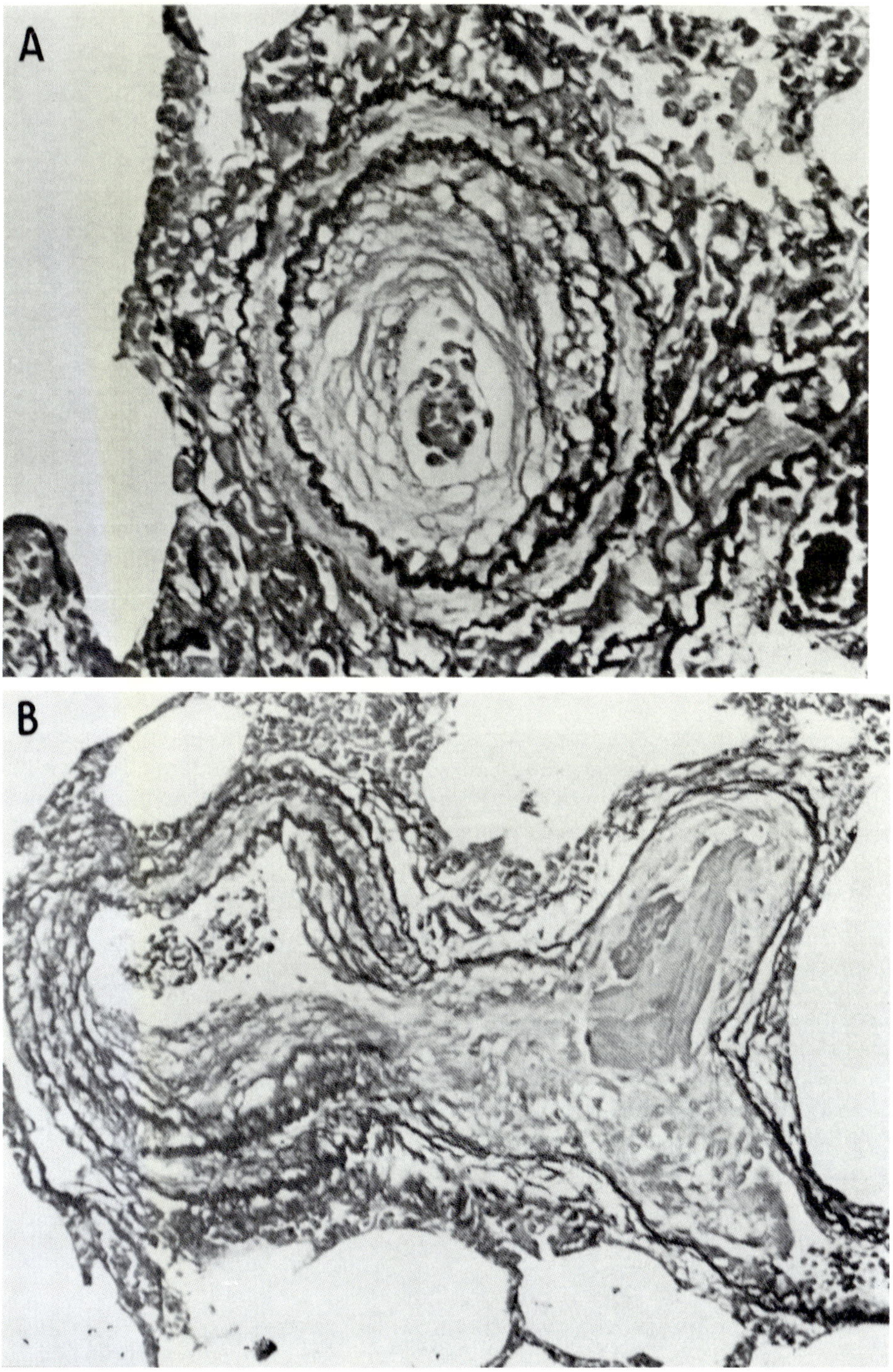

FIG. 7. *A*, Muscular pulmonary artery from patient with primary pulmonary hypertension with a history of ingestion of aminorex. The media is thickened with concentric fibroelastic tissue with narrowing of the lumen. *B*, Plexiform lesion in muscular pulmonary artery (same case as in *A*). (Reproduced by permission, from Kay, J. M., Smith, P., Health, D.: Aminorex and the pulmonary circulation. *Thorax 26:* 262–276, 1971.)

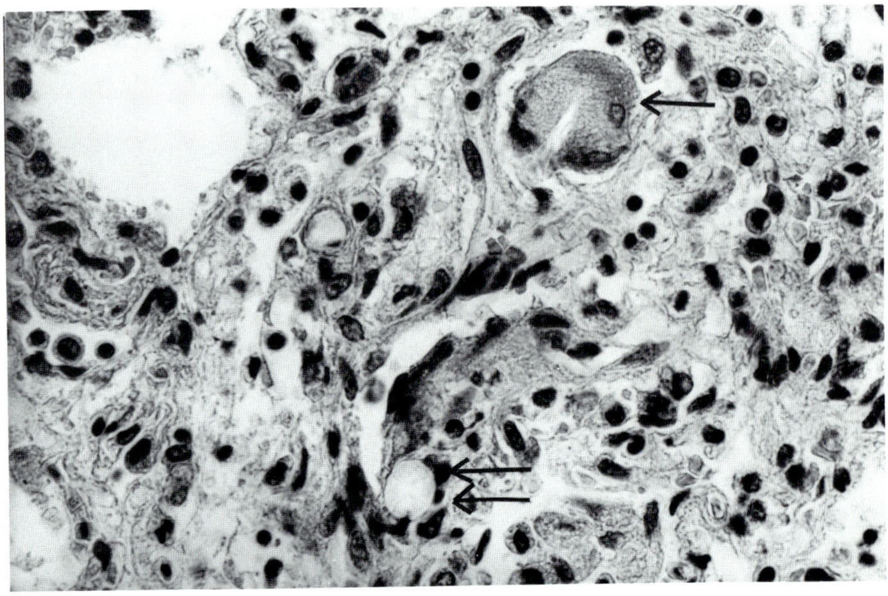

FIG. 8. Found at autopsy, talc granuloma from a narcotic addict shows a giant cell containing talc (*arrow*) and a large starch particle identified by polarized light (*double arrow*).

been recognized for more than 50 years. The subject of asthma and hypersensitivity was extensively reviewed by Samter and Beers[101] and Giraldo, Blumenthal, and Spink.[44] The syndrome of nasal polyps, eosinophilia, and asthma occurs in approximately 50% of ASA-sensitive patients.[112] Small doses of ASA are required to elicit symptoms and all patients that are sensitive react within 2 hours after oral ingestion. The bronchospasm is readily reversible after administration of a bronchodilator. ASA has also been reported to cause skin eruption, angioedema, rhinitis, purpura, angina pectoris, and recurrence of pustular psoriasis.[44]

The pathogenesis of ASA-induced bronchospasm is unknown. Recent work demonstrated that ASA, indomethacin, and other analgesics selectively inhibit bronchodilator prostaglandin synthesis.[116] This correlates with their ability to produce bronchoconstriction, and the severity of the bronchoconstriction is dose-related. If the synthesis or release of bronchodilator prostaglandins is inhibited, this would allow the action of the bronchoconstrictor (PGF2α) prostaglandin to go unopposed and result in bronchospasm.

Other drugs, including indomethacin, flufenamic acid, mefenamic acid (Ponstan), aminopyrine, benzoic acid derivatives, phenylbutazone, and tartrazine (a common food additive)[44, 63, 101, 103, 106, 112] are also associated with hypersensitivity and bronchospasm in ASA-sensitive patients.

A subgroup of drugs including acetaminophen (Paracetamol), dextropropoxyphene (Darvon), and pentazocine (Talwin) may also produce bronchospasm but are often used as analgesic substitutes in ASA-sensitive patients because the incidence of bronchospasm is lower.[33] Some of these have been shown to be weaker prostaglandin synthetase inhibitors than aspirin and this may account for the difference in activity.[33]

RESPIRATORY MUSCLE PARALYSIS

Muscular paralysis is produced by a wide variety of pharmacologic agents that are used extensively in clinical medicine, especially in the area of anesthesia. Some drugs, however, are not usually associated with neuromuscular blockade and hypoventilation. Many aminoglycoside and polypeptidic antibiotics, including neomycin, streptomycin, kanamycin, gentamycin, polymixin A, polymixin B, colistin, and viomycin are in this category.[95] One of the most potent polypeptidic antibiotic neuromuscular blockers is polymixin B.[3] The duration of neuromuscular blockade is dose-related. Neostigmine and calcium chloride antagonize the neuromuscular blockade produced by some of these antibiotics. Respiratory muscle paralysis occurs most often in (1) patients with renal failure unable to excrete the agent; (2) use of another muscle relaxant at the time of general anesthesia; (3) parenteral administration; (4) overdosage, usually accidental; and (5) patients with neuromuscular disease (myasthenia gravis).[95]

PLEURAL DISEASE

Pleural effusions complicating drug therapy are frequently associated with drugs producing the SLE-like syndrome. Two other medications, nitrofurantoin and methysergide, are also associated with the development of pleuritis and effusions.

Nitrofurantoin produces effusions only in the acute type of reaction with the rapid onset of fever, chills, dyspnea, alveolar-interstitial infiltrates, and eosinophilia.[39, 53, 92] Methysergide causes inflammatory fibrosis within the retroperitoneal space, endocardium, and pleura.[50, 69] The onset is insidious, 6 months to several years after starting the medication, and begins with cough and dyspnea. Pleural thickening and/or chronic effusions are seen on X-ray, and pleural biopsy reveals marked fibrotic thickening with an overlying layer of nonspecific inflammatory exudate consisting of lymphocytes and plasma cells. Discontinuation of the drug is usually the only treatment necessary, although steroids have been used in resistant cases.

MISCELLANEOUS

The pulmonary effects of Dilantin have been described in the literature since 1959 when Moore[82] reported that 87% of a group of subjects on Dilantin developed X-ray changes in the pulmonary parenchyma. He described increased bronchovascular markings occasionally resembling diffuse interstitial fibrosis. Subsequent studies refuted these findings,[79, 77] but all of these studies used only the chest X-rays to evaluate pulmonary changes. Hazlett, Ward, and Madison[54] studied pulmonary function changes in Dilantin therapy and found that a significant proportion developed physiologic impairment of pulmonary gas exchange with an increased incidence in those subjects starting the medication before 8 years of age. Although the pulmonary histologic appearance has not been documented, one case with both liver and pulmonary involvement showed noncaseating granulomatous hepatitis with dense periportal infiltration with eosinophils. Previous cases have also shown a systemic vasculitis and peripheral eosinophilia with depressed serum complement levels, suggesting an immune-complex injury.

TABLE 4. DRUG-INDUCED LUNG DISEASE

Drug	DAD*	Pulmonary edema	Hypersensitivity		SLE*	Pulmonary hypertension	Bronchospasm in ASA-sensitive patients	Muscle paralysis	Pleural disease	Miscellaneous
			with eosinophilia	without eosinophilia						
Aminorex						X				
Aminosalicylic acid			X		X					
Anticoagulants										X
Anticonvulsants					X					X
Azathioprine (Imuran)				X						
Baygon (Propoxur)		X								
Bleomycin	X									
Bromocarbamide		X								
Busulfan	X									
Chlorambucil	X									
Chlorpropamide			X							
Colchicine				X						
Colistin								X		
Corticosteroids										X
Cyclophosphamide	X									
Dextran		X								
Dilantin					X					X
Disodium chromoglycate (Intal)			X							
Gentamycin								X		
Gold			X	X						
Griseofulvin					X					
Guanoxan					X					
Heroin (opiates)		X								
Hexamethonium	X									
Hydralazine			X		X					
Hypaque		X								
Imipramine			X							
Indomethacin							X			
Isoniazid (INH)			X		X					
Isoguinazepon					X					
Mecamylamine (Inversine)			X							

Mefenamic acid (Ponstan)							X		
Melphalan (Alkeran)	X								
Mephenesin (Tolserol)			X						
Methotrexate	X			X					
Methyldopa					X				
Methysergide (Sansert)	X								X
Methylthiouracil					X				
Neomycin								X	
Nitrofurantoin (acute & chronic)	X		X						X
Oral contraceptives					X				
Paracetamol (Acetaminophen)							X		
Paraquat	X								
Paraminosalicylic acid (PAS)			X		X				
Penicillamine				X					
Penicillin			X		X				
Pentazocine (Talwin)		X					X		
Phenylbutazone		X			X		X		
Ethchloryinol (Placidyl)		X							
Polymixin A & B								X	
Procainamide					X				
Procarbazine			X	X					
Propoxyphene (Darvon)		X					X		
Reserpine					X				
Salicylates		X					X		
Salicylazosulfapyridine			X						
Streptomycin					X			X	
Sulfonamides			X		X				
Tartrazine							X		
Tetracycline					X				
Thiazides		X							
Talc (injected)						X			
Viomycin								X	

* DAD, diffuse alveolar damage; SLE, systemic lupus erythmatosus.

Dilantin is also associated with the drug-induced SLE syndrome in which pleural effusions are seen, as well as with the pseudolymphoma syndrome in which both hilar and or mediastinal adenopathy are found.[100]

Corticosteroids, as well as being an important factor in the development of opportunistic infections, also have a more direct effect on the respiratory system. Mediastinal lipomatosis due to the redistribution of reserve fat may mimic other mediastinal diseases and result in unnecessary surgery.[68] The increased fat content in the mediastinum causes a smooth symmetrical widening of the upper mediastinum without pressure effect on the trachea. The fact that these patients are always Cushingoid clinically and often have a related increase in the pericardial fat pad may help to make the diagnosis.

Anticoagulants can cause bleeding into the lungs, mediastinum or pleural space.[89]

Oral contraceptives are related to the development of collagen diseases[13] as well as being controversially implicated in thromboembolic disease.[38] Any unexplained pulmonary symptoms in a female taking oral contraceptives should raise the possibility of drug-induced thromboembolism.

In this discussion we have attempted to compile the available information on drug-induced lung disease and present it using a classification system based on clinical and pathologic criteria. Table 4 consists of a summary of this information.

REFERENCES

1. Adamson, I. Y. R., and Bowden, D. H.: The pathogenesis of bleomycin-induced pulmonary fibrosis in mice. *Am. J. Pathol. 77:* 185–198, 1974.
2. Adamson, I. Y. R., Bowden, D. H., and Wyatt, J. P.: Oxygen poisoning in mice. Ultrastructural and surfactant studies during exposure and recovery. *Arch. Pathol. 90:* 463–472, 1970.
3. Adamson, R. H., Marshall, F. N., and Long, J. P.: Neuromuscular blocking properties of various polypeptide antibiotics (26154). *Proc. Soc. Exp. Biol. Med. 105:* 494–497, 1960.
4. Alarcón-Segovia, D.: Drug-induced lupus syndromes. *Mayo Clinic Proc. 44:* 664–681, 1969.
5. Alarcón-Segovia, D.: Drug-induced antinuclear antibodies and lupus syndromes. *Drugs 12:* 69–77, 1976.
6. Alarcón-Segovia, D., and Alarcón, D. G.: Pleuro-pulmonary manifestations of systemic lupus erythematosus. *Dis. Chest 39:* 7–17, 1961.
7. Ali, N., and Banks, T.: Pentazocine addiction causing bacterial endocarditis and pulmonary embolism. *Chest 64:* 762–763, 1973.
8. Bäck, O., Lundgren, R., and Wiman, L-G.: Nitrofurantoin-induced pulmonary fibrosis and lupus syndrome. *Lancet 1:* 930, 1974.
9. Belin, R. P., Shea, M. A., Stone, N. H., and Griffen, W. O.: Iodoliposputosis following lymphangiography. Report of a case. *Dis. Chest 48:* 543–544, 1965.
10. Bell, R. J. M.: Pulmonary infiltration with eosinophils caused by chlorpropamide. *Lancet 1:* 1249–1250, 1964.
11. Bhat, K. S. S., Anderson, K. R., and Stewart, R. D. H.: Lung disease associated with methotrexate therapy. *Aust. N. Zeal. J. Med. 4:* 277–280, 1974.
12. Bogartz, L. J., and Miller, W. C.: Pulmonary edema associated with propoxyphene intoxication. *JAMA 215:* 259–262, 1971.
13. Bole, G. G., Jr., Friedlaender, M. H., and Smith, C. K.: Rheumatic symptoms and serological abnormalities induced by oral contraceptives. *Lancet 1:* 323–326, 1969.
14. Bone, R. C., Wolfe, J., Sobonya, R. E., Kerby, G. R., Stechschulte, D., Ruth, W. E., and Welch, M.: Desquamative interstitial pneumonia following chronic nitrofurantoin therapy. *Chest 69 (Suppl.):* 296–297, 1976.
15. Bowden, D. H., and Adamson, I. Y. R.: Reparative changes following pulmonary cell injury. Ultrastructural, cytodynamic, and surfactant studies in mice after oxygen exposure. *Arch.*

Pathol. 92: 279–283, 1971.

16. Bowden, D. H., and Wyatt, J. P.: Lung injury and repair: A contemporary view. *Pathology Annual, 1970,* edited by Sommers, S. C., pp. 279–307.
17. Brettner, A., Heitzman, E. R., and Woodin, W. G.: Pulmonary complications of drug therapy. *Radiology 96:* 31–38, 1970.
18. Broderick, T. W., Reinke, R. T., and Goldman, E.: Salicylate-induced pulmonary edema. *Am. J. Roentgenol. 127:* 865–866, 1976.
19. Bron, K. M., Baum, S., and Abrams, H. L.: Oil embolism in lymphangiography; Incidence, manifestations, and mechanisms. *Radiology 80:* 194–202, 1963.
20. Burgher, L. W., Kass, I., and Schenken, J. R.: Pulmonary allergic granulomatosis: A possible drug reaction in a patient receiving cromolyn sodium. *Chest 66:* 84–86, 1974.
21. Byrd, R. B., and Schanzer, B.: Pulmonary sequelae in procaine amide induced lupus-like syndrome. *Dis. Chest 55:* 170–172, 1969.
22. Byrne-Quinn, E., and Grover, R. F.: Aminorex (Menocil) and amphetamine: Acute and chronic effects on pulmonary and systemic haemodynamics in the calf. *Thorax 27:* 127–131, 1972.
23. Cameron, J. D.: Pulmonary edema following drip-infusion urography. Case report. *Radiology 111:* 89–90, 1974.
24. Chiu, C. L., and Gambach, R. R.: Hypaque pulmonary edema. A case report. *Radiology 111:* 91–92, 1974.
25. Clarysse, A. M., Cathey, W. J., Cartwright, G. E., and Wintrobe, M. M.: Pulmonary disease complicating intermittent therapy with methotrexate. *JAMA 209:* 1861–1864, 1969.
26. Codling, B. W., and Chakera, T. M. H.: Pulmonary fibrosis following therapy with melphalan for multiple myeloma. *J. Clin. Pathol. 25:* 668–673, 1972.
27. Constantinidis, K. A.: Letter: Eosinophilic pneumonia: An unusual side effect of therapy with salicylazosulfapyridine. *Chest 70:* 315–316, 1976.
28. Crystal, R. G. (moderator), Fulmer, J. D., Roberts, W. C., Moss, M. L., Line, B. R., and Reynolds, H. Y.: NIH Conference: Idiopathic pulmonary fibrosis. Clinical, histologic, radiographic, physiologic, sintagraphic, cytologic, and biochemical aspects. *Ann. Intern. Med. 85:* 769–788, 1976.
29. David, P. R., and Burch, R. E.: Pulmonary edema and silacylate intoxication. *Ann. Intern. Med. 80:* 553–554, 1974.
30. Davidson, J. W.: Pulmonary complications of lymphography (letter). *N. Eng. J. Med. 285:* 237, 1971.
31. Davies, D., and MacFarlane, A.: Fibrosing alveolitis and treatment with sulphasalazine. *Gut 15:* 185–188, 1974.
32. Davies, P. D. B.: Drug-induced lung disease. *Br. J. Dis. Chest 63:* 57–70, 1969.
33. Delaney, J. C.: The diagnosis of aspirin idiosyncrasy by analgesic challenge. *Clin. Allergy 6:* 177–181, 1976.
34. Denman, E. J., and Denman, A. M.: The lymphocyte transformation test and gold hypersensitivity. *Ann. Rheum. Dis. 27:* 582–589, 1968.
35. Doniach, I., Morrison, B., and Steiner, R. E.: Lung changes during hexamethonium therapy for hypertension. *Br. Heart J. 16:* 101–108, 1954.
36. Eastmond, C. J.: Diffuse alveolitis as complication of penicillamine treatment for rheumatoid arthritis. *Br. Med. J. 1:* 1506, 1976.
37. Eastwood, M.: Sulphasalazine-induced lung disease. *Lancet 2:* 659–660, 1974.
38. Elgee, N. J.: Medical aspects of oral contraceptives. *Ann. Intern. Med. 72:* 409–418, 1970.
39. Fiegenberg, D. S., Weiss, H., and Kirshman, H.: Migratory pneumonia with eosinophilia associated with sulfonamide administration. *Arch. Intern. Med. 120:* 85–89, 1967.
40. Fraimow, W., Wallace, S., Lewis, P., Greening, R. R., and Cathcart, R. T.: Changes in pulmonary function due to lymphangiography. *Radiology 85:* 231–241, 1965.
41. Frand, U. I., Shim, C. S., and Williams, M. H., Jr.: Methadone-induced pulmonary edema. *Ann. Intern. Med. 76:* 975–979, 1972.
42. Geddes, D. M., and Brostoff, J.: Pulmonary fibrosis associated with hypersensitivity to gold salts. *Br. Med. J. 1:* 1444, 1976.
43. Geller, M., Kriz, R. J., Zimmerman, S. W., Flaherty, D. K., and Dickie, H. A.: Penicillin-associated pulmonary hypersensitivity reaction and interstitial nephritis. *Ann. Allergy 37:* 183–190, 1976.

44. Giraldo, B., Blumenthal, M. N., and Spink, W. W.: Aspirin intolerance and asthma. A clinical and immunological study. *Ann. Intern. Med. 71:* 479–496, 1969.
45. Glauser, F. L., Powers, D., Fischer, P., Egan, P., Smeltzer, D., Lewis, J., Smith, W. R., and Morton, M.: Pulmonary tissue concentrations of ethchlorvynol after intravenous injection. *Am. Rev. Resp. Dis. 115:* 83–88, 1977.
46. Glauser, F. L., Smith, W. R., Caldwell, A., Hoshiko, M., Dolan, G. S., Baer, H., and Olsher, N.: Ethchlorvynol (Placidyl®)-induced pulmonary edema. *Ann. Intern. Med. 84:* 46–48, 1976.
47. Goldstein, R. A., and Janicki, B. W.: Immunologic studies in nitrofurantoin induced pulmonary disease. *Med. Ann. D.C. 43:* 115–119, 1974.
48. Gough, J. H., Gough, M. H., and Thomas, M. L.: Pulmonary complications following lymphography: With a note on technique. *Br. J. Radiol. 37:* 416–421, 1964.
49. Gould, V. E., and Miller, J.: Sclerosing alveolitis induced by cyclophosphamide. Ultrastructural observations on alveolar injury and repair. *Am. J. Pathol. 81:* 513–530, 1975.
50. Graham, J. R.: Cardiac and pulmonary fibrosis during methysergide therapy for headache. *Am. J. Med. Sci. 254:* 1–12, 1967.
51. Graham, J. R., Suby, H. I., LeCompte, P. R., and Sadowsky, N. L.: Fibrotic disorders associated with methysergide therapy for headache. *N. Eng. J. Med. 274:* 359–368, 1966.
52. Gurtner, H. P., Gertsch, M., Salzmann, C., Scherrer, M., Stucki, P., and Wyss, F.: Häufen sich die primär vasculären formen des cornischen cor pulmonale? *Schweizerische Medizinische Wochenschrift 98:* 1579–1589, 1968.
53. Hailey, F. J., Glascock, H. W., Jr., and Hewitt, W. F.: Pleuropneumonic reactions to nitrofurantoin. *N. Engl. J. Med. 281:* 1087–1090, 1969.
54. Hazlett, D. R., Ward, G. W., Jr., and Madison, D. S.: Pulmonary function loss in Diphenylhydantoin therapy. *Chest 66:* 660–664, 1974.
55. Heard, B. E., and Cooke, R. A.: Busulphan lung. *Thorax 23:* 187–193, 1968.
56. Hill, R. N., Spragg, R. G., Wedel, M. K., and Moser, K. M.: Adult respiratory distress syndrome associated with colchicine intoxication. *Ann. Intern. Med. 83:* 523–524, 1975.
57. Horowitz, A. L., Friedman, M., Smith, J. I., Yagoda, A., LaMonte, C., and Watson, R. C.: The pulmonary changes of bleomycin toxicity. *Radiology 106:* 65–68, 1973.
58. Hrnicek, G., Skelton, J., and Miller, W. C.: Pulmonary edema and salicylate intoxication. *JAMA 230:* 866–867, 1974.
59. Israel, H. L., and Diamond, P.: Recurrent pulmonary infiltration and pleural effusion due to nitrofurantoin sensitivity. *N. Engl. J. Med. 266:* 1024–1026, 1962.
60. Israel, K. S., Brashear, R. E., Sharma, H. M., Yum, M. N., and Glover, J. L.: Pulmonary fibrosis and nitrofurantoin. *Am. Rev. Resp. Dis. 108:* 353–356, 1973.
61. Jones, G. R., and Malone, D. N. S.: Sulphasalazine-induced lung disease. *Thorax 27:* 713–717, 1972.
62. Jones, S. E., Moore, M., Blank, N., and Castellino, R. A.: Hypersensitivity to procarbazine (Matulane ®) manifested by fever and pleuropulmonary reaction. *Cancer 29:* 498–500, 1972.
63. Juhlin, L., Michaëlsson, G., and Zetterström, O.: Urticaria and asthma induced by food-and-drug additives in patients with aspirin hypersensitivity. *J. Allergy Clin. Immunol. 50:* 92–98, 1972.
64. Kaplan, A. I., and Sabin, S.: Dextran 40: Another cause of drug-induced noncardiogenic pulmonary edema. *Chest 68:* 376–377, 1975.
65. Katzenstein, A-L. A., Bloor, C. M., and Liebow, A. A.: Diffuse alveolar damage—The role of oxygen, shock, and related factors. A review. *Am. J. Pathol. 85:* 210–228, 1976.
66. Kay, J. M., Smith, P., and Heath, D.: Aminorex and the pulmonary circulation. *Thorax 26:* 262–270, 1971.
67. Koehler, P. R., Meyers, W. A., Skelley, J. F., and Schaffer, B.: Body distribution of ethiodol following lymphangiography. *Radiology 82:* 866–871, 1964.
68. Koerner, H. J., and Sun, D. I-C.: Mediastinal lipomatosis secondary to steroid therapy. *Am. J. Roent. Rad. Ther. Nucl. Med. 98:* 461–464, 1966.
69. Kok-Jensen, A., and Lindeneg, O.: Pleurisy and fibrosis of the pleura during methysergide treatment of hemicrania. *Scand. J. Resp. Dis. 51:* 218–222, 1970.
70. Kravis, T. C., Ahmed, A., Brown, T. E., Fulmer, J. D., and Crystal, R. G.: Pathogenic mechanisms in pulmonary fibrosis. Collagen-induced migration inhibition factor production and cytotoxicity mediated by lymphocytes. *J. Clin. Invest. 58:* 1223–1232, 1976.
71. Lacovino, J. R., Leitner, J., Abbas, A. K., Lokich, J. L., and Snider, G. L.: Fatal pulmonary

reaction from low doses of bleomycin. An idiosyncratic tissue response. JAMA 235: 1253–1255, 1976.

72. Lee, S. L., and Chase, P. H.: Drug-induced systemic lupus erythematosus: A critical review. *Sem. Arthr. Rheum. 5:* 83–103, 1975.
73. Lewman, L. V.: Fatal pulmonary hypertension from intravenous injection of methylphenidate (ritalin) tablets. *Human Pathol. 3:* 67–70, 1972.
74. Liebow, A. A., and Carrington, C. B.: The eosinophilic pneumonias. *Medicine 48:* 251–285, 1969.
75. Litt, M.: Eosinophils and antigen-antibody reactions. *Ann. N. Y. Acad. Sci. 116:* 964–985, 1964.
76. Littler, W. A., and Ogilvie, C.: Lung function in patients receiving busulphan. *Br. Med. J. 4:* 530–532, 1970.
77. Livingston, S., Whitehouse, D., and Pauli, L. L.: Study of the effects of diphenylhydantoin sodium on the lungs. *N. Engl. J. Med. 264:* 648–651, 1961.
78. Löbel, H., Machtey, I., and Eldror, M. Y.: Pulmonary infiltrates with eosinophilia in an asthmatic patient treated with disodium cromoglycate. *Lancet 2:* 1032, 1972.
79. Low, N. L., and Yahr, M. D.: The lack of pulmonary fibrosis in patients receiving diphenylhydantoin. *JAMA 174:* 1201–1202, 1960.
80. Lundgren, R., Bäck, O., and Wiman, L. G.: Pulmonary lesions and autoimmune reactions after long-term nitrofurantoin treatment. *Scand. J. Resp. Dis. 56:* 208–216, 1975.
81. Malmquist, J., Trell, E., Torp, A., and Lindström, C.: A case of drug-induced(?) pulmonary hypertension. *Acta Med. Scand. 188:* 265–272, 1970.
82. Moore, M. T.: Pulmonary changes in hydantoin therapy. *JAMA 171:* 1328–1333, 1959.
83. Nesbit, M., Krivit, W., Heyn, R., and Sharp, H.: Acute and chronic effects of methotrexate on hepatic, pulmonary, and skeletal systems. *Cancer 37:* 1048–1057, 1976.
84. Nevins, M., Berque, S., Corwin, N., and Lyon, L.: Phenylbutazone and pulmonary oedema (letter). *Lancet 2:* 1358, 1969.
85. Podoll, L. N., and Winkler, S. S.: Busulfan lung. Report of two cases and review of the literature. *Am. J. Roent. Radium Ther. Nucl. Med. 120:* 151–156, 1974.
86. Presant, S., Knight, L., and Klassen, G.: Methadone-induced pulmonary edema. *Canad. Med. Assoc. J. 113:* 966–967, 1975.
87. Reichlin, S., Loveless, M. H., and Kane, E. G.: Loeffler's syndrome following penicillin therapy. *Ann. Intern. Med. 38:* 113–120, 1953.
88. Repo, U. K., and Nieminen, P.: Pulmonary infiltrates with eosinophilia and urinary symptoms during disodium cromoglycate treatment. A case report. *Scand. J. Resp. Dis. 57:* 1–4, 1976.
89. Reussi, C., Schiavi, J. E., Altman, R., Yussem, E. E., and Rouvier, J.: Unusual complications in the course of anticoagulant therapy. *Am. J. Med. 46:* 460–463, 1969.
90. Robin, E. D., Carey, L. C., Grenvik, A., Glauser, F., and Gaudio, R.: Capillary leak syndrome with pulmonary edema. *Arch. Intern. Med. 130:* 66–71, 1972.
91. Robin, E. D., Cross, C. E., and Zelis, R.: Pulmonary edema. *N. Engl. J. Med. 288:* 239–246, 292–304, 1973.
92. Robinson, B. R.: Pleuropulmonary reaction to nitrofurantoin. *JAMA 189:* 239–240, 1964.
93. Rodman, T., Fraimow, W., and Myerson, R. M.: Löffler's syndrome: Report of a case associated with administration of mephenesin carbamate (Tolseram). *Ann. Intern. Med. 48:* 668–674, 1958.
94. Roeckel, I. E.: Pathologic alterations in the lung following use of immunosuppressant agents. *Ann. Clin. Lab. Sci. 3:* 212–218, 1973.
95. Rosenow, E. C., III: The spectrum of drug-induced pulmonary disease. *Ann. Intern. Med. 77:* 977–991, 1972.
96. Rosenow, E. C., III, DeRemee, R. A., and Dines, D. E.: Chronic nitrofurantoin pulmonary reaction. Report of five cases. *N. Engl. J. Med. 279:* 1258–1262, 1968.
97. Rubin, G., Baume, P., and Vandenberg, R.: Azothioprine and acute restrictive lung disease. *Aust. N. Zeal. J. Med. 3:* 272–274, 1972.
98. Rubio, F. A., Jr.: Possible pulmonary effects of alkylating agents. *N. Engl. J. Med. 287:*
99. Salisbury, B. G., Tate, C. F., Jr., and Davies, J. E.: Baygon-induced pulmonary edema. *Chest 65:* 455–457, 1974.
100. Saltzstein, S. L., and Ackerman, L. V.: Lymphadenopathy induced by anticonvulsant drugs and mimicking clinically and pathologically malignant lymphomas. *Cancer 12:* 164–182, 1959.
101. Samptor, M., and Beers, R. R.: Intolerance to aspirin. *Ann. Intern. Med. 68:* 975–983, 1968.
102. Samuels, M. L., Johnson, D. E., Holoye, P. Y., and Lanzotti, V. J.: Large-dose bleomycin

therapy and pulmonary toxicity. A possible role of prior radiotherapy. *JAMA 235:* 1117–1120, 1976.
103. Santiago, B. M., Jr., and Klaustermeyer, W. B.: Acute respiratory failure secondary to indomethacin in an aspirin-intolerant asthmatic patient. *Ann. Allergy 37:* 138–141, 1976.
104. Seyer, J. M., Hutcheson, E. T., and Kang, A. H.: Collagen polymorphism in idiopathic chronic pulmonary fibrosis. *J. Clin. Invest. 57:* 1498–1507, 1976.
105. Sigihara, H., Hagedorn, M., Bottcher, D., Neuhof, H., and Mittermayer, Ch.: Interstitial pulmonary edema following bromocarbamide intoxication. *Am. J. Pathol. 75:* 457–472, 1974.
106. Smith, A. P.: Response of aspirin-allergic patients to challenge by some analgesics in common use. *Br. Med. J. 2:* 494–496, 1971.
107. Sostman, H. D., Matthay, R. A., Putman, C. E., and Walker Smith, G. J.: Methotrexate-induced pneumonitis. *Medicine 55:* 371–388, 1976.
108. Sovijärvi, A. R. A., Lemola, M., Stentius, B., and Idänpään-Heikkilä, J.: Nitrofurantoin-induced acute, subacute and chronic pulmonary reactions. A report of 66 cases. *Scand. J. Resp. Dis. 58:* 41–50, 1977.
109. Staub, N. C.: "State of the Art" Review. Pathogenesis of pulmonary edema. *Am. Rev. Resp. Dis. 109:* 358–372, 1974.
110. Steinberg, A. D.: Pulmonary edema following ingestion of hydrochlorothiazide. *JAMA 204:* 825–827, 1968.
111. Steinberg, A. D., and Karliner, J. S.: The clinical spectrum of heroin pulmonary edema. *Arch. Intern. Med. 122:* 122–127, 1968.
112. Stenius, B. S. M., and Lemola, M.: Hypersensitivity to acetylsalicylic acid (ASA) and tartrazine in patients with asthma. *Clin. Allergy 6:* 119–129, 1976.
113. Sternlieb, I., Bennett, B., and Scheinberg, I. H.: D-Penicillamine-induced Goodpasture's syndrome in Wilson's disease. *Ann. Intern. Med. 82:* 673–676, 1975.
114. Sturner, W. Q., and Garriott, J. C.: Deaths involving propoxyphene. A study of 41 cases over a two-year period. *JAMA 223:* 1125–1130, 1973.
115. Symmers, W. St. C.: The occurrence of angiitis and of other generalized diseases of connective tissues as a consequence of the administration of drugs (with a note on drug allergy as a cause of thrombotic purpura). *Proc. Roy. Soc. Med. 55:* 20–28, 1962.
116. Szczeklik, A., Gryglewski, R. J., and Czerniawska-Mysik, G.: Relationship of inhibition of prostaglandin biosynthesis by analgesics to asthma attacks in aspirin-sensitive patients. *Br. Med. J. 1:* 67–69, 1975.
117. Szwed, J. J.: Pulmonary angiothrombosis caused by "blue velvet" addiction. *Ann. Intern. Med. 73:* 771–774, 1970.
118. Teppo, A-M.: Haltia, K., and Wager, O.: Immunoelectrophoretic "tailing" of albumin line due to albumin-IgC antibody complexes: A side effect of nitrofurantoin treatment? *Scand. J. Immunol. 5:* 249–261, 1976.
119. Thurlbeck, W. M., and Thurlbeck, S. M.: Pulmonary effects of paraquat poisoning. *Chest 69 (Suppl.):* 276–280, 1976.
120. Topilow, A. A., Rothenberg, S. P., and Cottrell, T. S.: Interstitial pneumonia after prolonged treatment with cyclophosphamide. *Am. Rev. Resp. Dis. 108:* 114–117, 1973.
121. Tuchman, H.: Löffler's reaction to para-aminosalicylic acid. *Am. Rev. Tuber. 70:* 171–175, 1954.
122. Weg, J. G., and Harkleroad, L. E.: Aberrations in pulmonary function due to lymphangiography. *Dis. Chest 53:* 534–540, 1968.
123. Whitcomb, M. E.: Drug-induced lung disease. *Chest 63:* 418–422, 1973.
124. Wilson, I. C., Gambill, J. M., and Sandifer, M. G.: Loeffler's syndrome occurring during imipramine therapy. *Am. J. Psychiatr. 119:* 892–893, 1963.
125. Winterbauer, R. H., Wilske, K. R., and Wheelis, R. F.: Diffuse pulmonary injury associated with gold treatment. *N. Engl. J. Med. 294:* 919–921, 1976.
126. Yagoda, A., Mukherji, B., Young, C., Etcubanas, E., Lamonte, C., Smith, J. R., Tan, C. T. C., and Krakoff, I. H.: Bleomycin, an antitumor antibiotic. Clinical experience in 274 patients. *Ann. Intern. Med. 77:* 861–870, 1972.
127. Zyroff, J., Slovis, T. L., and Nagler, J.: Pulmonary edema induced by oral methadone. *Radiology 112:* 567–568, 1974.

Chapter 3

Pathology of Adult Respiratory Distress Syndrome*

PHILIP C. PRATT

This syndrome, consisting of rapidly progressive deterioration of pulmonary gas transfer and reduction in pulmonary compliance, has been recognized with increasing frequency during recent years.[27] It occurs in patients with a severe acute initial problem, sometimes pulmonary but often extrapulmonary, who survive this episode but then develop respiratory dysfunction which often progresses inexorably, despite vigorous and elaborate therapy, with death following in from two to six or more weeks. Reported initiating processes have included viral pneumonitis,[7, 27] massive trauma as in battle wounds or automobile accidents,[4, 15] cutaneous burns,[18] parturition[13, 23] drowning,[25] acute central nervous system disease with associated pulmonary edema,[10] extensive or prolonged surgical procedures especially with cardiopulmonary bypass,[24] severe pyogenic systemic infection,[13] hemorrhage,[15] and unsuccessful suicidal hanging.[8]

The clinical syndrome usually begins after a period of partial or sometimes apparently complete recovery from the initial process. The improved status may continue for at least several hours to one, two, or even four days.[1] Then evidence of respiratory impairment appears with the patient aware of dyspnea, and blood gas analysis revealing hypoxemia. Therapy for this usually involves administration of oxygen with or without ventilatory assistance. If the process progresses, such assistance inevitably becomes necessary. High and increasing pressures needed to produce an adequate tidal volume indicate decreasing pulmonary compliance.[1] Positive end-expiratory pressure (PEEP) is often used and usually permits some reduction in inhaled oxygen concentration.[1, 22] Some patients begin to improve at this point and may recover. Others continue to show diminishing compliance and increasing hypoxemia despite increasing concentrations of oxygen until death occurs from respiratory failure, usually after 10–40 days.[1] Chest X-rays at the time of onset of respiratory distress usually show bilateral patchy "alveolar" infiltrates. PEEP often results in reduction of these shadows and recovery may be complete.[22] If not, the shadows increase again and become confluent; before death the lungs appear diffusely consolidated.[1]

The etiology and pathogenesis of this clinical syndrome remain obscure. As

* Supported in part by Contract No. NO1-HR-52946 from the National Heart, Lung and Blood Institute.

already noted, the original problems can scarcely be thought to have a common pathway since they range from trauma to viral infections. Metabolic damage during hypoperfusion could be proposed for many cases but a period of hypoperfusion has not been present in all. In many cases large volumes of intravenous fluids have been administered and hypervolemia has been proposed as an important factor;[15] again this cannot be shown to have occurred in all cases. Lung damage by mechanical ventilation has also been suggested since virtually every patient has had this form of therapy; however, several efforts to demonstrate that such ventilation produces lung damage have failed.[2, 14] It appears probable that many different mechanisms can lead to the onset of delayed respiratory distress.

Despite this wide range of initiating problems and the probable variety of mechanisms leading to the onset of respiratory distress, a remarkable feature of the syndrome is the homogeneity of the morphologic changes found in the lungs at autopsy.[13] The intent of the following sections is to illustrate this homogeneity and to present the author's conclusions as to the reasons for it.

The illustrative material is derived from patients who have died following treatment in medical or surgical intensive care units of both local hospitals and others for which the author is a consultant. Careful records and thorough control of the therapy were maintained during treatment. For the purpose of the present report the author has studied tissues from a series of 35 autopsied cases from such units. For comparison, 5 cases with dypsnea but no elaborate therapy will also be summarized.

MATERIALS AND METHODS

Cases included in the study had been treated with all available modalities including respirators and PEEP. Each received oxygen at a mean concentration above 50%. The sequential evolution of morphologic lesions with time will be reviewed.

The tissue used for the study consists of at least one block of peripheral lung tissue from each lobe considered by the prosector to be representative of the general appearance. Tissue blocks were fixed in formalin, embedded in paraffin, sectioned at 6 μ, and stained with hematoxylin-eosin and Masson trichrome stains.

Light microscopic observations were recorded in tabular form indicating extent and severity of lesions on a scale from 0–3. Each of a series of 18 separate types of lesion was recorded individually for the section from each lobe. All observations were made and recorded before examination of the clinical summary or gross protocol. Subsequently, these records were examined and used to reach a final evaluation of the underlying illness, its duration, the duration of respiratory failure and therapy, and the major cause of death. To date, 35 treated cases have been recorded and evaluated according to these procedures.

A second group of cases has also been reviewed. These were patients who had one or another of the various initiating episodes which often lead to the respiratory distress syndrome with oxygen therapy, intubation, PEEP, and other maneuvers. However, these patients did not receive such therapy, for various reasons, and thus can serve as "controls" for the treated cases.

The circumstances in these five cases are summarized briefly in order of increasing duration of dyspnea.

Case 1: A 54-year-old man had nutritional cirrhosis and esophageal varices. Massive hemorrhage had been successfully treated on two occasions. He returned to the hospital with a third episode which had been in progress for several hours. He was *in extremis* from shock and died within 8 hours after arrival at the emergency room. He had received 35 units of blood and died on the operating table during laparotomy.

At autopsy the lungs (700 and 490 grams) showed congestion and moderate edema but no hyaline membranes.

Case 2: A 53-year-old man was discovered, by friends, in his bed at home with second and third degree burns covering about 30% of his body, including the chest, back, and face. The bed was partially consumed by fire. Apparently the fire had occurred while the patient was alone and may have gone out spontaneously. The man had last been seen 3 days previously. The burns appeared to be of this age.

The patient was brought to the hospital comatose, dehydrated, and in shock. The arterial Po_2 on arrival was 42 mm Hg. Despite hydration, intubation, and 40% oxygen, he died within hours after arrival.

At autopsy the lungs (540 and 490 grams) showed early bronchopneumonia, contained soot suspended in bronchial mucus, and there was evidence of aspiration of gastric contents. The alveolar septa were thin and no hyaline membranes were seen.

Case 3: A 54-year-old man had carcinoma of the eosphagus. He refused surgery but remained in the hospital. After 2 months he developed gangrene of one foot, which was treated by amputation. Postoperatively he was noted to be dyspneic but, because of patient refusal, nothing was done except for a few intermittent positive-pressure breathing treatments. He survived with progressive dyspnea for 6 days and died in respiratory failure.

At autopsy the lungs (960 and 640 grams) showed edema and plugging of many small bronchi by mucus. There was no pneumonia. In addition, alveolar septa were thin and no hyaline membranes were seen.

Case 4: A 57-year-old man had recurrent glioblastoma multiforme. He had had significant neurologic deficits following the first resection and the family requested that elaborate therapy be withheld. The patient had increased intracranial pressure and pulmonary edema and was dyspneic. Because of the request the patient received no therapy and virtually no laboratory studies were done; blood gas tensions were not obtained. It is clear that his condition was stable during a two-week course. Finally, the patient became febrile and dyspnea worsened. He died in respiratory failure one week later.

At autopsy the lungs (830 and 700 grams) were extensively consolidated by pneumonia and contained abscesses. No hyaline membranes or fibrosis were present, even in areas least involved by the pneumonia (see Fig. 9).

Case 5: A 60-year-old man had nutritional cirrhosis and massive ascites producing dyspnea. The patient also had moderate pulmonary emphysema. Treatment consisted of aspiration of the ascites, which partially relieved the dyspnea although both recurred in a few days. The patient survived for 18 days with dyspnea constantly present. Finally, aspiration of gastric contents occurred and the patient died shortly thereafter.

At autopsy the lungs (460 and 350 grams) were virtually normal except for moderate centrilobular emphysema, and were without septal thickening, hyaline membranes, or fibrosis.

SEQUENTIAL EVOLUTION OF RESPIRATORY DISTRESS LESIONS

The evolution of lesions with time in the series of treated cases is presented in Figures 1 to 8. The legends provide detailed descriptions of the morphology, which is briefly summarized here.

From the first few days to about one week after the beginning of therapy for respiratory failure, the changes consisted mainly of thickened alveolar septa showing edema and capillary congestion. Eosinophilic amorphous deposits (hyaline membranes) were present in all cases. These were always more prominent

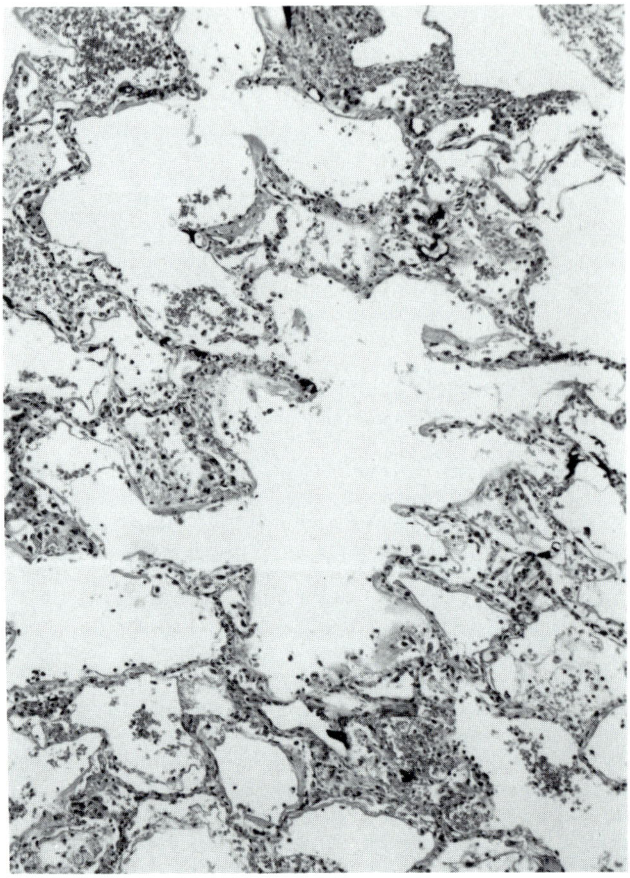

FIG. 1. An 18-year-old patient with automobile trauma. Respiratory failure was treated for 5 days. The field shows longitudinal sections through several alveolar ducts. Intervening alveolar spaces contain mild leukocytic infiltration indicating early pneumonia. Alveolar septa are generally slightly thicker than normal. Thin hyaline membranes are recognizable along the alveolar ducts, especially at the tips of projecting alveolar septa. Compare with Figure 9, a case with pneumonia but no oxygen therapy. × 100.

in the alveolar ducts than in adjacent alveoli and appeared first at the tips of septa which project into the lumens of the alveolar ducts. From about 1–2 weeks the above changes persisted and hyaline membranes became thicker and more extensive. Towards the end of the second week fibroblasts appeared in the vicinity of the most prominent hyaline membranes and slight collagen deposition was noted. Also during the second week, adjacent alveoli often showed partial or complete lining by cuboidal epithelial cells. Beyond two weeks, fibrosis became progressively more prominent.

This fibrosis occurred in a rather characteristic pattern, superficially reminiscent of organized pneumonia. However, after examination of multiple cases, it was noted that the fibrosis usually followed a branching, ramifying pattern similar to the distribution of alveolar ducts. Intervening alveoli, between the fibrosed ducts, were small but still patent and still showed cuboidal epithelial

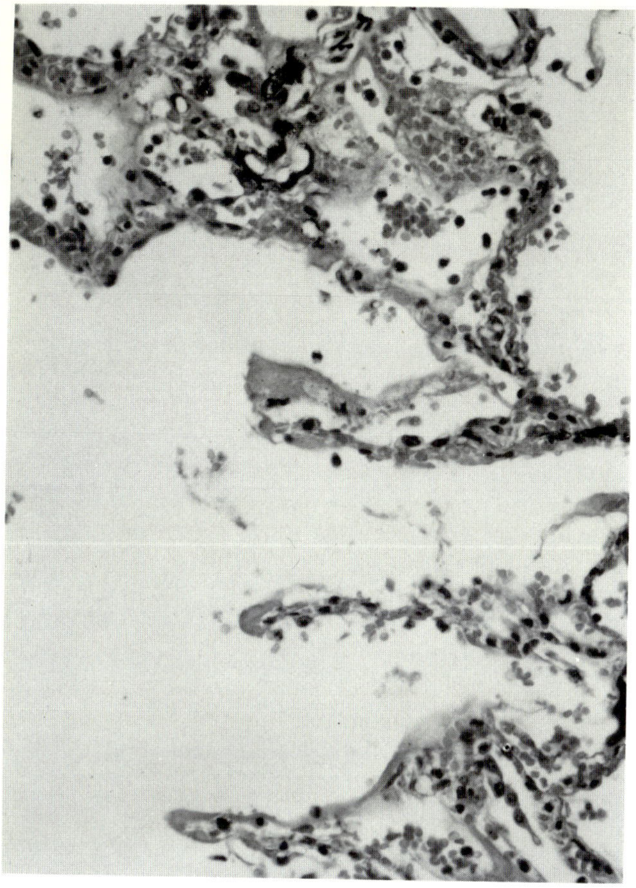

FIG. 2. Same case as Figure 1. This higher magnification shows the hyaline membranes at the tips of projecting septa and extending downward into the alveolar spaces × 250.
250.

lining and slight septal fibrosis. In subsequent discussion this lesion will be termed alveolar duct fibrosis. Further search revealed the progressive steps from the presence of a few strands of collagen along a duct, to a continuous layer, to partial and then complete filling of the lumen by fibrosis.

Still another observation arose from recognition of alveolar duct fibrosis. When pyogenic infection involves such alveolar ducts the appearance is easily mistaken for microabscess formation; in fact, several lesions had originally been recorded as abscesses. Finally, in cases where pulmonary hemorrhage occurred terminally, the partially fibrosed ducts with red cells in the lumen could easily be misinterpreted as abnormal blood vessels with initimal or adventitial fibrosis. Indeed at least one report does illustrate an "abnormal vessel," which is probably an alveolar duct.[5]

DISCUSSION

Table 1 shows, for the 35 treated cases, the underlying disease class; the number of cases receiving therapy for up to one, from one to two, and more

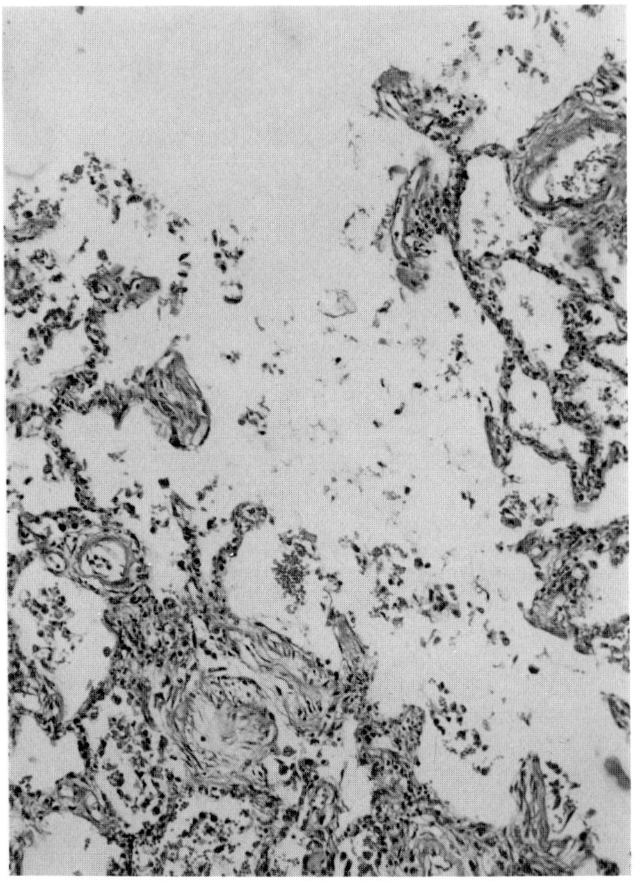

FIG. 3. A 50-year-old patient with massive gastrointestinal hemorrhage. Respiratory failure was treated for 9 days. An alveolar duct extends across the field from top to bottom. Hyaline membranes and also fibroblasts and collagen can be seen at the tips of several projecting septa. The fibrosis also extends into the alveolus at the lower center. × 100.

than two weeks; and the number of cases with hyaline membranes alone, or with alveolar duct fibrosis. It is noted in this table that none of the 10 cases in which death occurred within the first week had any alveolar duct fibrosis, although all of them had hyaline membranes. Between one and two weeks, 9 of 11 cases had alveolar duct fibrosis but in only one case was this thought to be the major factor responsible for death. Among 14 cases with duration longer than two weeks, 11 were considered to have died from progressive respiratory failure caused by alveolar duct fibrosis.

The table shows that the lesions found varied more closely with the duration of the treatment for respiratory impairment than with the original disease. Thus, while only one patient with viral pneumonitis showed hyaline membranes without any fibrosis, the fact that none of these cases died within the first week is probably the main reason for this. On the other hand, alveolar duct fibrosis was present in 22 of 25 cases surviving for longer than one week and was present in

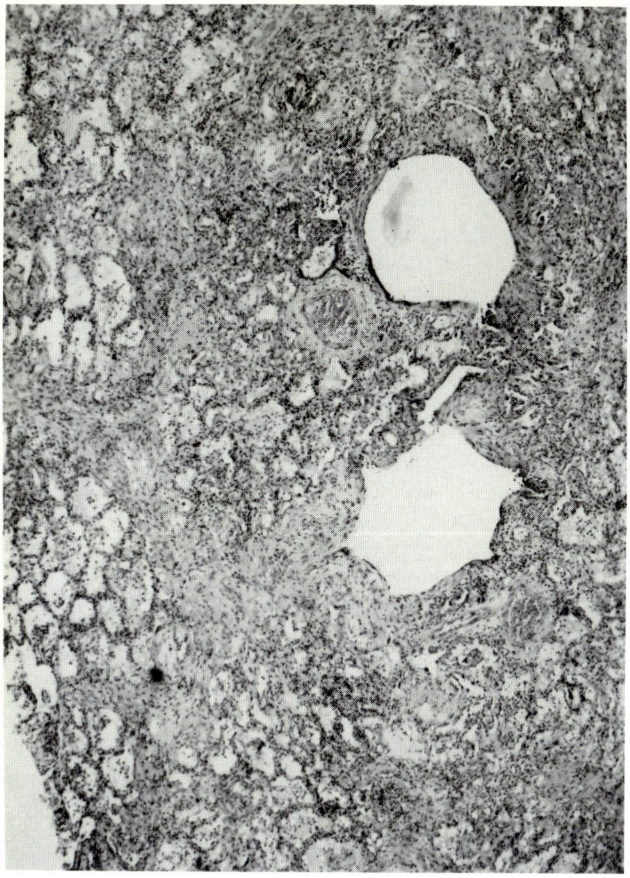

FIG. 4. A 23-year-old patient with probable suicidal narcotic drug overdose. Respiratory failure was treated for 12 days. The lumen of a bronchiole is seen above, and of the proximal portion of an alveolar duct, below. Extending towards the left from the duct lumen is a band of collagenous tissue and fibroblasts. Note that this band branches and extends towards the left lower corner and upwards across the left center. This branching sheet of fibrosis is distributed in the pattern of an alveolar duct. Note intervening alveoli with slightly thickened septa. × 40.

2 or more cases of each disease type except Goodpasture's syndrome. Neither patient with this disease survived the first week of respiratory failure.

The chi-square test of the changing distribution of cases with time gives a probability level of less than 0.01 ($\chi^2 = 39.9$; degrees of freedom = 4).

Two basic concepts can be proposed to explain the constancy of the morphologic appearance. First, it may be that the lung is capable of responding to various injuries in only a limited manner so that no matter what has caused diffuse damage the ultimate result, if damage is severe enough, will be diffuse interstitial fibrosis.[13] The second concept is that the underlying disease simply leads to the initiation of vigorous respiratory therapy which then continues to produce cell damage even though the patient may have recovered from the original process. The result would be that most or all of the changes observed at autopsy would be the result of the therapy. The uniformity of the morphology,

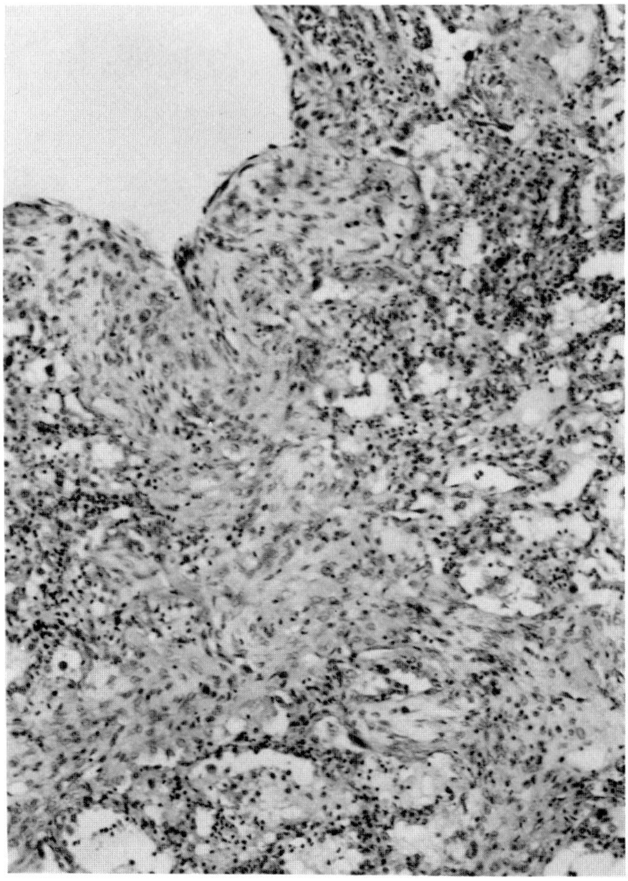

FIG. 5. Same case as Figure 4. The alveolar duct lumen is seen at top left. It is lined by a fibrous layer which is thicker and fills the duct lumen completely towards the center and bottom of the field. Alveolar spaces are clearly recognizable along the bottom and at the right. × 100.

despite varied underlying diseases, would then be logically expected. As noted in the introduction, most components of respiratory therapy (mechanical ventilation, intubation, PEEP) have not been shown to produce pulmonary damage in either man[2, 17, 20] or experimental animals.[14] Therefore the most likely responsible factor is the prolonged inhalation of increased concentations of oxygen.

Three major points can be made in support of this concept. First, it has long been known that oxygen is a toxic gas. For example, exposure of primates to high concentrations of oxygen produces all the changes noted in man, from hyaline membranes to interstitial fibrosis.[11, 12] This occurs even though the experimental animals are normal at the start, and not subjected to shock, infection or other initiating factors. Oxygen also produces lung lesions, although not always fibrosis, in all species tested.

The second point supporting the proposed concept relates to the tendency for lesions in the treated cases to be found earliest and to be most prominent along alveolar ducts. This location would be difficult to explain except in terms of the inhalation of a toxic gas. While some workers hold that gas is distributed to

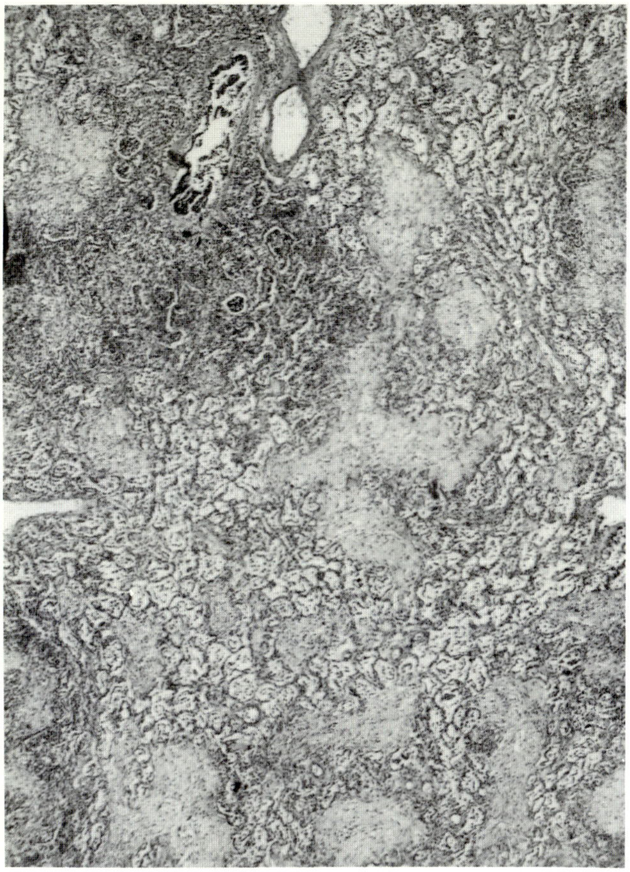

FIG. 6. A 15-year-old patient with eclampsia and Caesarean section. Respiratory failure was treated for 42 days. A bronchiole and arteriole are seen at top. The origin of the associated alveolar duct is not in this plane, but the branching sheet of fibrosis near the center of the field has the distribution of an alveolar duct. Intervening alveoli are rather small and all are lined by cuboidal epithelium. Septa are slightly thickened. × 30.

alveolar ducts and alveoli solely by diffusion, and is identical in concentration throughout the primary lobule,[3] there is reason to believe that during quiet respiration, mass to and fro movement of air does occur in alveolar ducts and alveoli.[26] The volume change in these structures is sufficient to bring the interface of newly inhaled gas to the level of the alveolar ducts.[26] Distribution of oxygen molecules from here to the distal alveoli would be by diffusion with counter-diffusion of carbon dioxide. It follows then that if an increased concentration of oxygen is inhaled, the alveolar ducts would be exposed to that concentration while more distal portions of the lobule would receive lower concentrations. Furthermore, the tips of the alveolar septa projecting into alveolar ducts would receive the most intense exposure of all. As illustrated in Figures 1 to 3, hyaline membranes first appear on these septa and fibrosis begins here also.

The third supporting point is based on the series of five untreated dyspneic patients. Each of these patients had dyspnea of sufficient degree that, except for

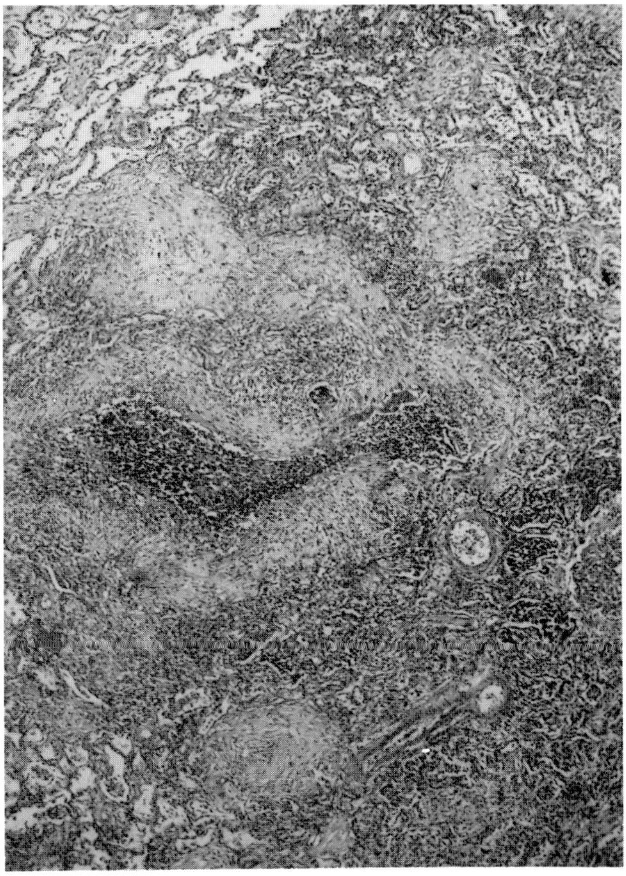

FIG. 7. Same patient as in Figure 6. In this field an alveolar duct with fibrosis extends horizontally from right to left. Its lumen is filled with leukocytes due to a terminal acute infection. This lesion could readily be misinterpreted as a microabscess. A branch of this duct, above, is completely filled by fibrosis. × 40.

accompanying circumstances, they would have received oxygen and other forms of therapy. Several of the clinical charts contain a specific comment that these therapies were considered and rejected. Cases 1, 2, and 3 had acute episodes (hemorrhagic shock, extensive burn with smoke inhalation, and surgery) which often are precipitating factors for the adult respiratory distress syndrome. It has been reported that each of these can produce hyaline membranes independently, although none were found in these specific examples. Cases 4 and 5 survived long enough so that, if treated, they might well have shown both hyaline membranes and fibrosis. In this connection, a previous report,[19] which also called attention to fibrosis involving alveolar ducts, included 12 patients treated with oxygen who did not develop the progressive respiratory distress syndrome but died as a result of their underlying process. At autopsy, hyaline membranes were found in 11 of the 12 cases.

While the 5 cases reported here can not be proposed in any strict sense as "controls" for the treated cases, they do constitute patients with acute episodes

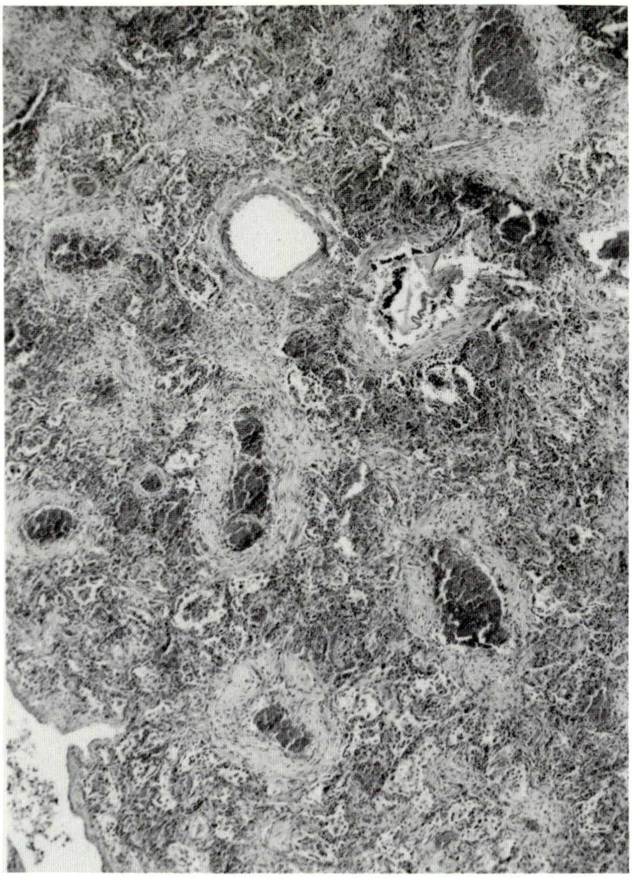

FIG. 8. A 33-year-old pregnant patient with respiratory viral infection. Respiratory failure was treated for 15 days; a hemorrhagic diathesis developed terminally. Several cross-sections of alveolar ducts with fibrosis can be seen. The lumen of each is filled with blood as are many adjacent alveoli. The thick-walled spaces with blood in the lumen could readily be misinterpreted as abnormal blood vessels with intimal and adventitial fibrosis. Note the normal artery to the left of the bronchiole in the upper center. × 40.

such as frequently eventuate in progressive adult respiratory distress syndrome. The fact that these patients did not show hyaline membranes or other initial morphologic phases of this process is, at the least, compatible with the concept that the morphologic changes seen at autopsy in treated cases are more the result of therapeutic efforts than they are of the initial disease.

It is likely that interstitial edema and even hyaline membranes are reversible since many patients who recover after showing evidences of the syndrome have been shown to have normal pulmonary function parameters.[1, 20, 21] On the other hand, unlysed fibrin has been shown to have binding sites with fibrobast cell membrane and may promote fibroblast growth.[16] Thus initiation or prolongation of hyaline membranes by oxygen exposure may be the major factor in the ultimate development of the interstitial and alveolar ductal fibrosis described.

The implications of the concept proposed here are not negative with regard

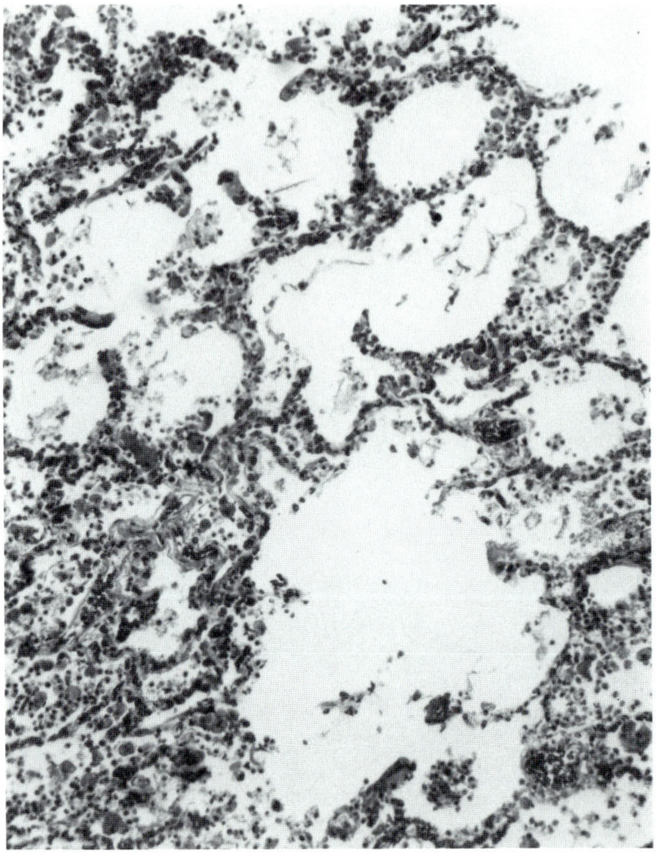

FIG. 9. A 57-year-old patient with recurrent glioblastoma multiforme. For clinical events, see the summary of case 4 under "Materials and Methods." There was extensive pneumonia, partly the result of aspiration of gastric contents. This field shows cross-sections of several alveolar ducts in an area less involved by pneumonia than most of the lung. It is in areas such as this that hyaline membranes and other lesions would be most prominent if vigorous therapy had been provided. Note that alveolar septa are thin, even those projecting into the ducts, and no membranes are present. × 100.

to therapeutic efforts with patients. The concept simply leads to the conclusion that any patient should be treated with the lowest possible concentration of oxygen for the shortest possible time. The patient's arterial Po_2 should be determined frequently, and a target pressure set, if cardiac output is adequate, at a level of about 50–70 mm Hg[22] rather than the normal level of about 75–100 mm Hg.[20] When the patient begins to improve the arterial O_2 will rise. As it does so, the inhaled concentration should be promptly reduced to restore the tension to the target range. In this way whatever toxic effect the oxygen may have in the specific patient will be minimized.

It would be helpful if one could identify a concentration of inhaled oxygen which could be considered "safe" for prolonged administration to any patient. At one time many workers assumed that 60% was probably innocuous; few, if any, would accept this today.[10] The variability between individuals in tolerance

TABLE 1

Underlying disease	Duration of therapy before death									Total Cases
	Up to 1 week			1–2 weeks			Over 2 weeks			
	A*	B	C	A	B	C	A	B	C	
Viral or pyogenic pneumonia				1	4	1		1	4	11
Trauma	3						1	1	2	7
Diabetes mellitus	1				1				2	4
Post surgery				1	1				1	3
Parturition	1								2	3
Goodpasture's syndrome	2									2
Other	3				2					5
Total	10	0	0	2	8	1	1	2	11	35

* *A,* number of cases with hyaline membranes but no ADF; *B,* number of cases with ADF present but not the major cause of death; *C,* number of cases with ADF as the major cause of death.

is such that this level could be innocuous for some patients while it would produce reaction in others. Susceptibility may also be influenced by the underlying disease process. The best conclusion, as already noted is that no patient should be exposed to any concentration higher than required to attain an acceptable arterial Po_2.

The mechanism of cell damage by oxygen is not fully established to the satisfaction of all workers. However, a fairly well accepted concept can be broadly summarized as follows[6]: Cell metabolism involves the stepwise reduction of oxygen to water with the addition of one electron at each step. The first step produces an oxygen molecule with a single negative charge, called superoxide, which is an oxygen "free radical." The next step produces hydrogen peroxide; the third produces another "free radical," the hydroxyl ion; and the fourth produces water. Free radicals are highly reactive molecules which tend to cause destructive, unregulated reactions with other organic molecules. For example, they break double bonds in certain organic molecules. This process can damage cell plasma membranes, mitochondria, and many enzymes. One such radical can initiate a chain reaction involving multiple molecules. Defense mechanisms exist, such as superoxide dismutase,[6] and presumably are adequate for ambient conditions. However, elevated oxygen concentrations result in a more rapid than normal production of free radicals. Since free radicals occur even during metabolism at ambient oxygen levels, it follows that any increase in oxygen concentration will cause them to increase. Thus, on the basis of mechanism, one should not expect that any elevated concentration of oxygen could be considered "safe."

It is not being suggested that oxygen should be withheld from any patient whose arterial oxygen tension cannot be maintained at an acceptable level without it. While the pathologist should perhaps refrain from offering specific therapeutic advice to the clinician, another point seems to follow logically from the above considerations. If the "acceptable" arterial oxygen tension is at about 50–60 mm Hg, then a patient at this level on room air probably does not need oxygen. A patient who achieves this level only by means of labored breathing should probably receive treatment by assisted ventilation using room air, rather than by the addition of oxygen to his environment. The author recognizes that this is the reverse of standard practice. However, as already noted, there is no evidence that mechanical ventilation *per se* produces lung damage, and therefore it is probably safer than increased oxygen concentration. Many patients, and perhaps most, can inhale moderately increased oxygen concentrations without developing progressive respiratory distress. At present there is no method to identify in advance those patients who will develop lung damage. Such a diagnostic test would be highly desirable.

SUMMARY

The morphology and sequential evolution of the pulmonary lesions in respiratory distress syndrome have been reviewed. Reasons have been presented to support the conclusion that these lesions are in the main produced by toxic effects of oxygen rather than the underlying disease process which initiated the episode of respiratory failure. The mechanism of oxygen toxicity has been briefly reviewed. The implication of these considerations is that in any patient with acute respiratory impairment, oxygen should be used as therapy only if it is required to prevent death from hypoxia and should be used in the lowest possible effective dose. As the patient improves and arterial oxygen tension rises this dose should be promptly reduced.

REFERENCES

1. Ashbaugh, D. G., Bigelow, D. B., Petty, T. L., and Levine, B. E.: Acute respiratory distress in adults. *Lancet 2:* 319–323, 1967.
2. Barber, R. E., Lee, J. and Hamilton, W. K.: Oxygen toxicity in man. A prospective study in patients with irreversible brain damage. *N. Engl. J. Med 283:* 1478–1484, 1970.
3. Bouhuys, A.: Distribution of inspired gas in the lungs. *In Handbook of Physiology,* Section 3, *Respiration,* Vol. I., pp 715–733, Edited by Fenn, W. O. and Rahn, H. Washington, American Physiology Society, 1964.
4. Blaisdell, F. W., Lim, R. C., Jr., Stallone, R. J.: The mechanism of pulmonary damage following traumatic shock. *Surg. Gynecol. Obstet. 130:* 15–22, 1970.
5. Bonikos, D. S., Bensch, K. G., Northway, W. H., and Edwards, D. K.: Bronchopulmonary dysplasia: The pulmonary pathologic sequel of necrotizing bronchiolitis and pulmonary fibrosis. *Human Pathol. 7:* 643–666, 1976.
6. Crapo, J. D., and Tierney, D. F.: Superoxide dismutase and pulmonary oxygen toxicity. *Am. J. Physiol. 226:* 1401–1407, 1974.
7. Finckh, E. S., Bader, L.: Pulmonary damage from Hong Kong influenza. *Aust. N. Zeal J. Med 4:* 16–22, 1974.
8. Fischman, C. M., Goldstein, M. S., and Gardner, L. B.: Suicidal hanging: An association with the adult respiratory distress syndrome. *Chest 71:* 225–227, 1977.
9. Gould, V. E., Tosco, R., Wheelis, R. F., Gould, N. S., and Kapanci, Y.: Oxygen pneumonitis in man: Ultrastructural observations on the development of alveolar lesions. *Lab. Invest. 26:* 499–508, 1972.
10. Hyde, R. W., and Rawson, A. J.: Unintentional iatrogenic oxygen pneumonitis—Response to therapy. *Ann. Intern. Med. 7:* 517–531, 1969.
11. Kapanci, Y., Weibel, E. R., Kaplan, H. P., and Robinson, F. R.: Pathogenesis and reversibility of the pulmonary lesions of oxygen toxicity in monkeys. II: Ultrastructural and morphometric studies. *Lab. Invest. 20:* 101–118, 1969.
12. Kaplan, H. P., Robinson, F. R., Kapanci, Y., and Weibel, E. R.: Pathogenesis and reversibility of the pulmonary lesions of oxygen toxicity in monkeys. I: Clinical and light microscopic studies. *Lab. Invest. 20:* 94–100, 1969.
13. Katzenstein, A. L. A., Bloor, C. M., and Liebow, A. A.: Diffuse alveolar damage—The role of oxygen, shock, and related factors. *Am. J. Pathol. 85:* 210–228, 1976.

14. deLemos, R., Wolfsdorf, J., and Nachman, R.: Lung injury from oxygen in lambs: The role of artificial ventilation. *Anesthesiology 30:* 609–618, 1969.
15. Mills, M.: Pulmonary effects of nonthoracic trauma: The clinical syndrome. *J. Trauma 8:* 651–655, 1968.
16. Mosher, D. F.: Cross-linking of cold insoluble globulin by fibrin stabilizing factor. *J. Biol. Chem. 250:* 6614–6621, 1975.
17. Nash, G., Blennerhassett, J. B., and Pontoppidan, H.: Pulmonary lesions associated with oxygen therapy and artificial ventilation. *N. Engl. J. Med 276:* 368–374, 1967.
18. Nash, G., Foley, F. D., Langlinais, P. C.: Pulmonary interstitial edema and hyaline membranes in adult burn patients: Electron microscopic observations. *Human Pathol. 5:* 149–160, 1974.
19. Orell, S. R.: Lung pathology in respiratory distress following shock in the adult. *Acta Pathol. Microbiol. Scand.* (Sect. A.) *79:* 65–76, 1971.
20. Petty, T. L., and Ashbaugh, D. G.: The adult respiratory distress syndrome: Clinical features, factors influencing prognosis and principles of management. *Chest 60:* 233–239, 1971.
21. Pontoppidan, H., Geffin, B., and Lowenstein, E.: Acute respiratory failure in the adult. *N. Engl. J. Med. 287:* 743–752, 1972.
22. Pontoppidan, H., Wilson, R. S., and Rie, M. A.: Optimal respiratory therapy with special reference to patients who are candidates for extracorporeal membrane oxygenation randomization study. In *Artificial Lungs for Acute Respiratory Failure,* edited by Zapol, W. M., and Qvist, J. pp. 363–373, New York, Academic Press, 1977.
23. Pratt, P. C.: Personal observation.
24. Ratliff, N. B., Young, W. G., Jr., Hackel, D. B., Mikat, E., and Wilson, J. W.: Pulmonary injury secondary to extracorporeal circulation: An ultrastructural study. *J. Thorac. Cardiovasc. Surg. 65:* 425–432, 1973.
25. Rivers, J. F., Orr, G., and Lee, H. A.: Drowning: Its clinical sequelae and management. *Br. Med. J. 2:* 157–161, 1970.
26. Storey, W. F., and Staub, N. C.: Ventilation of terminal air units. *J. Appl. Physiol. 17:* 391–397, 1962.
27. Sutton, F. D., Hudson, L. D., and Petty, T. L.: Recognition and management of the adult respiratory distress syndrome. *Chest* (Suppl.) *66:* 345–465, 1974.

Chapter 4

Clinical-Pathologic Approach to Diffuse Infiltrative Lung Disease*

CHARLES B. CARRINGTON AND EDWARD A. GAENSLER

Clinicians recognize a group of chronic lung diseases with several features in common. Clinically, dyspnea is the predominant symptom, and on examination frequently the only finding is "dry rales." Radiographs generally show a diffuse "infiltration" by irregular lines, small nodules, or "ground glass" shadows. Physiologically, the abnormalities primarily affect oxygen exchange and result in hypoxemia, whereas the mechanics of breathing are little impaired. None of the names used to designate this group is entirely accurate. "Diffuse lung disease" does not exclude the much more common obstructive disorders which are also "diffuse" yet specifically excluded here. The term "interstitial" is misleading because most of these disorders also have intra-alveolar abnormalities, and in some the latter actually predominate. Finally, "alveolar-capillary block" does not correspond to recent interpretation of the pathophysiologic process involved. We believe that the term "chronic diffuse infiltrative" is the most appropriate, although it must be acknowledged that sometimes the disease is more or less localized and sometimes the distinction between "acute" and "chronic" is uncertain.

This group of disorders has received increasing attention in recent years, perhaps because of more liberal use of lung biopsy with the opportunity to study early and active rather than nonspecific end-stage disease. A growing interest in environmental lung disease and in immunologic disorders also may have focused attention on infiltrative lung disease. Finally, an increasing therapeutic armamentarium, including effective antibiotics, antiinflammatory agents, immunosuppressive drugs and pulmonary lavage, has stimulated a search for more precise diagnosis and a study of the natural history of these diseases. The proportion of these disorders among all of our referrals has increased each year, and the 1,234 cases now on file represent 21.2% of all referrals seen during the last 25 years (Table 1). Most likely, this experience has been weighted by our special interests.

This review will focus primarily on the diagnostic approach; and, in this context,

* This study was supported in part by Pulmonary SCOR Grant HL-15063, Program Project Grant HL-19717, and Career Award HL-1173 from the National Heart, Lung and Blood Institute, the United States Public Health Service, and the Sherrill A. Parsons Memorial Fund.

TABLE 1. DIFFUSE INFILTRATIVE LUNG DISEASE

	Total no.	With biopsy
Infections (3.2%)		
miliary tuberculosis	15	5
fungal and amoebic	10	2
viral?	14	2
"Allergic" reactions (3.1%)		
chronic eosinophilic pneumonia	30	21
asthma with infiltration and drug reactions	8	1
Malignant neoplasms (2.4%)		
leukemia and lymphoma	9	3
bronchoalveolar carcinoma	4	4
carcinomatosis, metastatic	16	7
Environmental diseases (24.8%)		
allergic alveolitis	15	5
silicosis, coal and graphite	65	21
asbestosis (excluding survey cases)	115	58
other silicates	17	4
berylliosis	63	16
toxic gases (NO_2, SO_2, Br, Cl) and "smoke"	31	2
Connective tissue disorders (7.9%)		
progressive systemic sclerosis	43	10
lupus erythematosus	26	2
rheumatoid lung	22	4
other or combined	7	2
Sarcoidosis (20.8%)	257	65
Interstitial pneumonias (12.8%)		
acute	7	6
usual	76	61
usual, due to radiation	24	6
desquamative	47	45
lymphocytic	4	4
Unusual specific disorders (3.8%)		
Wegener's granulomatosis	6	5
idiopathic hemosiderosis	3	3
Goodpasture's syndrome	5	5
pulmonary alveolar proteinosis	13	13
pulmonary alveolar microlithiasis	1	1
eosinophilic granuloma	15	15
tuberous sclerosis	1	1
lymphangioleiomyomatosis	3	3
Pulmonary vascular diseases (6.4%)		
arteriolitis	3	2
veno-occlusive	3	3
multiple emboli and idiopathic hypertension	73	12
Chronic passive congestion (1.9%)	23	7
Nonspecific reactions (5.8%)		
honeycombing, etiology?	18	16
focal fibrosis	22	20
primarily small airways disease	12	12
cystic fibrosis	10	2
primarily emphysema	3	3
aspiration (oil, blood, food)	4	4
normal lung	2	2
No diagnosis (7.2%)	89	5
	1,234	490

it will emphasize the expectations of the clinician with regard to histologic examination and the needs of the pathologist with regard to clinical information that may be helpful, indeed may be essential, to correct histologic interpretation.

The spectrum of disorders included in chronic diffuse infiltrative lung disease is very large and constantly growing. An alphabetic listing is not useful, and, therefore, for some years we followed an etiologic grouping suggested by Buechner.[4] With clarification of certain etiologies, description of new histologic patterns, characterization of allergic and immunologically mediated disorders, and the growing list of environmental lung diseases, we have recently used a classification based upon our experience (Table 1). This may form a useful framework for the following discussion although we will not specifically deal with the clinical and histologic features of each "entity" nor even of each major category.

DIAGNOSTIC APPROACH

In most instances the disease is discovered as the result of a chest roentgenogram obtained because of respiratory symptoms. Discovery was incidental to routine examination or because of symptoms suggestive of a systemic disorder in about 20% of cases.[14] The chief complaint in over one-half of our cases was dyspnea, sometimes with cough, expectoration, and weight loss, and less frequently with fever, night sweats, or other evidence of toxicity. Joint pains, with or without swelling and redness, was the only other relatively common chief complaint, occurring in about 6%, prominently in sarcoidosis and quite often in the interstitial pneumonias.[6]

The history is by far the most productive part of the examination and, in our earlier experience, has led to a diagnosis in 32% of all cases.[14] Apart from the conventional present, past, and family history, the most important aspect concerns environmental and occupational review. This should account for all materials worked on and for the tools and any intermediary compound used to facilitate the job, for example cutting oils, graphite, or talc.[13, 29, 30] Similar symptoms in other workers, the availability of masks, and frequent state inspections are important clues to potentially dangerous exposure. A review of recreational activities, hobbies, and geographic locations must be included here. The following case illustrates the importance of an occupational history accounting for every job, however brief, and also the importance of special stains.

Case 1: This 40-year-old policeman in a small town was first seen locally because of cough and dyspnea progressive for seven or eight years. Except for this, and some problems with a duodenal ulcer, he had been well and had worked for the police department since graduation from high school. Examination revealed diffuse dry rales with a close-to-the-ear sound and finger clubbing. Routine laboratory studies were all normal. The chest roentgenogram revealed the lungs to be somewhat reduced in volume. Additionally, there were fine irregular or linear markings at both bases, and the cardiac silhouette was indistinct (Fig. 1). A lung biopsy was interpreted as usual interstitial pneumonia (UIP) with honeycombing, and this diagnosis was confirmed by an authority on lung pathology.

About two years later the patient's physician attended our seminar on environmental lung disease. We mentioned a paper plant where, many years ago, cigarette filter paper had been made by mixing in a carding machine 85% acetate with 15% "Cape Blue" asbestos. Since then there has been a high prevalence of asbestosis among these workers even after brief exposure. The physician then recalled that this policeman had actually worked for 3 months at that same paper plant 17 years previously, but he had always worn a mask. Upon referral to us, this history was confirmed. Lung function studies showed marked lung volume restriction, slight impairment of flow attributed to a long smoking

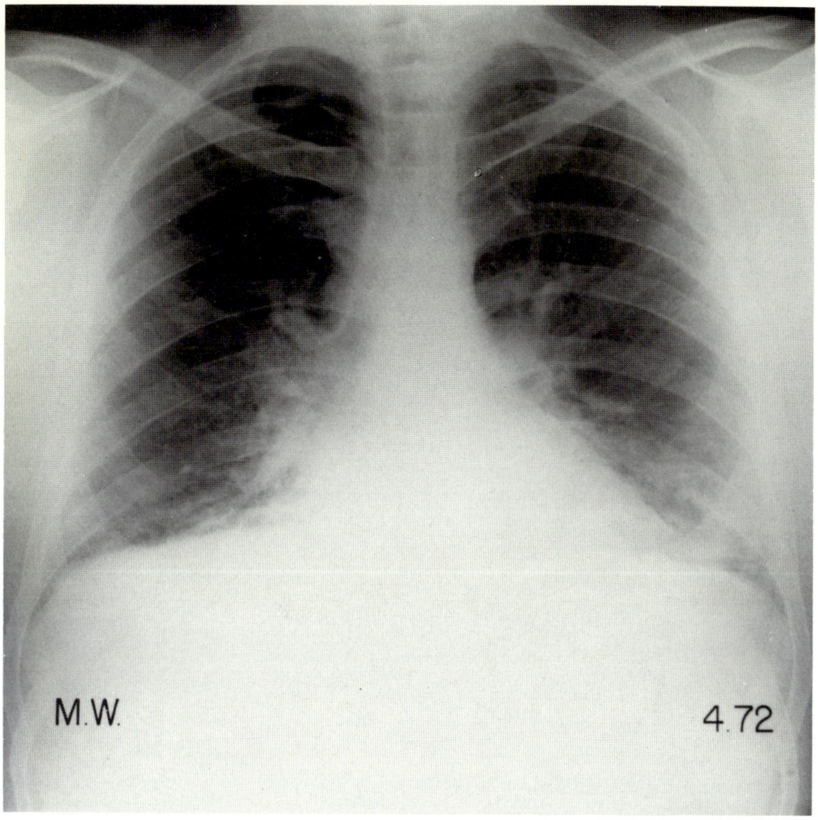

FIG. 1. Chest roentgenogram of patient #1. The lung volume is somewhat reduced and there is a fine linear or irregular infiltration causing the cardiac outline to become indistinct. Note the largely basal distribution of lesions and also the discrepancy between the relatively slight radiographic opacities and the marked functional (Table 2) and severe pathologic alterations (Fig. 2).

history, marked hypoxemia during slight exercise and a single breath diffusing capacity reduced to 46% of predicted (Table 2). The sections of lung tissue were reviewed. A chronic interstitial pneumonia of the usual pattern and some regions of endstage honeycombing were indeed present (Fig. 2). A moderate number of asbestos bodies were readily identified on recut sections stained for iron (Fig. 2, *inset*), although they were more difficult to find on sections stained with hematoxylin and eosin.

As this case illustrates, historical information is as important to the pathologist as it is to the clinician, since there are many ways in which the lung can be injured, but only a few stereotyped ways in which it can react. A few of these tissue reactions, such as the dust macule with or without fibrosis, are diagnostic of an environmental insult, especially when they contain abundant dust. Virtually all other lung reactions may or may not be related to the environment. For example, the sarcoid reaction may be "idiopathic" or it may result from exposure to beryllium; UIP may be "cryptogenic" (Case 4) or it may be caused by exposure to fibrous silicates (Fig. 2); and bronchiolitis obliterans may be the consequence of a viral pneumonia or it may result from acute or chronic exposure to oxides of nitrogen. Sometimes the pathologist is more familiar with the causes of occupational lung injury than the clinician, and then direct questions or those implied

Table 2. Lung Function Studies of Patients #1–#5*

	Case # 4/72		Case #2 4/75		Case #3					Case #4			Case #5 11/76	
					3/70	8/71	5/74	9/73		12/74	9/75 Rx	8/76 Rx		
FVC, % predicted	47			68	66	81	62	89		83	68	69	90	
FEV_1/FVC, %	70			75	87	81	62	86		86	87	89	85	
FEF 25–75, % predicted	26			35	117	97	94	114		132	111	114	97	
MVV, % predicted	50			85	116	122	111	61		72	65	81	110	
RV, % predicted	78			87	54	64	58	49		46	42	44	85	
TLC, % predicted	53			77	71	87	67	94		85	81	60	91	
RV/TLC, %	36			38	23	23	28	27		31	28	30	24	
Dsb, % predicted	42			37	39	53	40	64		55	41	46	69	
	Rest	Ex.	Rest	Ex.	Rest	Rest	Rest	Rest	Ex.				Rest	Ex.
$P(A\text{-}a)O_2$, torr	28	50	48	61				72	61				28	25
PaO_2, torr	81	60	64	46	70	76	78	42	65				80	89
$PaCO_2$, torr	34	35	35	35	45	38	34	36	27				33	34
Des, ml/min/torr	10	16	7	7				10	9				13	16

* Pulmonary terms and symbols from: A Report of the ACCP-ATS Joint Committee on Pulmonary Nomenclature, B. Burrows, Chairman, *Chest 67:* 583–593, 1975. FVC, forced vital capacity; FEV_1 forced expiratory volume in 1 second; FEV_1/FVC, FEV_1 expressed as a percentage of the FVC; FEF 25–75, forced expiratory flow rate between 25 and 75% of FVC; MVV, maximum voluntary ventilation; RV, residual volume; TLC, total lung capacity; RV/TLC, residual volume expressed as a percentage of total lung capacity; Dsb, single breath diffusing capacity; $P(A\text{-}a)O_2$, alveolar arterial oxygen gradient; PaO_2, partial pressure of oxygen in arterial blood; $PaCO_2$, partial pressure of carbon dioxide in arterial blood; Dss, steady state diffusing capacity.

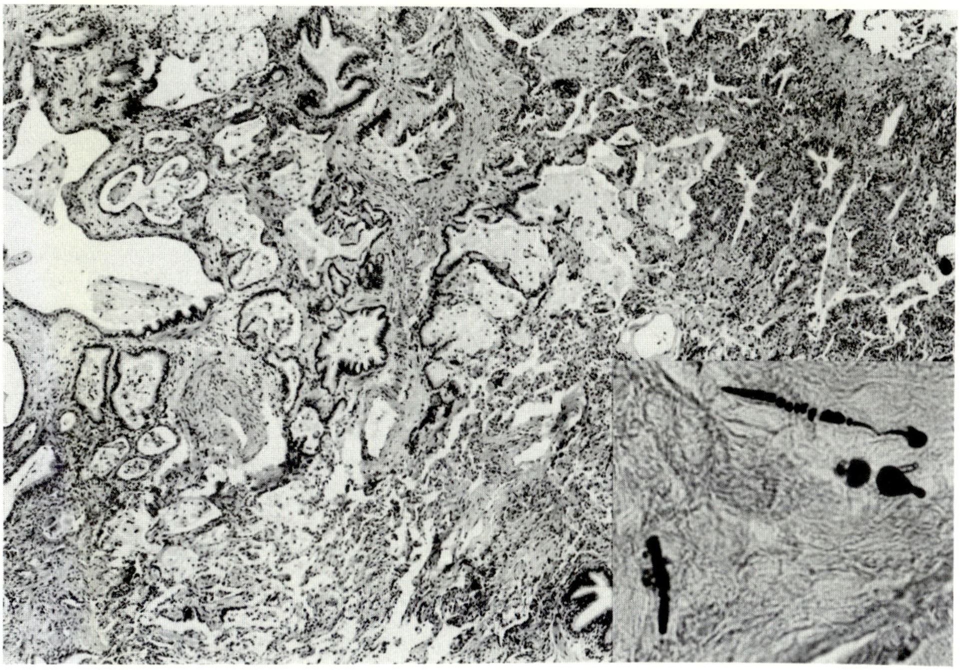

FIG. 2. Open lung biopsy from patient #1. Typical variegated interstitial pneumonia of "usual" pattern with changes ranging from cellular infiltrates to end-stage honeycombing. There is pooling of mucus in the large air spaces, and there is proteinaceous debris in some of the alveoli whose walls are infiltrated by a mixture of round cells. *Inset:* A few of the asbestos bodies, readily identified on recut sections, stained with a Prussian blue stain for iron.

by the tentative diagnoses may be of great help both in focusing the investigation and in stimulating renewed efforts when the original history was inadequate. Such questions are especially important when there is only a little dust in the lung tissue (Case 1) or when the histologic pattern is compatible with an environmental insult and there is no pathognomonic dust (Figs. 4 and 5). In such cases, the correct diagnosis can be made only with the aid of epidemiologic data.

The chest roentgenogram by definition should be abnormal. However, the pathologist consulted about a possible lung biopsy should be aware that the roentgenogram may be normal even when there is severe interstitial lung disease. This was true in 7.7% of our 508 patients who had lung biopsy, including patients with UIP, desquamative interstitial pneumonia (DIP), sarcoidosis, bronchiolitis obliterans, allergic alveolitis, asbestosis, and lymphangioleiomyomatosis.[11] As a corollary, in our experience the severity of radiographic infiltration correlates poorly both with physiologic abnormalities and with pathologic estimates of severity.[6, 17, 18] The following patient illustrates such a discrepancy in that the roentgenogram was always normal while there were a severe impairment of gas exchange and impressive lesions microscopically. This patient, like the first (Case 1), also illustrates the importance of taking a detailed environmental history, with noxious exposure here unrelated to occupation.

Case 2: This 46-year-old secretary and accountant saw her physician because of exertional dyspnea, a dry cough, and fatigue of two years' duration. Her symptoms improved during the summer and worsened each winter. Her history apparently was noncontributory, examination was not revealing, and the chest roentgenogram was normal. Nevertheless she was placed on corticosteroids and her condition improved. She discontinued therapy after one month because of depression and other side effects. Severe symptoms recurred during the next winter; and in March 1975 she saw her physician once more, now unable to perform simple household tasks or to walk more than 1 block without resting. Again examination and the roentgenograms were normal, but the Pa_{O_2} was only 44 torr at rest. When referred to us because of dyspnea and hypoxemia of unknown etiology, she confirmed that she had always been a secretary, had confined her activities to home and office and had never worked in a factory. Her chest roentgenogram was normal once more (Fig. 3), and clinical examination was not remarkable. Laboratory tests revealed a diffuse hyperglobulinemia and a rheumatoid factor titer of 1:2,560. Lung function studies revealed slight lung volume restriction, no obstructive impairment, and a screening diffusing capacity was reduced to 37% of predicted. Furthermore, she had severe hypoxemia with a Pa_{O_2} of only 46 torr during slight exercise (Table 2). Her open lung biopsy initially was interpreted as compatible with sarcoidosis. However, the fact that the miliary granulomata were randomly scattered rather than clustered along lymphatic vessels, and that an extensive interstitial infiltrate rich in plasma cells (Fig. 4), and an intense bronchiolitis were present (Fig. 5), suggested that a biologic dust sensitivity reaction should also be strongly considered.

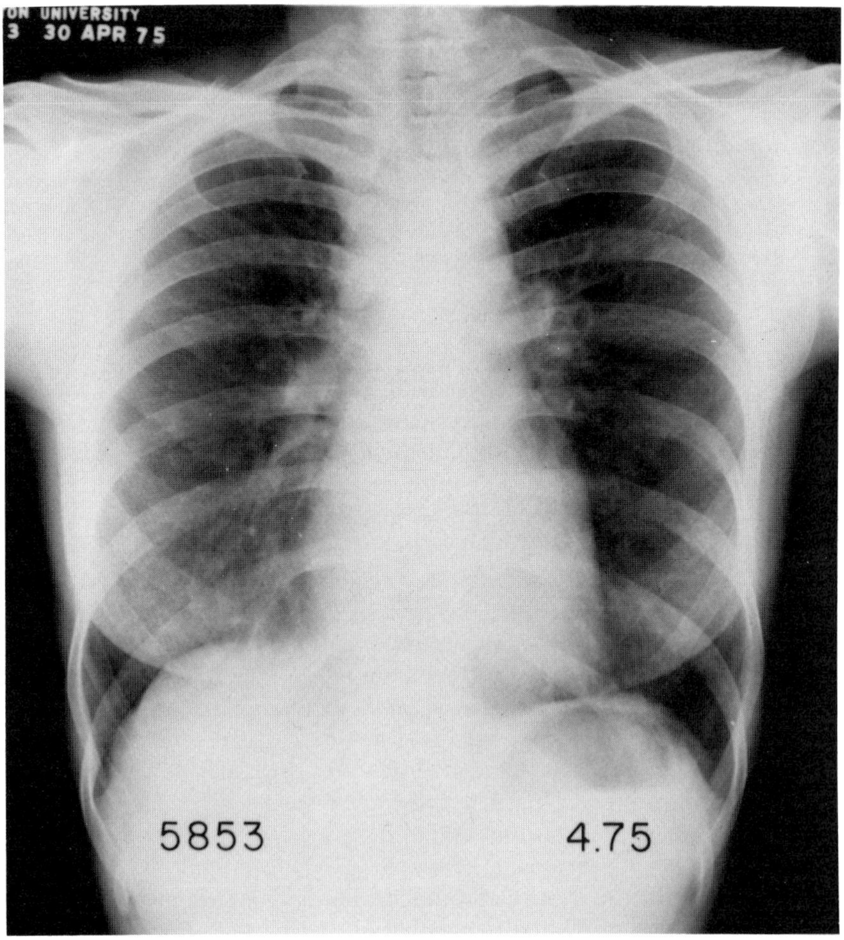

FIG. 3. The chest roentgenogram of patient #2 shows no abnormalities at a time when her Pa_{O_2} was only 48 torr (Table 2).

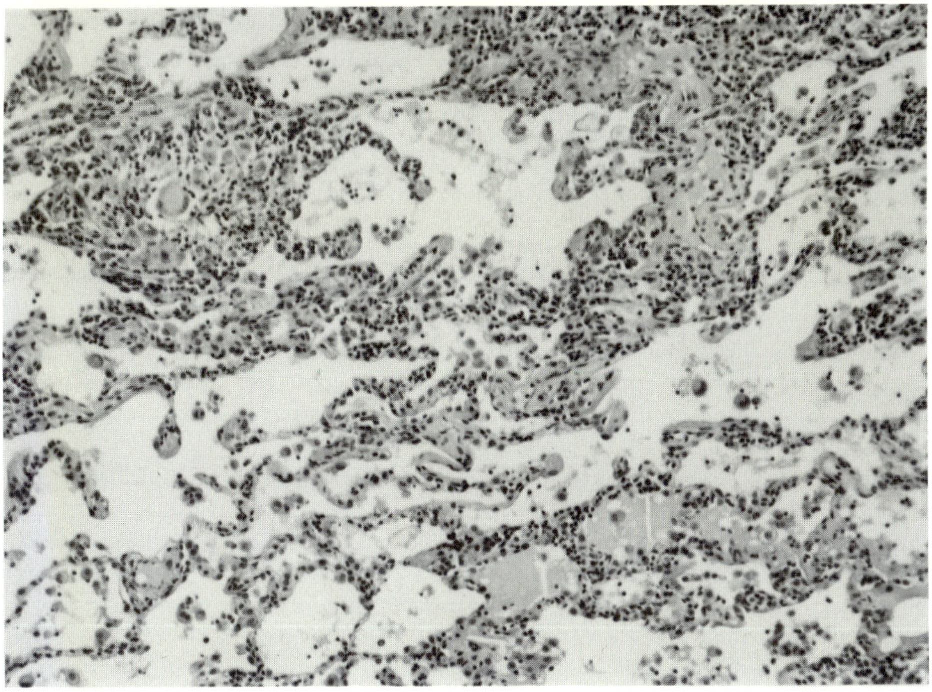

FIG. 4. Open biopsy of patient #2. Despite the normal roentgenogram there is a diffuse interstitial pneumonia rich in plasma cells. This somewhat overshadows the small granuloma.

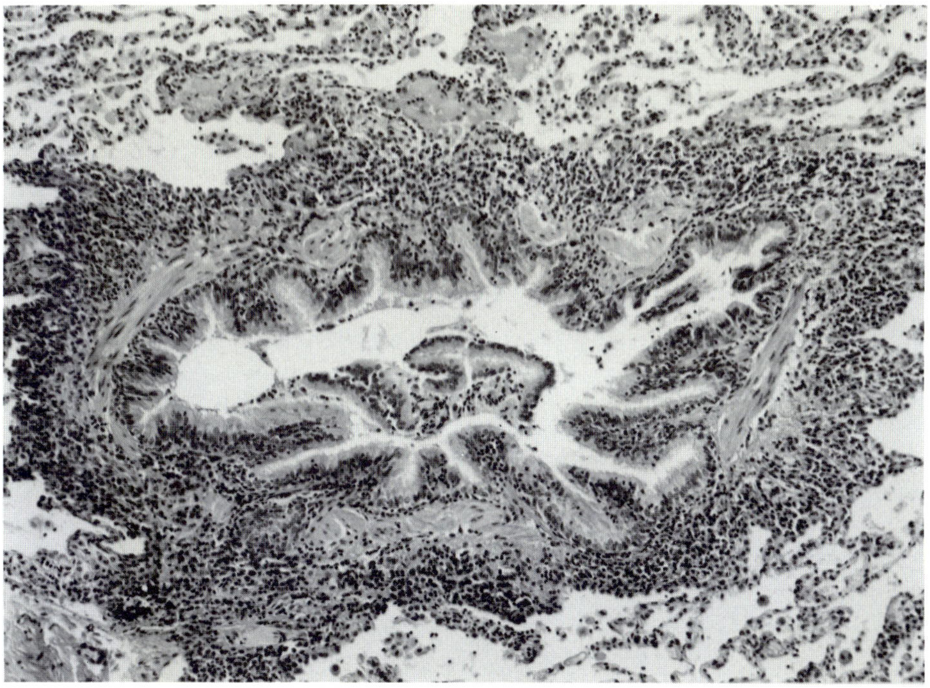

FIG. 5. Open biopsy of patient #2. There is an intense infiltration of this bronchiole by lymphocytes and plasma cells. The combination of a diffuse interstitial pneumonia, bronchiolitis, and miliary granulomata is suggestive of a biologic dust reaction although it is also compatible with idiopathic sarcoidosis.

As a result we reviewed her environmental history. She disliked animals and birds and had never done any farm or outdoor work. However, she minded the dryness of her home during the winter and therefore had had two humidifiers installed in series in the forced air heating system of her home. Culture of the humidifier water grew thermoactinomyces, *Penicillium cladosporium,* yeasts, and 6 unidentified fungi. The patient had positive serum precipitins to *Thermoactinomyces vulgaris, Micropolyspora faeni,* and Cladosporium; and double gel diffusion showed the strongest bands against the humidifier water. The diagnosis of allergic alveolitis was now confirmed; and dramatic improvement during the succeeding summer was sustained during the next winter, when the humidification system was removed. Indeed, her diffusing capacity more than doubled without specific therapy (Table 2).

This case also illustrates the nonspecificity of some tissue reactions. Nevertheless, the way in which the biopsy findings redirected the clinical investigation towards an environmental cause emphasizes the value of close collaboration between the clinician and the pathologist.

Radiographic opacities may consist of the linear or irregular markings[22] that are most often seen in interstitial pneumonias (Figs. 1, 12, and 14). Alternatively, they may be rounded, as in silicosis,[22] or "reticulo-nodular"—perhaps a combination of linear and rounded opacities—as is seen most often in granulomatous disorders.[7] Additionally, and most importantly, the entire lungs or parts thereof may have a "ground glass" appearance.[18] Such opacities have been referred to as "alveolar pattern" or "airlessness" and may indeed result from displacement of alveolar gas by cellular or amorphous debris, as in pulmonary edema, or from patchy or diffuse atelectasis. However, a similar ground glass pattern also may be seen when the alveoli are smaller than normal, as in full expiration, or, more pertinent, when all alveolar walls are diffusely thickened by cells and/or scars. Finally, a honeycomb pattern has been well described both from the radiologic[19] and from the pathologic standpoint;[20, 27] the significance of this "end-stage lung" is discussed below.

These various radiographic patterns, together with their predominant location, can be related statistically to certain pathologic entities, but in individual cases they are rarely diagnostic. A few exceptions include pulmonary alveolar microlithiasis, recognized by the sand-like appearance of the roentgenogram, or a ground glass pattern involving the lung periphery, which is virtually diagnostic for chronic eosinophilic pneumonia.[16] Other radiographic patterns may be diagnostic when supported by minimal clinical information, for example a reticulonodular pattern together with bilateral hilar adenopathy in young black persons represents a combination of findings diagnostic of sarcoidosis.

A review of previous radiographs often is the most revealing diagnostic procedure in the study of pulmonary disease. The pathologist should share in this information or ask for older films for an indication of the natural history of the disease. Most persons have had such roentgenograms during previous unrelated admissions, for insurance examinations or in connection with pre-employment screening. The time and expense involved in correspondence and travel to obtain such films is paltry compared to the alternatives of long hospitalization, extensive laboratory investigations, or, worse, discharge and later readmission with the hope of establishing the natural history prospectively. Recent films frequently enable differentiation of acute from chronic disease as discussed below; and films spanning many years often document the onset of diffuse lung disease many years before the appearance of symptoms. This is because the pulmonary reserve is very large; and, unlike airways obstruction, restrictive lung disease initially does not greatly increase the work of breathing.

Physical examination does not often aid in diagnosis. Dry rales with a "close-to-the-ear" sound or "cellophane rales" may be heard early during the course of interstitial disease but are quite nonspecific. We recorded such adventitious sounds in about 60% of our patients with UIP and asbestosis and in 20% with sarcoidosis.[10] Digital clubbing, exercise cyanosis, and signs of cor pulmonale merely are indicative of advanced disease. More specific findings, such as hepatosplenomegaly, enlarged lymph nodes and especially signs suggesting connective tissue disorders, are important leads to further examination. Careful cardiac examination may reveal the diffuse lung disease to be a consequence of heart disease, most often mitral stenosis.

Routine laboratory studies may be of interest in regard to kidney disease or anemia. Polycythemia generally is secondary and nonspecific as is a reversed albumin:globulin ratio or an elevated sedimentation rate. Eosinophilia suggests an allergic disorder or the presence of parasites. However, such allergic reactions as chronic eosinophilic pneumonia may be seen without eosinophilia,[16] while this finding is not uncommon in infections such as tuberculosis or coccidioidomycosis. Additionally, our routine studies have included screening for connective tissue disorders, although the results more often than not have been confusing rather than enlightening. More recently we have screened for precipitating antibodies to various biologic dust antigens.

There are other routine examinations that can be done quickly, inexpensively and painlessly. They include skin testing for anergy, tuberculosis, and fungal infections and especially repeated examination of the sputum by aerobic and anaerobic culture for bacteria and fungi as well as multiple cytologic examinations. Occasionally, a search for asbestos bodies or alveolar casts may be useful.

Physiologic examination, particularly of respiratory gas exchange, is useful in detecting diffuse infiltrative lung disease, especially if the chest roentgenogram is normal (Cases 2 and 5). Furthermore, such studies characterize the severity of the disease much more accurately than either clinical examination or the chest roentgenogram. Therefore, pulmonary function tests are useful for monitoring the natural course of disease and for evaluating the results of therapy. They are, however, not helpful for specific diagnosis, because the type of physiologic derangement observed is common to virtually all of the disorders shown in Table 1. The type of pathophysiology has been well described.[3, 28] Generally, there is no overt obstruction, and restriction of lung volumes is variable and usually is seen only in advanced disease. The characteristic abnormalities consist of diminution of diffusing capacity and increased alveolar-arterial oxygen pressure difference ($P(A\text{-}a)O_2$) resulting in hypoxemia (Table 2, Fig. 16). This is accompanied by alveolar hyperventilation and a compensated respiratory alkalosis stimulated perhaps by chronic hypoxemia or perhaps by excessive reflexes from the lung or other sites. The principal abnormality, hypoxemia, was attributed for years to a decrease of the diffusing capacity from thickening of the alveolar-capillary membrane.[3, 9, 28] More recently this theory has fallen into disrepute for the following four reasons: (1) The diffusing capacity of the lung membrane is so large that normally complete equilibration of oxygen partial pressure between alveolar gas and capillary blood occurs in only one-fourth the time available for gas exchange. Therefore, a marked reduction of diffusing capacity, say to one-half of normal, would not result in an alveolar-end capillary P_{O_2} "gradient"; yet such patients commonly have an elevated $P(A\text{-}a)_{O_2}$. From this it has been reasoned that the $P(A\text{-}a)_{O_2}$ must be due to postcapillary venous admixture rather than to impaired diffusing capacity.[12] (2) It has been shown that at least one-half of the total resistance to diffusion is caused by the slowness of the reaction rate of oxygen with hemoglobin,[31] and this is not altered by lung disease. (3) If impaired diffusion were the sole cause of an elevated $P(A\text{-}a)_{O_2}$, then this $P(A\text{-}a)_{O_2}$ would always increase with exercise, which causes an accelerated flow rate of blood through capillaries.[3, 28] Actually, in about one-third of our patients $P(A\text{-}a)_{O_2}$ decreased with exercise.[6] Finally, (4) the histologic picture evoked by the term "alveolar-capillary block"—a uniform thickening of the blood-gas barrier—is rarely seen. Occasionally, alveolar walls are uniformly lined by epithelial cells, and sometimes there are selected fields where the walls are diffusely thickened by cellular infiltration or amyloid. Except for such uncommon examples, microscopic examination rarely reveals lesions suggesting alveolar-capillary block. Most often there are focal solid lesions and much normal intervening lung tissue, as in sarcoidosis (Fig. 21) and silicosis; or sometimes the alveoli appear to be completely filled by granular debris or macrophages, as in proteinosis. Even in interstitial pneumonia, cellular thickening and fibrosis generally are quite uneven (Figs. 4, 7, 8, and 15). Sometimes the alveolar walls are thick, but the capillaries are seen to spiral around the periphery of the fibrous tissue, which then does not contribute to an increased diffusion distance. Thus, edema and cellular infiltration may not alter the thickness of the blood-air barrier, a possibility confirmed by electron microscopic studies discussed elsewhere in this monograph.[26] For all of these reasons, it is now assumed that hypoxemia in this group of disorders is largely the result of ventilation/perfusion discrepancies.[12, 35] Such mismatching of gas and blood is easily explained on histologic grounds considering the very uneven involvement in most cases and the predilection of some lesions for the broncho-vascular rays.[7] These ventilation-perfusion discrepancies undoubtedly fully explain hypoxemia at rest. During exercise, however, the contact time between alveolar gas and capillary blood is greatly reduced, especially in patients with a compromised pulmonary capillary bed. Then impaired diffusing capacity may well contribute to hypoxemia in some cases.

Financially or physically traumatic procedures: Many more elaborate diagnostic procedures have been performed almost routinely in the past. Indeed, until 1965 our consulting physicians generally would not permit lung biopsy until virtually all other "special procedures" had been exhausted and until several extrapulmonary sites had been biopsied. Thus, virtually all patients had gastrointestinal series, barium enemas, intravenous pyelograms, skeletal surveys and a variety of scans, ostensibly in search of a primary tumor that might be the source of diffuse pulmonary metastases. Conjunctivae, muscle, bronchial walls, and liver were biopsied routinely in search for sarcoidosis, and renal biopsy was not uncommon to rule out Wegener's granulomatosis, Goodpasture's syndrome, or neoplasm. Finally, supraclavicular triangle exploration and, more recently, mediastinoscopy [5] were used routinely until we demonstrated that these procedures had a yield of less than 1% in diffuse infiltrative disease without hilar adenopathy.[14] With this approach, the average interval between the discovery of infiltrative disease and diagnosis was 1.53 years,[15] often with multiple admissions and repetitive examinations; frequently patients were unemployable during this entire time. We found that extensive radiographic studies and extrapulmonary biopsies not only were not justifiable on the basis of cost-benefit analysis but also that the combined morbidity and mortality of all of these studies far exceeded that of open lung biopsy.[14, 15] Also, it should be noted that about one-third of the disorders listed in Table 1 do not have extrapulmonary manifestations nor do they lead to characteristic secretions.

All of these considerations have persuaded us that lung biopsy should be performed forthwith when: (1) chronicity has been demonstrated, generally by lesions persisting for more than one month; (2) there are no specific leads; and (3) the simple studies, including blood tests, sputum examination and skin reactivity, have been unrevealing. In the past, 39.7% of our 1,234 patients with diffuse infiltrative disease eventually came to open lung biopsy (Table 1).

PATHOLOGIC EVALUATION OF THE BIOPSY

Diagnosis from Histology and Accessory Data

The histologic features of the many diseases listed in Table 1 have been described previously and will not be repeated here. However, in approaching the differential diagnosis of such lesions, there are several broad categories and specific questions which should be considered, and the features listed in Table 3 merit assessment. In many cases, one can quickly decide whether a lesion is acute or chronic, interstitial or alveolar or both, granulomatous or not, exudative or organizing. Thus, a lesion dominated by hyaline membranes and proteinaceous debris is more likely to be an acute reaction. The presence of tumor, dust, or infectious agents is also easily decided in most cases, although a few simple aids such as special stains may be needed and cultures should *always* be done. We have made it a rule to scan all sections under polarized light; it may be mentioned in passing that birefringent crystals are readily missed without high intensity illumination. Special studies that may aid in analyzing dusts are discussed elsewhere in this monograph.[1]

The distribution of parenchymal lesions is sometimes a useful clue. For example, pneumoconioses, sarcoidosis, and malignant lymphoma are the only diseases in which the lesions commonly tend to concentrate along the lymphatic pathways. Similarly, noting whether a lesion is diffuse or focal and whether it is uniform throughout or highly variegated helps in making some diagnoses. Finally, it is important to note lesions of blood vessels and of conducting airways (in most biopsies this means bronchioles). It must then be decided whether these are the dominant lesions or simply components of a more diffuse reaction. Bronchiolitis obliterans, for example, may result from infection, toxic injury, or allergy; and the resolution of this differential depends more on the associated parenchymal changes than on the morphology of the bronchioles themselves.

It is worth noting that the significance of some of the features in Table 3 may

TABLE 3. HISTOLOGIC FEATURES ASSESSED IN DIFFUSE INFILTRATIVE LUNG DISEASE

A. Alveoli, small air spaces
- hyaline membranes
- proteinaceous exudates
- stasis of secretions
- epithelial regeneration
- hemorrhage
- hemosiderosis (macrophages)
- alveolar cell population (kind and number)
- organisms, inclusion bodies
- dust

B. Interstitium
- edema
- diffuse cell population
- localized lymphoid follicles
- dust
- granulomas, with or without necrosis
- destruction
- organization, fibrosis, honeycombing

C. Conducting Airways
- narrowing by mural or external lesions
- obstruction or obliteration by scar or mucus
- cellular infiltrates
- granulomas
- loss

D. Vessels
- diffuse hypertrophy, intimal proliferation
- thrombi, emboli
- fibrous obliteration
- angiitis

E. Tumor

be difficult to assess from the biopsy alone. The presence of widespread alveolar hemorrhage may be the only apparent lesion in an early stage of pulmonary hemosiderosis, but more often it is an irrelevant result of the trauma of the biopsy. Radiographic and hematologic data clarify this situation. Acute alveolar injury occasionally closely simulates pulmonary alveolar proteinosis. This observation has interesting implications in regard to the pathogenesis of such lesions. However, the practical problem of deciding the likely course and prognosis in such a patient is best resolved by evaluating the history and chest radiograph, since in these respects the usual form of proteinosis and acute alveolar injury are quite different. The need for epidemiologic data in interpreting the significance of a few dust particles has already been noted.

The relationship of honeycombing to diffuse infiltrative lung disease merits special comment. Honeycombing is a nonspecific end stage of a wide variety of pulmonary lesions which cause loss and revision of architecture with scarring.[19, 20, 27] When seen more or less diffusely, it is usually the result of some interstitial process. The honeycombing itself is not useful in identifying the original process, however, but merely indicates that it was destructive and scar-forming. The characteristic features and patterns of the active disease are increasingly obscured as the lesion progresses and the scars accumulate. The closer a lesion approaches the final common pathway of honeycombing, the more difficult it becomes to distinguish it from the other interstitial diseases which similarly organize (Fig. 6). Such progression to honeycombing is illustrated by a patient whose original biopsy had typical lesions of eosiniophilic granuloma (Fig. 7). When the patient died of respiratory failure two years later, the autopsy revealed only nonspecific honeycombing (Fig. 8).

Confidence of Diagnosis and Differential Diagnosis. In a classic case, the pathologist may be certain of the diagnosis, but often this certainty is diluted (1) by the lack of some components, that is, either when the lesion is mild and early or when it is severe but burned out and late; (2) by the presence of atypical features; (3) because the lesion is a rather nonspecific one such as noncaseating granuloma; or (4) because similar histologic findings have different significance when they are localized rather than diffuse. A DIP-like or UIP-like reaction is sometimes encountered adjacent to other focal lesions such as neoplasms or abscesses or even near the granulomas of histiocytosis X, and an early stage of UIP also may be mimicked by a resolving viral pneumonia. Sometimes one encounters relatively focal lesions which resemble UIP but which never progress to affect other parts of the lung. Even more commonly, end-stage honeycombing is encountered as the focal residue from a variety of processes such as healed necrotizing pneumonia. When such impostors of a diffuse interstitial process are met, it is invaluable to have available the physiologic and radiographic data to determine whether or not one is dealing with a widespread process. The pathologist can gain some help from reports by the radiologist, but actual inspection of films is preferable. This will give him a much better concept of the lung as a whole and of the extent, distribution, and character of the radiographic abnormalities which must be correlated and explained. The patient whose roentgenogram is shown in Figure 9 illustrates this problem. The biopsy from the solid nodular lesion (Fig. 10) suggests there is little normal lung, whereas the other biopsy (Fig. 11) implies there is only normal lung. This disparity is readily explained by examination of the roentgenogram.

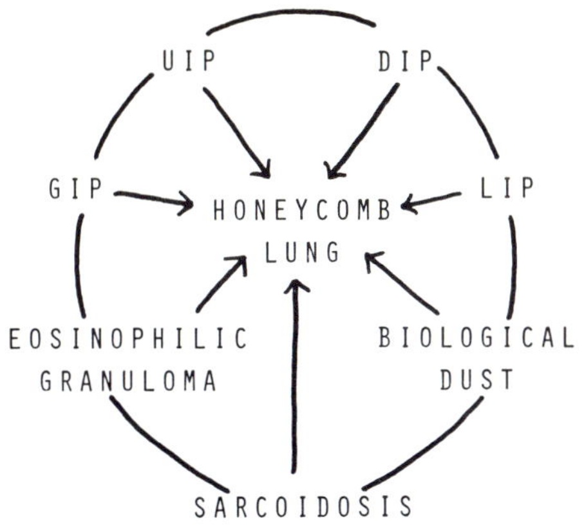

FIG. 6. Schematic representation of some of the pulmonary lesions which, in some patients, may progress to a nonspecific end-stage scarring or "honeycomb lung." The more closely the lesion approaches this final stage, the more difficult is recognition of the original pattern of reaction. *GIP, UIP, DIP,* and *LIP* = giant cell, usual, desquamative, and lymphocytic interstitial pneumonias. (Reproduced from *Chest 69:* 324, 1976.)

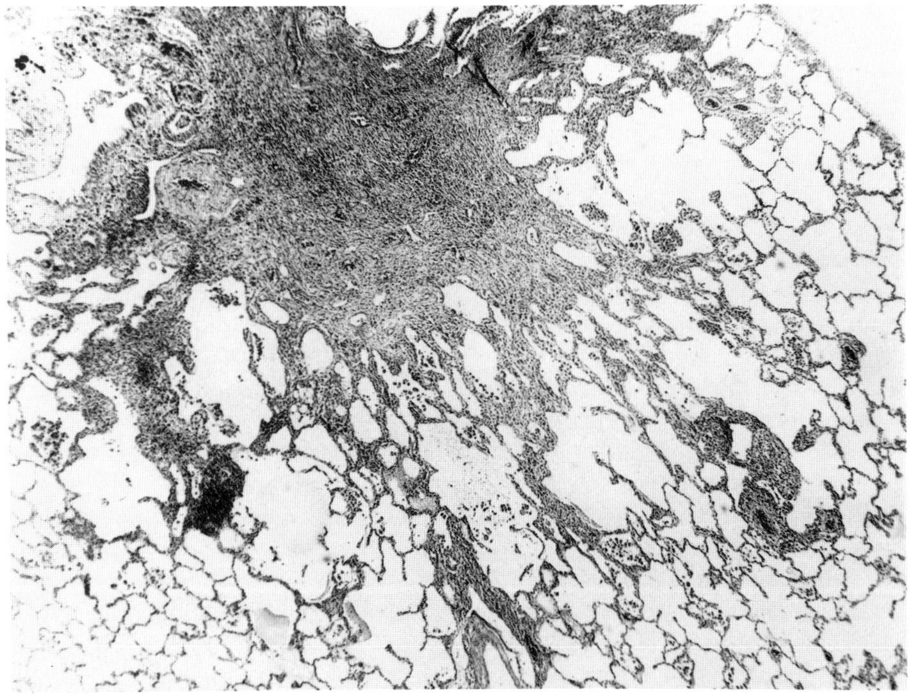

FIG. 7. Open lung biopsy from a 38-year-old dairy farmer who had a wedge resection because of progressive dyspnea. This has a classical focal interstitial lesion of eosinophilic granuloma, and under greater magnification the characteristic Langerhans histiocytes were easily identified. These same cells and a scattering of eosinophils infiltrate irregularly into adjacent alveolar walls.

Irreversible Change and Activity. In addition to rendering a diagnosis, it is important to estimate histologically the extent of destruction, fibrosis, and other irreversible damage and also the activity of the lesion. Both the diagnosis and the amount of irreversible damage affect the prognosis and the likely response to therapy. For example, a patient with UIP is not likely to do well with corticosteroid therapy irrespective of the extent of fibrosis, but a patient with DIP and mild fibrosis may well have arrest of his disease and even considerable improvement with such treatment.[6] In contrast, a patient with DIP at a stage of extensive fibrosis and honeycombing is unlikely to recover with steroids even though he has a disease which is usually responsive to such treatment. This is illustrated by the following case.

Case 3: A 56-year-old physician with tuberculosis first noted cough and exertional dyspnea in the fall of 1969. A chest roentgenogram had shown fine triangular densities and irregular markings in both cardiophrenic angles since 1966; in the spring of 1970 there was marked progression with reduction of lung volume and the irregular markings had become coarser and were now visible everywhere (Fig. 12). Functional impairment was also severe with marked restriction and a diffusing capacity of only 39% of predicted (Table 2). His tuberculin skin test had been positive for many years and now, treated with isoniazid, he failed to improve and therefore eventually consented to lung biopsy. The biopsy (Fig. 13) had many features characteristic of DIP but this process had progressed to a stage in which there was considerable interstitial fibrosis. This implied at best a limited potential for recovery on drug treatment and more likely only a possibility of arrest of the progression. He then received prednisone for about 1 year with some initial improvement, but this was not sustained (Table

2). In 1974 his physiologic studies were comparable to those 4 years earlier, dyspnea was unchanged, and the chest roentgenogram showed further increase of coarse irregular markings and some patchy ground glass densities.

Grading the activity of a lesion is also helpful in estimating prognosis. Thus, although UIP is a progressive disease in most patients, the rate of progression varies from barely perceptible to very rapid. The activity of the lesion, as indicated by cellular infiltrates, proteinaceous debris, epithelial regeneration, and fibroblasts, helps in predicting this course. The following case illustrates this correlation.

Case 4: This 68-year-old retired secretary was referred on 9/73 because of an abnormal chest roentgenogram obtained during an annual checkup. She had always been entirely well and had no complaints. When questioned about shortness of breath, she reported that she could climb two flights of stairs carrying all of her groceries without difficulty. She had never smoked, and no occupational exposure was reported. The chest roentgenogram showed striking coarse irregular linear opacities, most marked in the right mid and basal zones; and honeycombing was suspected (Fig. 14). The left diaphragm was elevated but not paralyzed, and the mediastinum was shifted to the right. The mass in the right hilar area was the ascending aorta. Interestingly, two and one years earlier, her chest films had exactly the same appearance.

Examination revealed bilateral dry rales. Usual skin tests, sputum examination, routine blood and urine tests, electro- and immunoelectrophoresis, LE preparations, and latex fixation were all negative or normal. Lung function studies revealed normal lung volumes and no obstruction. However, her single breath diffusing capacity was only 64% of predicted and there was severe hypoxemia with an exercise $P(A\text{-}a)O_2$ of 61 torr (Table 2).

A lung biopsy revealed a usual interstitial pneumonia (Fig. 15). There was a sparse interstitial cellular infiltrate in some regions and minimal proteinaceous exudate in the air spaces. In some foci

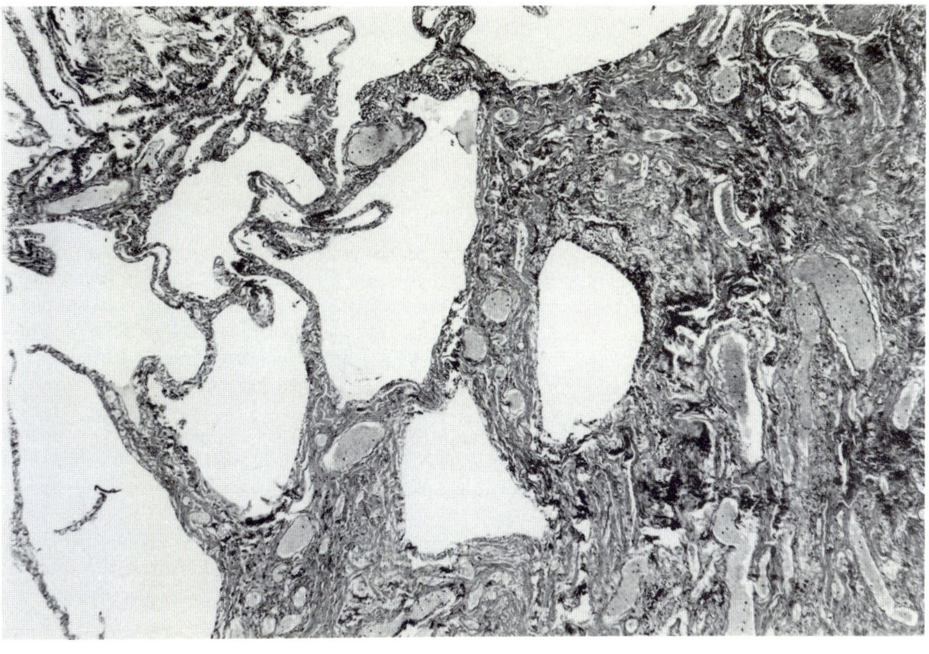

FIG. 8. Lung from autopsy of same patient as in Figure 7 who died from respiratory failure two years after biopsy. The lungs now have extensive honeycombing, and there is no longer any clue to the diagnosis of eosinophilic granuloma.

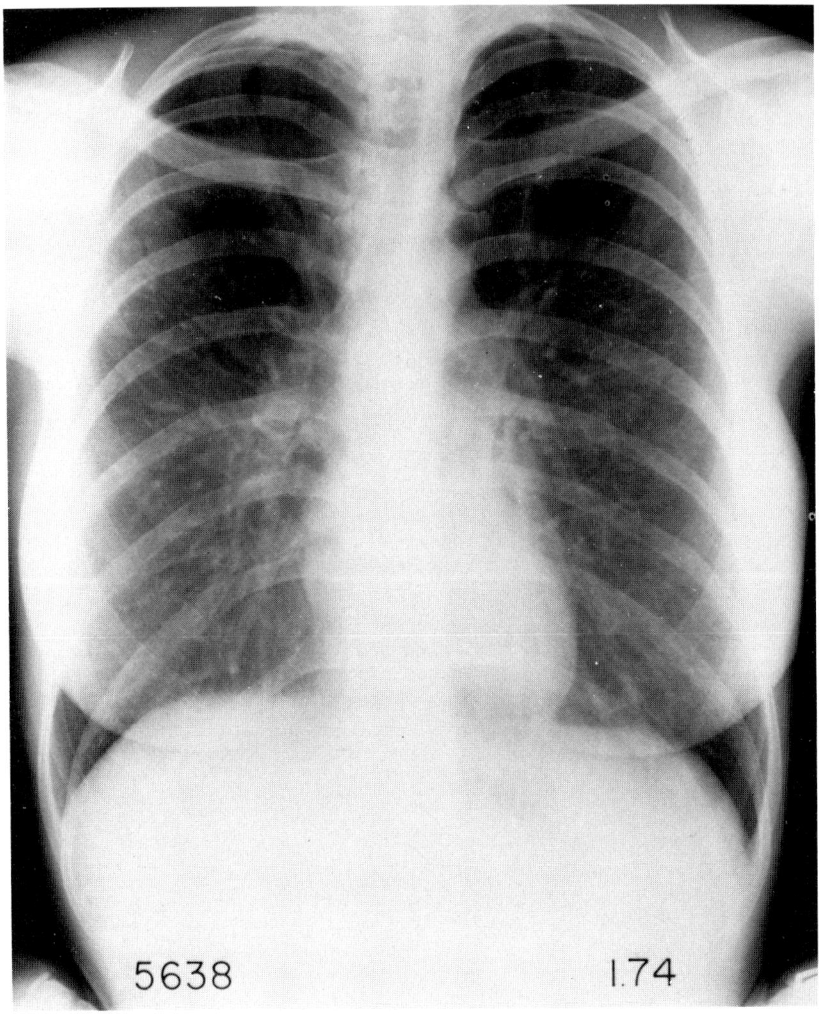

FIG. 9. Chest roentgenogram of a 28-year-old photographer's model who complained of marked weight loss. The film shows fine nodular infiltration apparently limited to both anterior segments of the upper lobes, more noticeable on the right. Lung function was entirely normal. A small anterior thoracotomy was performed with a preoperative diagnosis of talcosis because, for some years, she had sniffed cocaine cut with talc. Two biopsies were obtained, one from a hard nodulated mass in the anterior segment of the right upper lobe, and one from a normal-appearing middle lobe.

there was end stage fibrosis and fine honeycombing. Although the cellular components were sufficient to permit a diagnosis of UIP, the low degree of activity suggested that a relatively slow progression could be anticipated. Because of the histologic diagnosis, a favorable response to steroid therapy was thought to be unlikely.

During the next two years there was minimal deterioration of lung function (Table 2) but she developed slight dyspnea and a productive cough. Therefore prednisone was prescribed by her physician but three months and one year later lung function (Table 2) and the appearance of her roentgenogram had worsened considerably. Therapy was discontinued.

In summary, when evaluating a lung biopsy it is useful for the pathologist to know the history, radiographic appearance, and results of the pulmonary function tests. And it is important for the clinician to know the confidence with which the

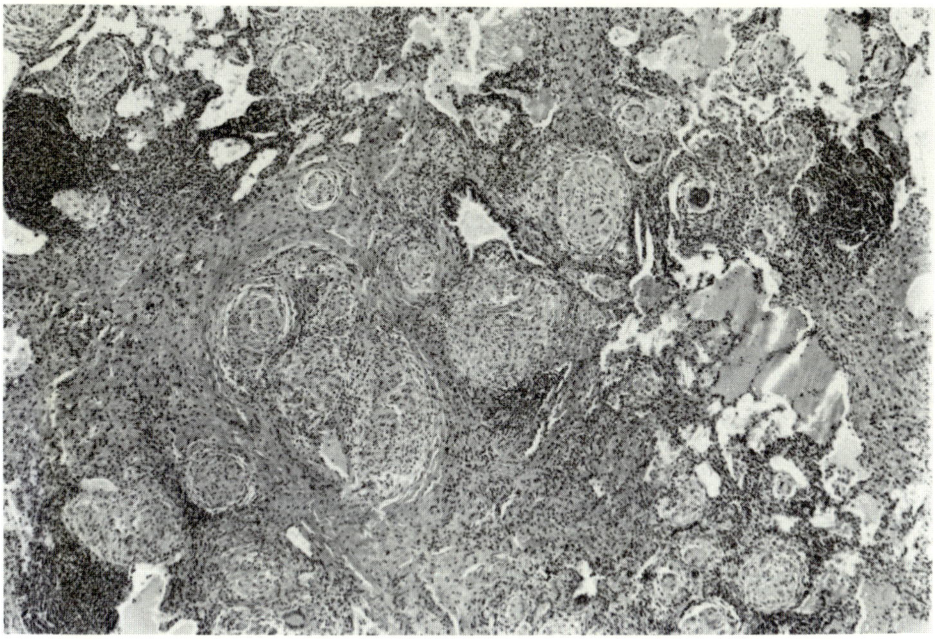

FIG. 10. The upper lobe biopsy from the patient in Figure 9. Most of the alveoli are obliterated by partly fibrotic, coalescent noncaseating granulomas typical of sarcoidosis. A bronchiole near the center is invaded and compressed by the granulomas. No extrinsic dust is seen, and none was identified by examination under bright polarized light. Compare with Figure 11.

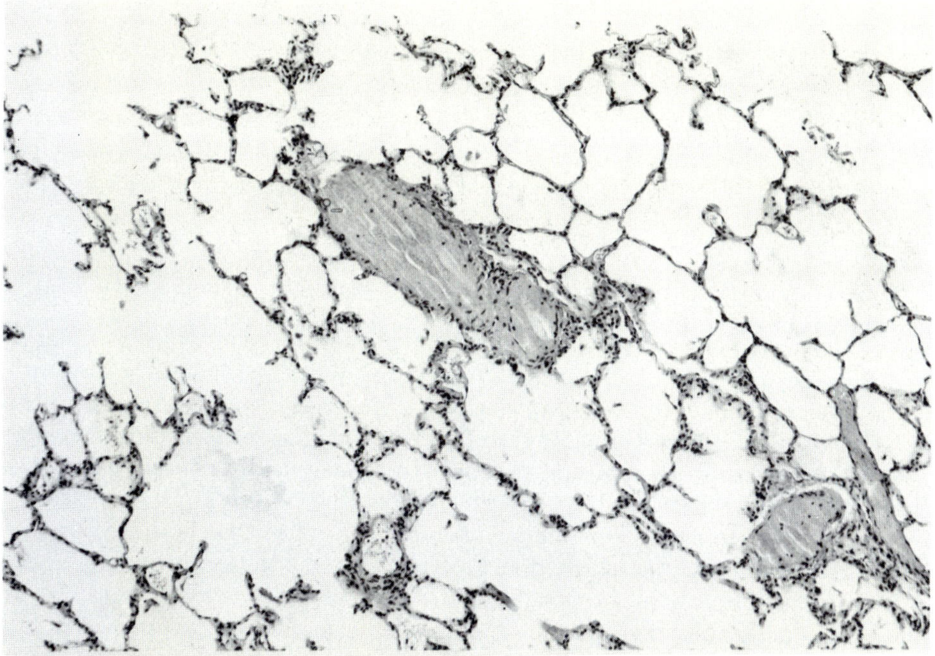

FIG. 11. The middle lobe biopsy from the patient in Figure 9. This is entirely normal. In this entire section there was but a single miliary granuloma, adjacent to a small venule in the pleura. Compare with Figure 10.

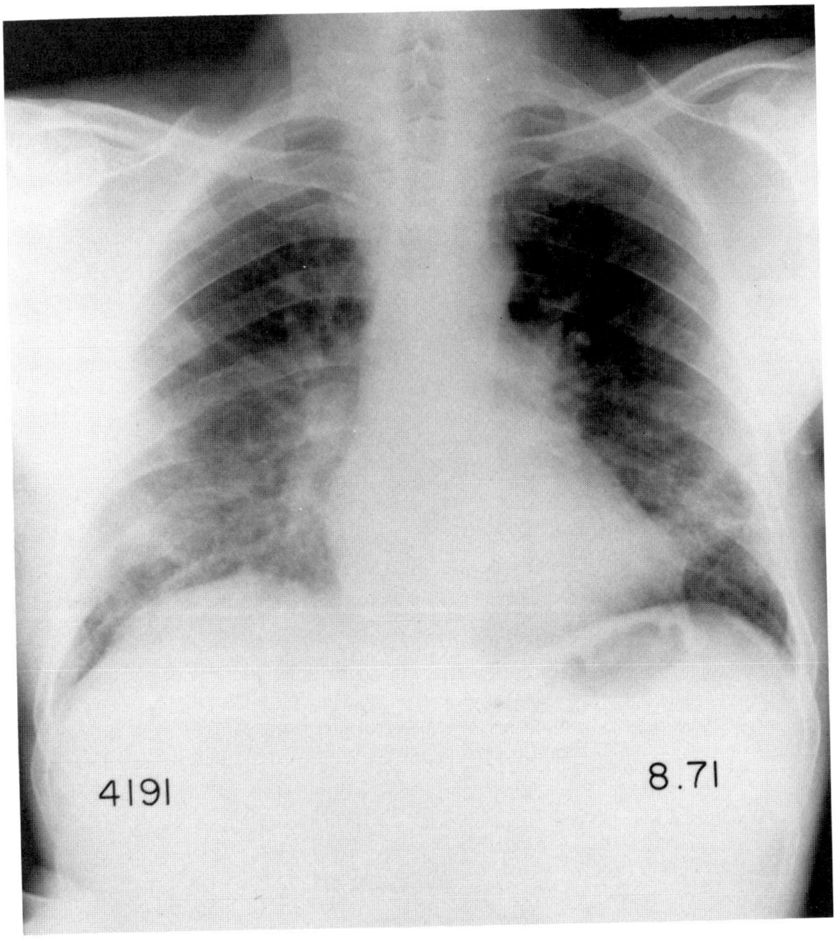

FIG. 12. Chest roentgenogram of patient #3 shortly after lung biopsy shows reduction in lung volume and moderately coarse, irregular lines distributed evenly throughout both lung fields. There are also a few patchy, "ground glass" opacities.

pathologist offers the diagnosis, the differential which was considered, the activity of the process, and the extent of tissue destruction and fibrosis.

Histologic Severity and Biopsy Quality: For assessing the severity of pulmonary disease in terms of diminished respiratory function, there are obviously better means than examination of a biopsy. Nevertheless, an estimate of this severity histologically serves a practical purpose. Conclusions regarding diagnosis, activity, permanent damage, and prognosis obviously will be sound only when the biopsy is representative. The degree to which this is true can be estimated by matching the histology to the pulmonary function and to the chest radiographs. In regard to abnormalities in function, both the type and the severity of the lesion should fit. Thus oxygen exchange at the parenchymal level is sensitive to interstitial infiltrates, alveolar destruction and usually to a small extent, by alveolar filling. A composite assessment of all of these should correlate closely with laboratory measurements of gas exchange (Fig. 16).[7,17,18] Air flow, on the contrary, is most sensitive to those lesions of emphysema, bronchitis, and bronchiectasis which cannot be assessed reliably from a lung biopsy. As described above, certain radiographic patterns are common in interstitial lung disease. The histologic findings should match the radiograph within certain limits, although it is true that some interstitial lesions may be found in patients with relatively normal radiographs. A mild interstitial infiltrate or irregular alveolar filling will not explain "cannon-ball" shadows on the radiograph, however, nor will the presence of a fibrocalcific granuloma or similar discrete nodule explain a diffuse haziness or reticular pattern. A marked disparity between the histology and the pulmonary function or the radiograph should raise doubt that the biopsy is representative and, accordingly, doubt that its interpretation is meaningful. Obviously the quality and validity of the biopsy are affected by the choice of procedure, the selection of biopsy site, and the subsequent handling of the tissue removed.

TECHNICAL CONSIDERATIONS OF LUNG BIOPSY

Open Lung Biopsy

This procedure was rarely performed before 1945 and then only by formal postero-lateral thoracotomy.[15] In 1949 Klassen[25] suggested a small thoracotomy. This simpler and briefer operation greatly increased the scope and usefulness of open biopsy, made it available to much sicker patients, and reduced the morbidity and possibly also the mortality.[15] It called for local anesthesia and resection of a

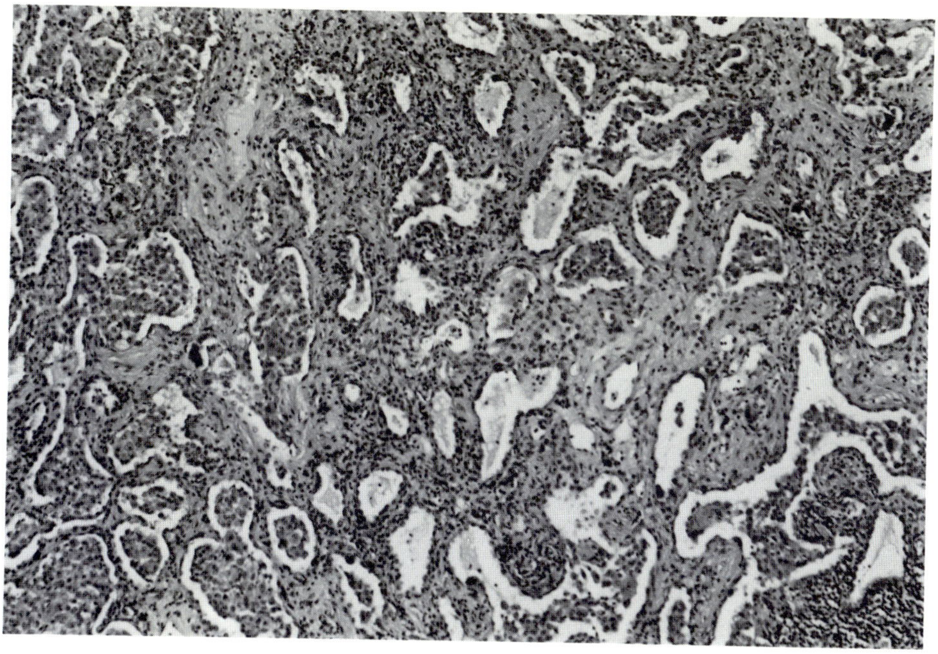

Fig. 13. Open lung biopsy from patient #3. The typical features of desquamative interstitial pneumonia are clearly seen. Note, however, that there is considerable scarring of some alveolar walls, and in some foci the normal architecture is obscured.

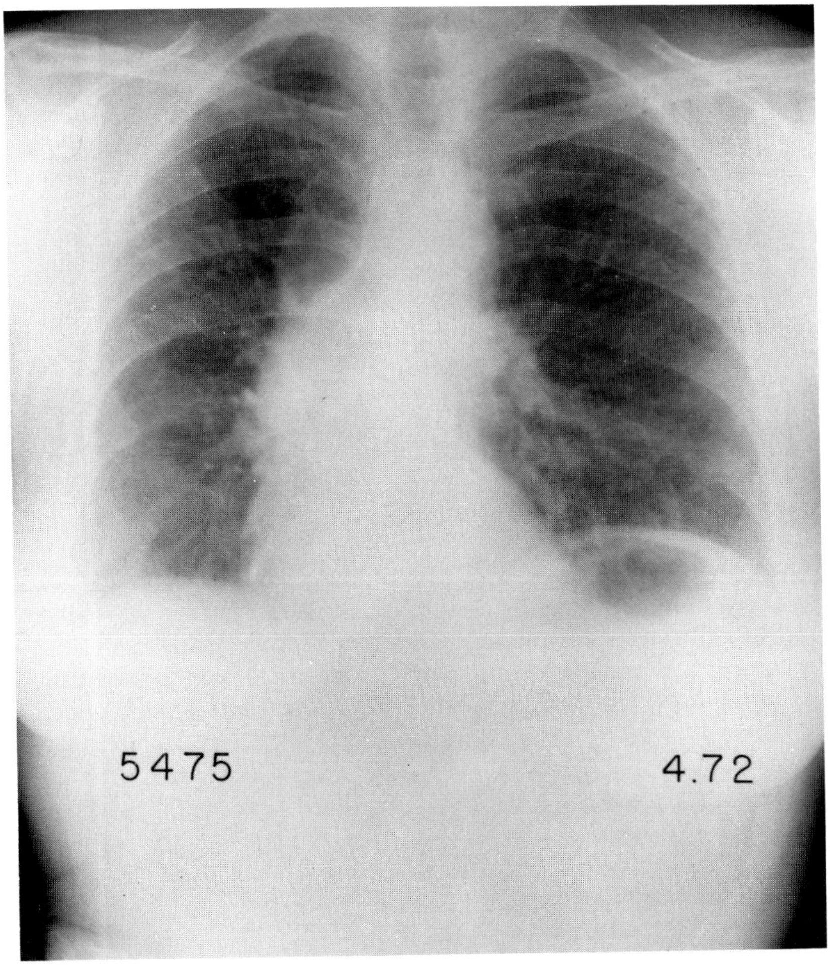

FIG. 14. Chest roentgenogram of patient #4. There is a diffuse, coarse linear or irregular infiltration, most marked in the right midlung region. Honeycombing is suspected. The left diaphragm is elevated but not paralyzed and the mediastinum is shifted to the right. The bulge at the right hilus is the ascending aorta.

small segment of rib; a portion of the lung was forced through the incision by positive pressure to avoid pneumothorax after excision.

Our own technique, used since 1952, is quite different and was designed for minimal trauma while permitting exploration and optimal choice and preservation of lung tissue. General endotracheal anesthesia is mandatory for control of inflation; local anesthesia has been associated with a much higher mortality and morbidity.[34] The anesthetic of choice is one that permits rapid intubation, is short-acting so that the patient is fully conscious at the end of the procedure, is not a respiratory depressant and permits administration of increased inspired oxygen concentration. Muscle relaxation is not required.

The incision is 4–7 cm long depending upon the thickness of the chest wall, and its location is dictated by the distribution of the disease. With diffuse involvement, we prefer an approach originally suggested by Chamberlain[8] for mediastinal exploration in the second interspace anteriorly, beginning medially just lateral to the sternum and internal mammary artery. This approach permits inspection and possible biopsy of the anterior aspect of the upper lobe, the entire middle lobe, and the superior and anterior segments of the lower lobe. The anterior mediastinum and hilus from the midportion of the superior cava to the superior pulmonary vein are easily exposed for inspection and possible node biopsy. Parenthetically, we also prefer this incision for mediastinal exploration, because, unlike the neck incision of mediastinoscopy,[5] it is not visible in clothing and permits better exposure and hemostasis. In patients with infiltration apparently limited to the lower lung regions and in young women, the incision is made in the fold of the breast such that it is not visible with a brassiere or a bikini. The breast tissue is retracted upwards for a thoracic incision in the 4th interspace. This interspace may be too low in patients with very small fibrotic lungs.

The lung is allowed to collapse, and the thoracic cavity is explored. Enlarged lymph nodes or pleural lesions are biopsied. An infant-size Tuffier retractor is then placed between the ribs and the reinflated lung is inspected and palpated as far as is possible.

For biopsy, a region of lung is selected with apparently average involvement. If various parts of the lung appear or feel quite differently, then two biopsies of the more and of the less involved areas can be obtained. Generally, the most severely involved areas are avoided, because they may show nothing but nonspe-

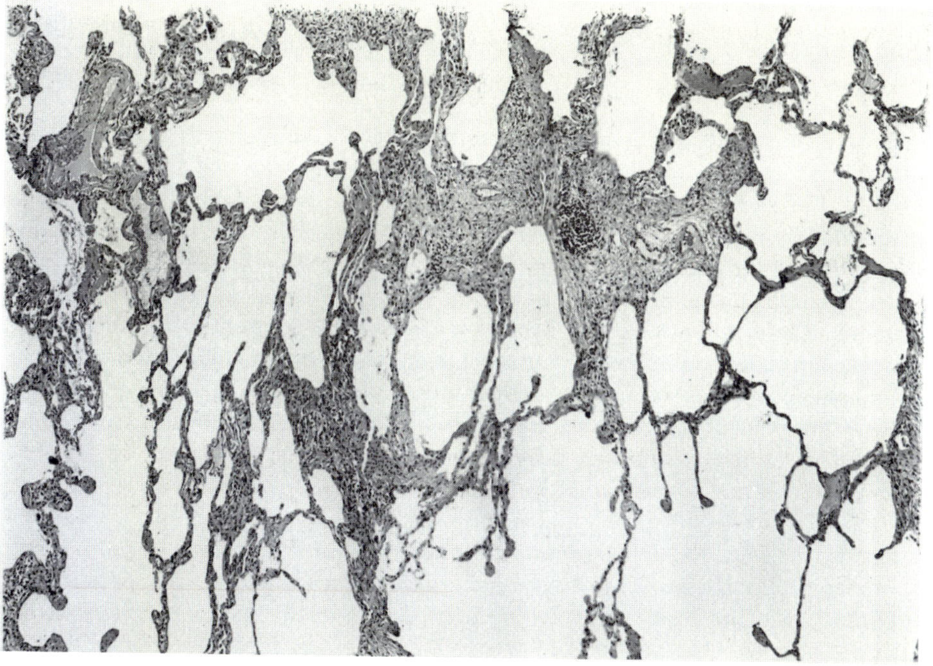

FIG. 15. Open lung biopsy from patient #4. A few alveolar walls are normal, and some are badly scarred. In others there is a definite but sparse infiltrate of monocytes, lymphocytes, and plasma cells. Proteinaceous exudates are virtually absent. This was interpreted as relatively inactive UIP.

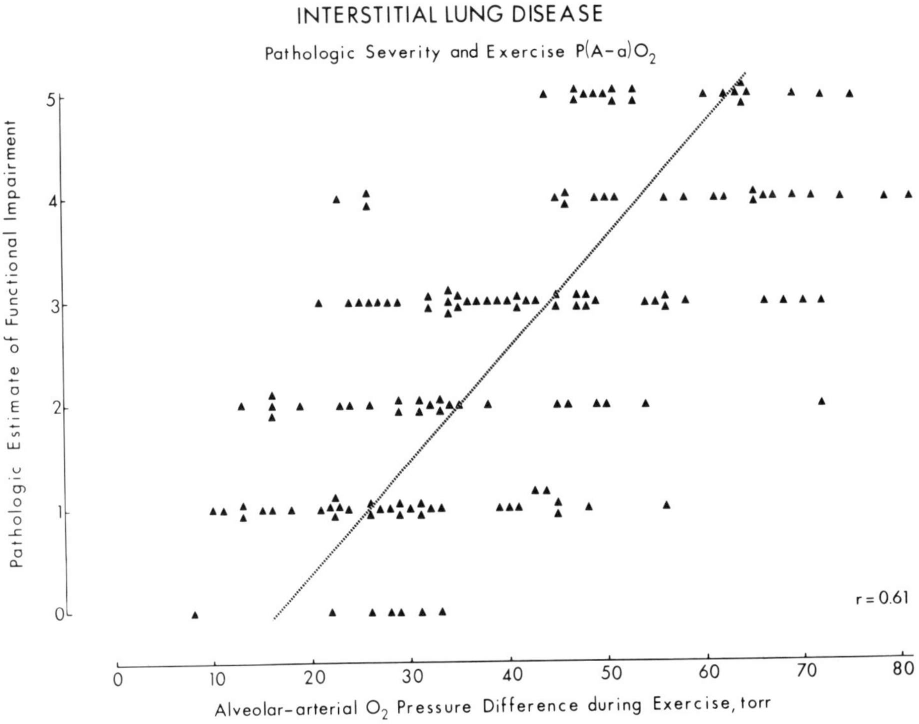

FIG. 16. Relationship of the pathologic estimate of functional impairment, graded from 0 (none) to 5 (worst), with functional impairment as measured by the alveolar-arterial O_2 pressure difference during exercise just before lung biopsy in 137 patients with diffuse infiltrative lung disease ($r = 0.61$, $P < 0.01$).

cific honeycombing. If one is to err it is better to do so in the direction of lesser rather than greater involvement. Unusual solitary nodules are avoided, because usually they show a healed fibrous focus or a healed granuloma that is irrelevant to the diffuse disease. Most surgeons prefer for biopsy the tip of the middle lobe or of the lingular segment, because these are easily delivered into the wound and but a single clamp is needed to delineate the tissue to be resected. This is poor economy of time, because these narrow dependent portions of the lung often show lesions that are not representative and hence should be avoided.

The selected lung margin is delineated for a distance of 4–5 cm, two stay sutures are placed, the lung is inflated until it just fills the thoracic cavity and a triangular segment is delineated by two narrow clamps. Two-thirds of the specimen is excised and immediately dropped into 10% buffered formalin within a few seconds. This procedure traps a maximum amount of air in the lung, and therefore atelectasis is minimal. Preservation of lung tissue in this fashion is most helpful to the pathologist as illustrated by Figures 17 and 18. In this patient with bronchiectasis the lung was fully inflated, and the tip of the middle lobe was clamped across. One-half of the wedge was fixed in formalin immediately as described above (Fig. 17). The other one-half was handed to the nurse "for pathology." It was duly wrapped in a moist sponge and eventually made its way to the refrigerator, from whence it was collected in the afternoon and processed in routine fashion (Fig. 18). The promptly fixed portion was sufficiently expanded that the individual alveolar walls—all normal—could easily be seen. In the other sample there was so much irregular atelectasis that it was difficult to determine if the alveolar walls were normal or not.

The remaining third of the specimen is then excised. About one-third of this is submitted routinely for aerobic and anaerobic cultures for bacteria, mycobacteria, and fungi. Disposition of the remaining tissue depends upon indications and special interests. Chemical analysis for toxic substances generally requires at least 3–5 gm. Tissue also may be stored for biochemical studies or frozen for immunologic studies. Generally, we immediately place a small portion under glutaraldehyde, cut it into several 1-mm^3 blocks and store it for electron microscopy.

The tissue underneath the clamps is closed with a continuous interlocking "cobbler's" suture, the clamps are removed and the wound is oversewn with an interlocking over and over stitch. The suture line is then tested under warm saline with an endotracheal pressure from 20–30 cm H_2O.

A small No. 18–22 French catheter is placed laterally in the incision and attached to an underwater seal, and the wound is closed in layers while the patient is recovering. The importance of drainage cannot be overemphasized. It is virtually impossible to close lung absolutely airtight. A resulting small pneumothorax is of no consequence to a person with nearly normal lungs. However, if the vital capacity and the pulmonary capillary bed are already severely reduced,

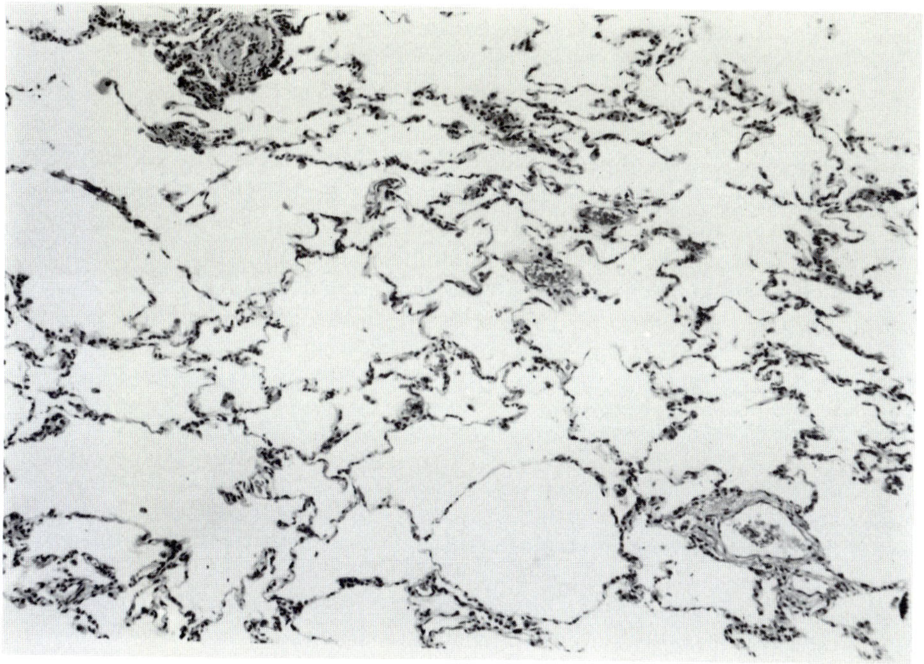

FIG. 17. Wedge from the normal part of lung from patient who underwent a lobectomy because of bronchiectasis. This sample, resected with the lung fully inflated, was immersed in formalin within seconds as described in the text. The individual alveolar walls and other architectual features are easily distinguished, and are all normal. Compare with Figure 18.

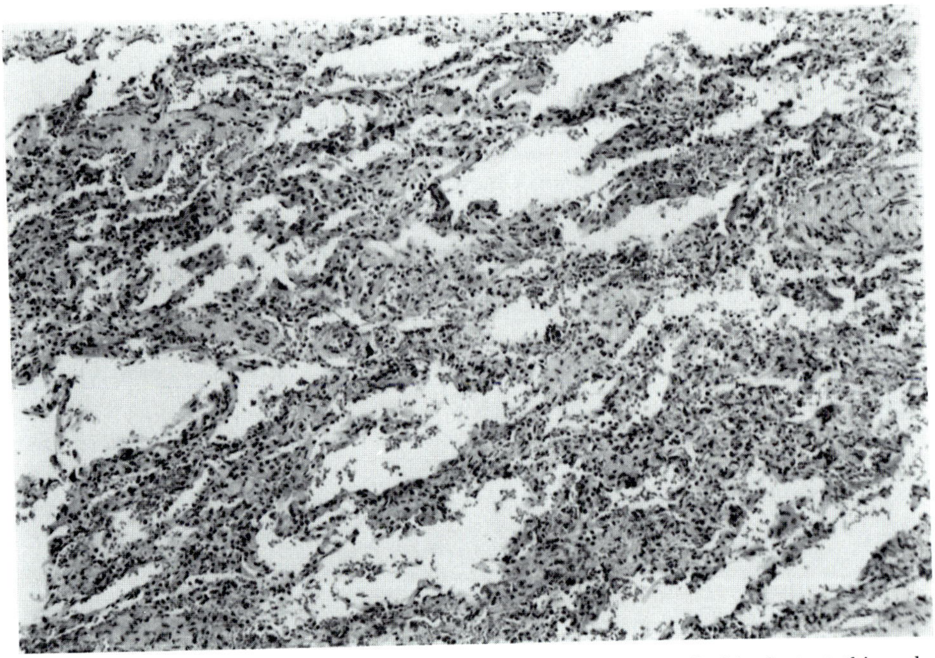

FIG. 18. Same patient as in Fig. 17, and *same magnification*. As described in the text, this wedge was taken immediately adjacent to the biopsy in Figure 17, but this sample was wrapped in a saline-moistened sponge and refrigerated before fixation. Many alveoli are collapsed, and it is much more difficult to determine whether or not the alveolar walls are normal. The only real difference between the two samples, however, was the way in which they were handled after resection.

then even a small pneumothorax is poorly tolerated. In series where this precautionary drainage was omitted, mortality and morbidity have been excessive.[23]

Postoperatively, oxygen may be given to hypoxic patients with appropriate monitoring, and mobilization is begun immediately. If the roentgenographic appearance is satisfactory, the tube is removed after 24 hours; and, generally, discharge is possible on the 3rd or 4th postoperative day.

Following this procedure for 25 years we have lost only one patient following 490 open biopsies. This single death occurred more than 20 years ago on the 13th postoperative day in a patient with advanced carcinomatosis and multiple pulmonary emboli.

CLOSED LUNG BIOPSY

Review of the diagnostic criteria for many diffuse infiltrative lung diseases reveals a strong reliance on histologic patterns, especially for the chronic lesions for which there is no histologically demonstrable causative agent. Hence the preference of many lung pathologists for open lung biopsies, the size of which facilitates pattern recognition. Nevertheless, there are some situations in which other biopsy techniques are sufficient; and then, because of the speed with which they are arranged, minimal hospitalization and cost, and perhaps lower morbidity, they are even preferable. Thus, in an attempt to identify an infectious agent such as pneumocystis carinii in the appropriate clinical setting, a closed biopsy may obviate the need for a thoracotomy. Similarly, the finding by a closed lung biopsy of lymphangitic carcinomatosis or numerous noncaseating granulomata typical in all aspects of sarcoidosis is quite adequate for diagnosis. The following case illustrates the value of transbronchial lung biopsy.

Case 5: A 27-year-old white electronics repair manager had infectious hepatitis in 1969. He recovered uneventfully and since then had had annual examinations including a chest roentgenogram. The films were normal until 1977 when a very fine diffuse infiltration was noted. This consisted of tiny rounded opacities of less than 1 mm in diameter which could be seen only on close inspection (Fig. 19). Although entirely asymptomatic, he was referred to us for evaluation. Upon arrival three weeks later, his film was normal both with high and low kilovoltage techniques and with several different exposures (Fig. 20). The history, including a detailed account of environment, physical examination, and routine laboratory studies were all unremarkable. Skin tests for histoplasmosis,

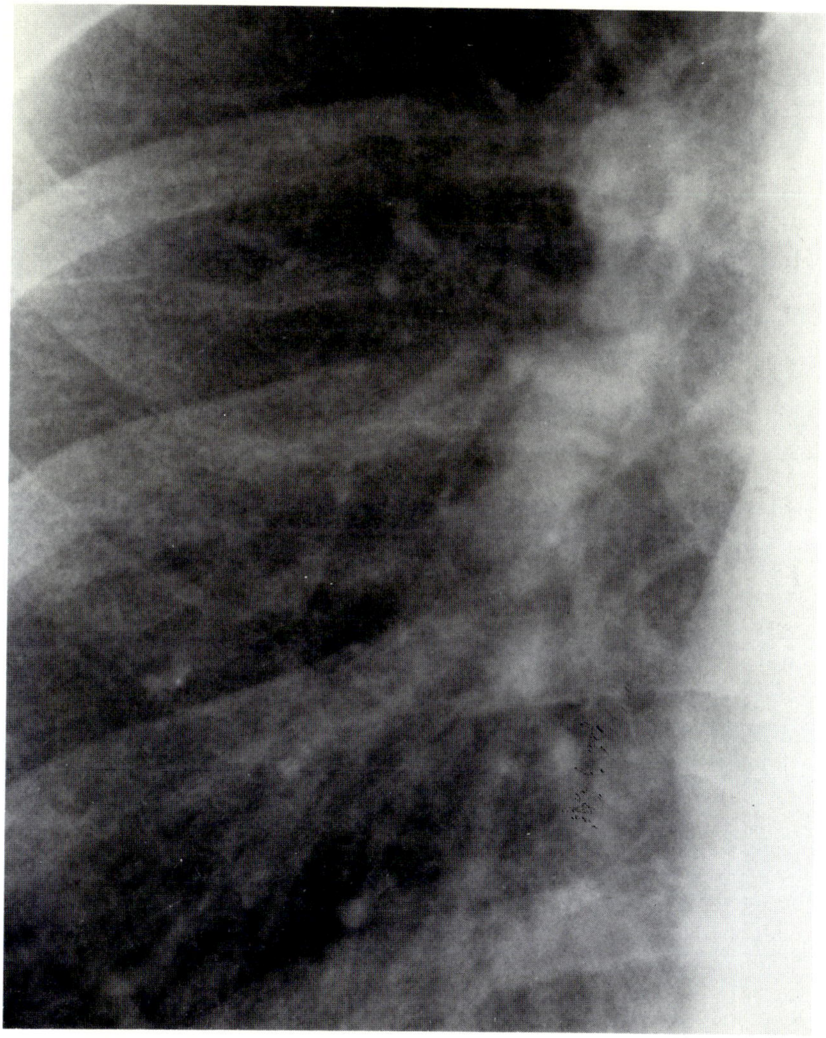

FIG. 19. Detail of chest roentgenogram of patient #5 obtained during routine health examination shows a delicate diffuse infiltration which, on close inspection, consists of tiny rounded opacities each apparently less than 1 mm in diameter.

coccidioidomycosis, candida, and PPD were negative. Urine, blood counts, protein electrophoresis, and serum calcium, phosphorous, and uric acid were also normal. LDH 5 was elevated to 20% suggesting hepatocellular damage. Serum precipitins for thermophylic bacteria and fungi were negative. Lung function studies showed normal lung volumes and air flow. However, the screening single breath diffusing capacity was only 60% of predicted, and the steady state diffusing capacity failed to rise during exercise (Table 2). A transbronchial biopsy revealed many coalescent miliary, non-necrotizing sarcoid granulomas (Fig. 21). These involved a small bronchus and a bronchiole, but there was no other bronchitis or bronchiolitis in these two small conducting airways. Most of the alveolar walls between granulomas were normal, but a few had a minimal round cell infiltrate. There was a tendency for the granulomas to concentrate near small blood vessels, *i.e.*, along lymphatic routes. Because the biopsy was so typical of sarcoidosis, an open biopsy was not believed to be necessary.

It must again be emphasized, however, that the presence of a few granulomas is not specific, and the diagnosis of sarcoidosis must be made with consideration

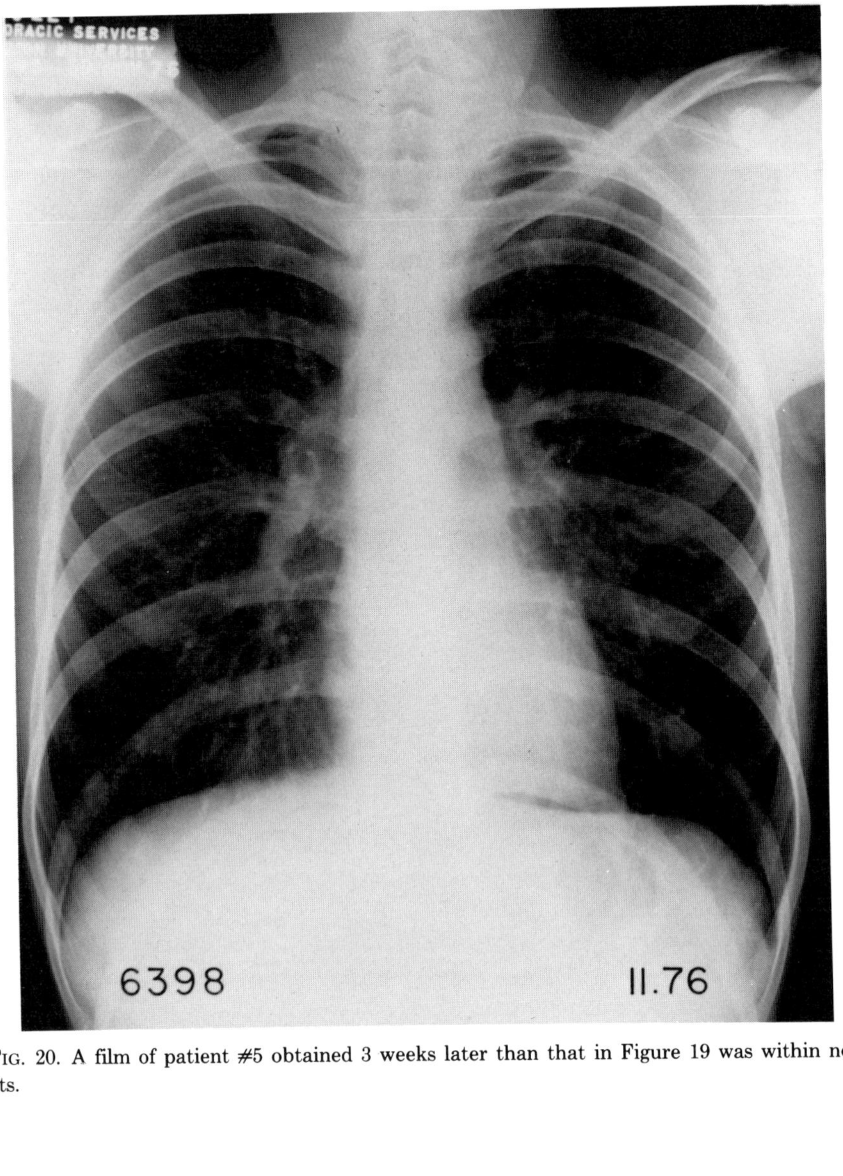

FIG. 20. A film of patient #5 obtained 3 weeks later than that in Figure 19 was within normal limits.

of the rest of the histologic features and the clinical setting (Case 2). Both the transthoracic and transbronchial approaches have been employed for closed biopsy.

Transthoracic Needle Biopsy. A variety of needles such as those described by Vim Silverman[24] and electric drill driven needles[32] have been used for core biopsy of lung tissue for the diagnosis of diffuse infiltrative lung disease. The literature suggests, and our experiences confirm, that this procedure entails a higher mortality than open lung biopsy because of several complications, including bleeding, tension pneumothorax, massive hemoptysis, and especially air embolism,[36] which are not encountered with open biopsy. The procedure thus entails all the disadvantages of a small specimen selected without thoracic inspection but not the advantages of lower morbidity; and, therefore, it should be avoided.

Transbronchial Biopsy. This procedure was first performed through a rigid bronchoscope[2] but gained popularity only with the advent of the fiberoptic bronchoscope.[21] The design of the larger of these instruments permits introduction of a tiny forceps. This is advanced to the periphery of the lung either by measurement or by fluoroscopic control. The instrument is then withdrawn slightly, the patient is asked to expire while the forceps are opened and several biopsies are obtained in this fashion. The fragments of tissue are tiny, usually 1 mm, and rarely up to 3 mm in diameter; but several specimens can be obtained. Mortality and morbidity in several series have been very low,[33, 37] but have not been finally evaluated. The procedure has the great advantage that it can be performed under topical anesthesia, thus not requiring expensive operating room time; and also hospitalization is shortened. Studies comparing diagnostic yield of

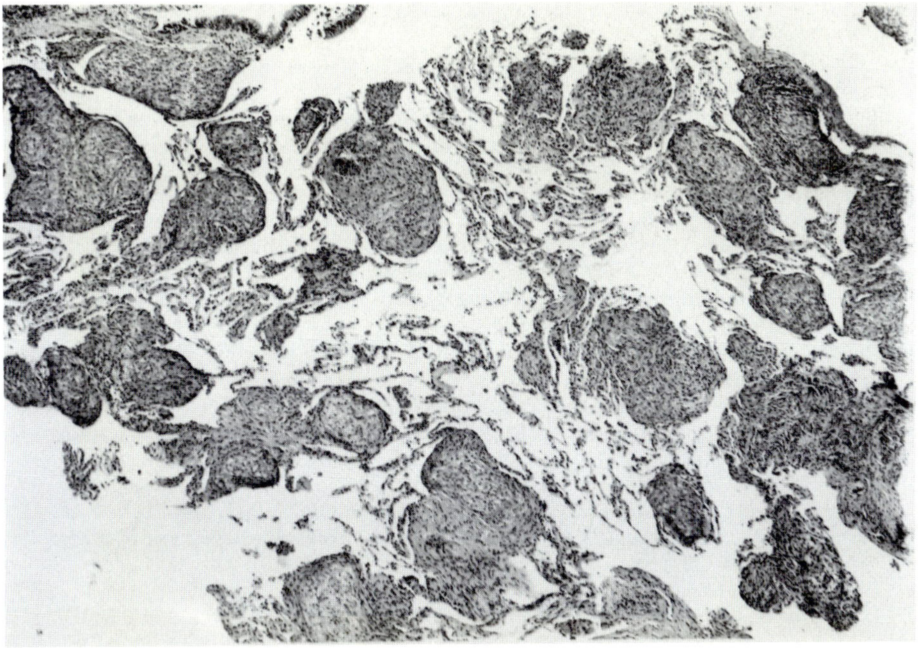

FIG. 21. Transbronchial biopsy from patient #5. There are many small, coalescent noncaseating granulomas, one of which involves the wall of a small bronchus. This is typical of sarcoidosis.

transbronchial and open biopsy are in progress, and the definitive place for the transbronchial procedure is not established. The diagnosis of UIP or interstitial fibrosis is especially foolhardy with a specimen obtained by transbronchial biopsy. Many patients with old or current bronchitis—which, unfortunately, includes a large part of our population—have changes confined to peribronchial alveoli which simulate UIP when no other alveoli are sampled. We have seen several instances where such a diagnosis from a transbronchial biopsy was invalidated by study of tissue subsequently obtained by open biopsy or at autopsy. We have seen another example where a transbronchial biopsy failed to confirm a clinical diagnosis of chronic eosinophilic pneumonia with an atypical roentgenogram because the bronchial and nearby parenchymal changes were indistinguishable from those which could be expected solely from the patient's underlying asthma. An open biopsy resolved this question and confirmed the original clinical impression. Thus there are still a variety of situations in which open biopsy is necessary. When this technique is chosen, proper site selection, inflation, and immediate fixation greatly enhance the value of that part of the specimen used for routine microscopy.

REFERENCES

1. Abraham, J. L.: Recent advances in pneumoconiosis: The responsibility of pathologists in etiologic diagnosis (see Chapter 6 of this volume).
2. Andersen, H. A., and Fontana, R. S.: Transbronchioscopic lung biopsy for diffuse pulmonary diseases: Technique and results in 450 cases. *Chest 62:* 125–128, 1972.
3. Austrian, R., McClement, J. H., Rinzetti, A. D., Jr., Donald, K. W., Riley, R. L., and Cournand, A.: Clinical and physiologic features of some types of pulmonary diseases with impairment of alveolar-capillary diffusion. The syndrome of "alveolar-capillary block." *Am. J. Med. 11:* 667–685, 1951.
4. Buechner, H. A.: The differential diagnosis of miliary diseases of the lungs. *Med. Clin. N. Am. 43:* 89–112, 1959.
5. Carlens, E.: Mediastinoscopy: A method for inspection and tissue biopsy in the superior mediastinum. *Dis. Chest 36:* 343–352, 1959.
6. Carrington, C. B., Gaensler, E. A., Coutu, R. E., FitzGerald, M. X., and Gupta, R. G.: Usual and desquamative interstitial pneumonia. *Chest 69:* 261–263, 1976 (Abstr.).
7. Carrington, C. B., Gaensler, E. A., Mikus, J. P., Schachter, A. W., Burke, G. W., and Goff, A. M.: Structure and Function in Sarcoidosis. 7th International Conference on Sarcoidosis and other Granulomatous Disorders, *Ann. N. Y. Acad. Sci. 278:* 265–283, 1976.
8. Chamberlain, J. M.: Discussion of "mediastinoscopy." *J. Thorac. Cardiovasc. Surg. 49:* 20, 1965.
9. Comroe, J. H., Forster, R. E., DuBois, A. B., Briscoe, W. A., and Carlsen, E.: *The Lung: Clinical Physiology and Pulmonary Function Tests,* pp. 111-139, Chicago, Year Book Medical Publishers, Inc., 1962.
10. Epler, G. R., Gaensler, E. A., and Carrington, C. B.: Rales in interstitial lung disease: Clinical, pathologic and physiologic correlations. *Br. J. Dis. Chest* (in press).
11. Epler, G. R., Mikus, J. P., McLoud, T. C., Carrington, C. B., and Gaensler, E. A.: Normal chest roentgenograms in chronic interstitial and pulmonary vascular disease. *Am. Rev. Resp. Dis. 115:* suppl: 104, 1977.
12. Finley, T. N., Swenson, E. W., and Comroe, J. H., Jr.: The cause of arterial hypoxemia at rest in patients with "alveolar-capillary block syndrome." *J. Clin. Invest. 41:* 618–622, 1962.
13. FitzGerald, M. X., Carrington, C. B., and Gaensler, E. A.: Environmental lung disease. *Med. Clin. N. Am. 57:* 593–622, 1973.
14. Gaensler, E. A.: Diagnostic techniques in diffuse or miliary lung diseases. Experience with 381 patients, In *Advances in Cardiopulmonary Diseases.* Vol. III, pp. 81-122. Edited by Banyai, A. L., and Gordon, B. L. Chicago, Year Book Medical Publishers, 1966.
15. Gaensler, E. A., Ball-Moister, M. V., and Hamm, J.: Open-lung biopsy in diffuse pulmonary disease. *N. Engl. J. Med. 270:* 1319–1331, 1964.

16. Gaensler, E. A., and Carrington, C. B.: Peripheral opacities in chronic eosinophilic pneumonia: The photographic negative of pulmonary edema. *Am. J. Roentgenol. 128:* 1-13, 1977.
17. Gaensler, E. A., Carrington, C. B., Coutu, R. E., and FitzGerald, M. X.: Radiographic-physiologic-pathologic correlations in interstitial pneumonias. In *Alveolar Interstitium of the Lung.* International Symposium, Paris, 1974. *Prog. Resp. Res. 8:* 223–241, Basel, S. Karger, 1975.
18. Gaensler, E. A., Carrington, C. B., Coutu, R. E., Tomasian, A., Hoffman, L., and Smith, A. A.: Pathological, physiological and radiological correlations in the pneumoconioses. *Am. NY Acad. Sci. 200:* 574-607, 1972.
19. Genereux, G. P.: The end-stage lung: Pathogenesis, pathology and radiology. *Radiology 116:* 279–289, 1975.
20. Heppleston, A. G.: The pathology of honeycomb lung. *Thorax 11:* 77–93, 1956.
21. Ikeda, S., Yanai, N., and Ishikawa, S.: Flexible bronchofiberscope. *Keio J. Med. 17:* 1–18, 1968.
22. Jacobson, G., Lainhart, W. S. (eds.): ILO U/C 1971 international classification of radiographs of the pneumoconioses. *Med. Radiogr. Photogr. 48:* 65–76, 1972.
23. Jefferson, F. R. III, Lawton, B. R., Myers, W. O., et al.: Open pulmonary biopsy: 19-year experience with 416 consecutive operations. *Chest 69:* 43–47, 1976.
24. Jones, F. L.: A comparison of trephine and Franklin-Silverman needles for percutaneous lung biopsy. *Am. Rev. Resp. Dis. 109:* 625–629, 1974.
25. Klassen, K. P., Anlyan, A. J., and Curtis, G. M.: Biopsy of diffuse pulmonary lesions. *Arch. Surg. 59:* 694–704, 1949.
26. Kuhn, C.: Ultrastructure and cellular function in the distal lung (see Chapter 1 of this volume).
27. Liebow, A. A., and Carrington, C. B.: The interstitial pneumonias, In *Frontiers of Pulmonary Radiology,* Edited by Simon, M., Potchen, E. J., and LeMay, M. pp. 102–141. New York, Grune & Stratton, 1969.
28. Marks, A., Cugell, D. W., Cardigan, J. B., and Gaensler, E. A.: Clinical determination of the diffusion capacity of the lungs. Comparison of methods in normal subjects and patients with "alveolar-capillary block" syndrome. *Am. J. Med. 22:* 5–73, 1957.
29. Morgan, W. K. C., and Seaton, A.: *Occupational Lung Diseases.* Philadelphia, W. B. Saunders, Co., 1975.
30. Parkes, W. R.: *Occupational Lung Disorders.* London, Butterworth & Co., Ltd., 1974.
31. Roughton, F. J. W., and Forster, R. E.: Relative importance of diffusion and chemical reaction rates in determining rate of exchange of gases in the human lung, with special reference to true diffusing capacity of pulmonary membrane and volume of blood in the lung capillaries. *J. Appl. Physiol. 11:* 290–302, 1957.
32. Steel, S. J., and Winstanley, D. P.: Trephine biopsy of the lung and pleura. *Thorax 24:* 576–584, 1969.
33. Suratt, P. M., Smiddy, J. F., and Gruber, B.: Deaths and complications associated with fiberoptic bronchoscopy. *Chest 69:* 747–751, 1976.
34. Theodos, P. A., Allbritten, F. F., Jr., and Breckenridge, R. L.: Lung biopsy in diffuse pulmonary disease. *Dis. Chest 27:* 637–638, 1955.
35. Wagner, P. D., Dantzker, D. R., Dueck, R., dePolo, J. L., Wasserman, K., and West, J. B.: Distribution of ventilation-perfusion ratios in patients with interstitial lung disease. *Chest 69:* 256–257, 1976.
36. Westcott, J. L.: Air embolism complicating percutaneous needle biopsy of the lung. *Chest 63:* 108–110, 1973.
37. Zavala, D. C.: Diagnostic fiberoptic bronchoscopy: Techniques and results of biopsy in 600 patients. *Chest 68:* 12–19, 1975.

Chapter 5

The Immunopathologic Basis of Hypersensitivity Pneumonitis

PETER A. WARD, ROBERT M. SENIOR, AND SOLON COLE

Hypersensitivity pneumonitis (HPN) is a form of diffuse lung disease that is the result of immunologic events provoked most often by an inhaled antigen. As with other immunologic responses, HPN only occurs after prior contact with the sensitizing agent and its provocation is antigen-specific; unrelated antigens will not trigger the reaction. For the purposes of this discussion, HPN will be considered synonomous with extrinsic allergic alveolitis and farmer's lung disease. This brief review will describe the clinical and diagnostic features of HPN and discuss some of the pathologic and immunologic aspects of HPN developed from studies in humans and experimental animals.

CLINICAL FEATURES

From a clinical standpoint, HPN can be divided into acute, subacute, and chronic categories.[22] The acute form refers to a viral pneumonia-like illness that typically occurs after an intense antigen inhalation in a highly sensitive individual. Symptoms begin within a few hours after antigen exposure, reaching maximum severity at 6–12 hours; spontaneous resolution of the fever and malaise is usually complete in 1–2 days, but cough, rales and radiographic abnormalities may last for weeks. Unless a careful medical history is obtained, acute HPN may not be diagnosed, since it has features typical of other acute lung diseases, especially infectious pneumonias, which occur with considerably more frequency.

In individuals who experience more mild reactions, or when there is less intense exposure to antigen, only a mild febrile respiratory illness may occur that the patient tolerates without seeking medical attention. Some individuals experience repetitive (even daily) bouts of acute HPN before the causative agent is recognized.

Low grade, but repeated, inhalation of antigen extending over weeks, months or years may lead to gradually progressive dyspnea and exercise intolerance without intervening pneumonia-like episodes. In these forms of HPN, which can be considered subacute or chronic, the radiographic and physiologic patterns are indistinguishable from chronic, diffuse interstitial lung disease due to a multitude of causes. As is the case with acute HPN, the subacute and chronic forms of HPN often resolve if further contact with the antigen is avoided.[1] In some patients, however, the duration and intensity of exposure produce severe, irreversible changes in lung structure. Respiratory failure with cor pulmonale and right ventricular failure may develop in these individuals.

An ever-increasing number of antigens capable of triggering HPN has been identified. Table 1 lists a few of the many types of HPN and the responsible sources of antigen. Among the causes of HPN are fungi and thermotolerant bacteria to which even city dwellers without exotic occupations may be exposed. Humidifiers in forced air units (including air conditioners and heating units) are often contaminated with micro-organisms.[7] Exposure to avian antigens among bird fanciers is another cause of HPN among the urban population. In these individuals, the subacute and chronic forms of HPN are most common. With reliable and sensitive immunodiagnostic tests, it is likely that HPN will become much more frequently diagnosed.

The diagnosis of HPN is usually made as a result of a suggestive history and exclusion of other causes for the pulmonary disease. In the acute forms, especially in the setting of occupations known to be associated with HPN, diagnosis is not difficult. On the other hand, the subacute and chronic forms are easily misdiagnosed. Initially, HPN may not even be considered in the differential diagnosis.

Simple laboratory tests to confirm a diagnosis of HPN are lacking (see below). Currently, proof of HPN requires: (1) reproducing an acute HPN episode by aerosol challenge with antigen, and (2) resolution of symptoms when the patient avoids contact with antigen. The use of aerosol challenge to diagnose HPN has not gained wide acceptance in North America because methods and reagents have not been well standardized, and there are medical-legal concerns. Lung biopsy is a procedure that may suggest HPN. Supplementing conventional microscopy with immunofluorescent techniques may identify the putative antigen in the tissues as well as the possible presence of immune complexes.[7]

HISTOLOGIC ASPECTS

The microscopic features of HPN are varied and appear to be highly dependent on the time of biopsy in relation to the onset of the illness. A lung biopsy done within a few days after an antigen aerosol is given to susceptible individuals shows a neutrophil-rich infiltrate involving alveolar septae, alveolar spaces and small airways, along with alveolar edema. In addition, there may be neutrophil infiltration of vascular walls, primarily of veins.[11] However, lung biopsies are seldom obtained soon after acute exposure to antigen. Usually, tissue is obtained

TABLE 1. ETIOLOGIC BASES OF SOME EXAMPLES OF HYPERSENSITIVITY PNEUMONITIS

Clinical description	Responsible agent
Farmer's lung	Thermophilic actinomycetes in mouldy hay
Maple bark disease	*Cryptostroma corticale* in wood pulp
Bagassosis	Thermophilic actinomycetes in sugar cane
Malt worker's disease	*Aspergillus clavatus* in barley
Humidifier lung	Thermophilic actinomycetes
Sauna taker's disease	*Pullularia* sp. in cedar wood
Sequoiosis	*Pullularia* sp.
Pigeon breeder's disease	Pigeon dropping extract
Wood pulp worker's disease	*Alternaria* sp.

from patients who have undiagnosed, persistant, diffuse pulmonary disease. In these individuals, the histopathologic changes range from diffuse interstitial infiltrates of chronic inflammatory cells, interstitial fibrosis and organizing alveolitis,[6, 12, 23] to the presence of epithelioid granulomas with giant cells (Fig. 1 and 2). There is seldom confusion with sarcoidosis. The granulomas are less well formed and are fewer in HPN. In addition, linear doubly refractile material and empty spaces are often encountered in the giant cells, when present. An important distinguishing feature is the presence of chronic interstitial inflammation in the alveolar walls between the granulomas in HPN. This finding is usually absent in sarcoidosis. There seems little doubt that if exposure to antigen is repeated and prolonged, reactive individuals will develop diffuse pulmonary fibrosis. Thus, the spectrum of morphologic changes in HPN is broad, and no single feature or collection of morphologic changes is diagnostic or etiologically indicative.

IMMUNOLOGIC APPROACHES FOR DIAGNOSIS

Immunopathologic studies in HPN have involved challenge of susceptible individuals by both skin and airway routes with subsequent application of immunofluorescent examination of biopsy material, in an attempt to demonstrate immunologic reactants.[11, 25] British investigators especially have been active in employing antigen challenge, using a variety of antigens. Their experience has suggested that skin testing is not particularly useful because there is a high frequency of reactivity to intradermally injected test materials in normal control

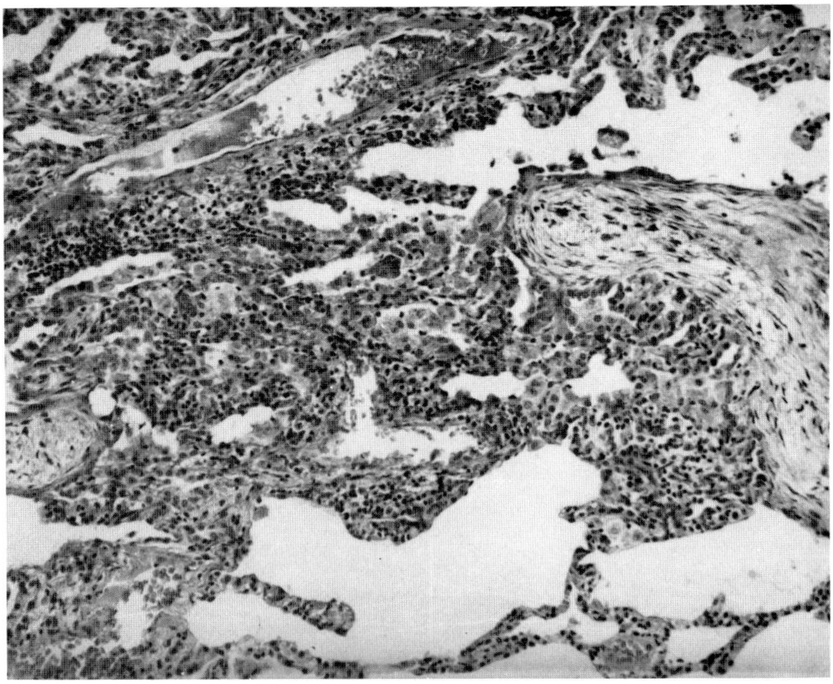

FIG. 1. Lung biopsy from a patient with farmer's lung disease. There is an interstitial infiltrate of chronic inflammatory cells (lymphocytes and monocytes) and an organizing alveolitis.

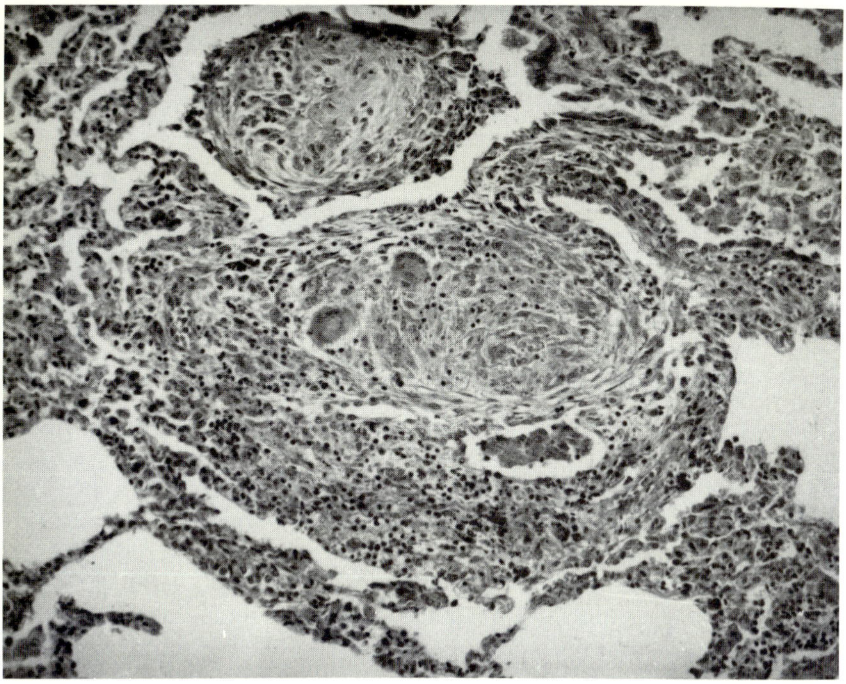

FIG. 2. Lung biopsy from a different patient with farmer's lung disease. Epithelioid granulomas with giant cells are present. Evidence of an interstitial infiltrate similar to that described in Figure 1 is also present.

persons.[17] Moreover, the skin reactions in control individuals often are not distinguishable either qualitatively or quantitatively from patients with HPN. On the other hand, aerosol challenge is useful in demonstrating tissue reactivity and helping to establish a diagnosis since control subjects do not react. In spite of clear-cut pulmonary reactions following aerosol challenge with antigen, there is not yet a satisfactory explanation of the immunologic mechanism of the pulmonary inflammatory response.

Apart from *in vivo* challenges with antigen, many studies have entailed examination of serum to demonstrate if an individual is reactive to a putative antigen of HPN.[2, 8, 15, 18] With few exceptions, serologic testing has included double diffusion in agar to demonstrate the presence of a precipitating antibody to antigen. As with skin testing, the usefulness of measuring precipitating antibody is severely limited by the fact that serums from nearly 50% of asymptomatic, clinically healthy, matched controls also show evidence of precipitating antibody. A high titer of antibody with a decline after resolution of symptoms may, however, be supportive of a diagnosis of HPN caused by the respective antigen.

Another approach to the measurement of immune responsiveness in HPN has been the quantitation of lymphocyte reactivity.[5, 9] In one form, this entails quantitating the incorporation of ^{3}H-thymidine into lymphocytes, reflecting changes in DNA metabolism during blastogenic transformation induced by antigen. A more revealing, but also more difficult approach is the detection of elaborated lymphokines from stimulated lymphoid cells. Migration inhibitory factor activity (MIF) is the "flagship" lymphokine and is the most often measured activity. It is the lymphokine for which most information exists. Peripheral blood lymphocytes from patients with HPN will, after several days of contact with antigen in culture, produce MIF activity that is usually detected in a second step involving migration inhibition of guinea pig macrophages. Production of MIF is a sensitive, specific indicator of lymphocyte reactivity. Whether it will be more reliable and more discriminating for the diagnosis of HPN remains to be determined. This will require vigorously detailed studies of carefully selected patients with definite HPN and appropriately matched controls.

A new observation in HPN is that a significant number of patients with HPN (due to *Microsporum faeni*), show greatly increased percentages of lymphocytes (50–70%) in the total population of cells retrieved from pulmonary lavage, compared with fewer than 20% of all cells being lymphocytes in lavages from normal controls and patients with other inflammatory lung diseases (with the exception of sarcoidosis).[19] To what extent these lymphocytes are antigen-reactive and whether they are actively producing lymphokines *in vivo* is unanswered. Thus, leukocyte differential counts in lavage fluids obtained from patients with undiagnosed diffuse interstitial lung disease may be worthwile. This finding is of special interest because lymphocytes can be frozen and later thawed, with retention of viability. Storage of lymphocytes for subsequent immunologic study represents a potentially important use of material obtained from lung lavage.

Preliminary studies have suggested that immunogenetic factors may be associated with HPN. In one report prevalance of the HL-A8 haplotype was five-fold greater in patients with HPN, compared with the frequency of this haplotype in the control population.[10] However, these data can only be regarded as suggestive, since too few cases have been studied. Even if it is shown that associations exist between HLA haplotype and HPN, this information still will not resolve diagnostic problems, nor explain the pathogenesis of HPN.

EXPERIMENTAL MODELS

Much work has been done to develop an experimental animal model of HPN. Rabbits, rats, guinea pigs, and monkeys have been immunized by a variety of methods with a variety of antigens, including extracts from thermophilic fungi and pigeon droppings.[3, 4, 13, 16, 20, 21] Following challenge with antigens, it has not been possible to obtain a reaction that clearly resembles HPN, but the studies have been useful if only in emphasizing the complexity of the problem. It has been found, for example, that, depending on the immunization regimen (route of administration of antigen, use of adjuvants, frequency of immunization), even with the same antigen the qualitative and the quantitative aspects of both humoral and cellular immune responses vary considerably. Similarly, the histopathologic changes in the lungs of experimental animals may display a variety of abnormalities ranging from alveolar and interstitial infiltrates of neutrophils, to chronic inflammatory cellular infiltrates. When complete Freund's adjuvant is used in the immunization protocol, epithelioid granulomas are often found in lungs of animals challenged with antigen by aerosol inhalation. However, Freund's adjuvant alone causes development of diffuse pulmonary granulomas, a fact that renders difficult the interpretation of experiments employing this adjuvant and makes extrapolations to human HPN questionable.

A major problem arises when attempts are made to assemble both clinical and experimental observations into a single, integrated scheme that would explain the pathogenesis of HPN. The rapid onset of pulmonary changes in reactive patients after antigen challenge by inhalation would seem to exclude a cell mediated (lymphocyte) immune type of mechanism. However, since cell-mediated immune reactions in lungs are not understood, interpretation of the clinical studies is difficult. It is probably fair to say, however, that the inability of drugs which block the release of anaphylactic mediators to influence the onset of lung reactions in aerosol-challenged and susceptible individuals strongly argues against an anaphylactic (IgE) mediated reaction.[17]

It has been demonstrated that the lung is susceptible to injury by immune complexes, in a manner analogous to the mechanism by which vessels are damaged by immune complexes.[14, 24] This entails the requirements for complement and neutrophils. The acute pulmonary reactions, caused by passive immunization of rats with antibody followed by exposure to antigen, feature a severe hemorrhagic alveolitis with large numbers of neutrophils in alveolar spaces. The destructive inflammatory reaction fails to develop if the complement system is blocked or if neutrophils are not available. Rather similar findings have been reported in a model of active sensitization in guinea pigs.[21] These reactions appear to be mediated by the same factors that are requisite for the development of hemorrhagic vasculitis in the reversed passive Arthus reaction in the skin.[21]

Active immunization of rabbits over a prolonged period (several months) with daily injections of large amounts of antigen produces the classical model of "chronic serum sickness." In addition to the well known glomerular lesions, these animals also develop diffuse pulmonary interstitial infiltrates of mixed inflammatory cells. By fluorescent microscopy, immune complexes are present in the interstitium and in capillary walls (in subendothelial and subepithelial locations).[4] In some animals, diffuse interstitial fibrosis and fibrin deposits have been demonstrated in the lungs. Pulmonary granulomas are not a feature in this animal model.[16, 20]

Passive transfer of serum or lymphocytes in various animal species has been done to try to define the nature of immunoreactants needed for challenged animals to mount a reaction that parallels HPN. Serum transfer does not appear to be particularly effective.[3] At best, challenged animals pretreated with serum develop hemorrhagic infiltrates with an admixture of inflammatory cells. The lesions are focal and nonprogressive. It is worth noting that, in a large effort over the past two decades to define the pathogenesis of immune complex-induced glomerulonephritis, there has not been a single convincing report in which passive administration of immune complexes has reproduced the glomerular lesions that are found in actively immunized and challenged animals. Thus, the lack of positive results in the serum transfer experiments must be considered in this historical perspective.

Transfer of sensitized lymphoid cells followed by aerosol challenge with antigen has resulted in the development of pulmonary lesions that consist of focal, diffuse infiltrates of chronic inflammatory cells. Although definitive conclusions are not possible, it seems reasonable to assume from the transfer studies that the presence of precipitating antibody alone is not sufficient to cause pulmonary histopathologic changes resembling those seen in HPN.

CONCLUSION

It is still not possible to present a satisfactory account of the immunopathologic basis of HPN. We do not know if the pulmonary pathophysiologic changes and the histopathologic features of HPN reflect a single immunologic mechanism, or if there are multiple mechanisms simultaneously or sequentially at play (*e.g.,* immune complex-induced and cell mediated tissue injury), or even if there are several independent pathways leading to the same common result. The data at hand would suggest that more than one mechanism is operative, with cell-mediated immunity having an important role. Clearly, further experimental work has to be done to lay the basis for an understanding of this form of immunologically induced lung injury. At the same time, more sensitive and relevant parameters of the immune response will have to be employed in clinical investigations to improve diagnostic accuracy. The availability of lung lavage material from HPN patients may be a major step in this direction. Until these problems are resolved, HPN represents a puzzling disease.

REFERENCES

1. Allen, D. H., Williams, G. V., and Woolcock, A. J.: Bird breeder's hypersensitivity pneumonitis: Progress studies of lung function after cessation of exposure to the provoking antigen. *Am. Rev. Resp. Dis. 114:* 555–566, 1976.
2. Barboriak, J. J., Sosman, A. J., and Reed, C. E.: Serological studies in pigeon breeder's disease. *J. Lab. Clin. Med. 65:* 600–604, 1965.
3. Bice, D. E., Salvaggio, J., and Hoffman, E.: Passive transfer of experimental hypersensitivity pneumonitis with lymphoid cells in the rabbit. *J. Allergy Clin. Immunol. 58:* 250–262, 1976.
4. Brentjens, J. R., O'Connell, D. W., Pawlowski, I. B., Hsu, K. C., and Andres, G. A.: Experimental immune complex disease of the lung. The pathogenesis of a laboratory model resembling certain human interstitial lung diseases. *J. Exp. Med. 140:* 105–125, 1974.
5. Caldwell, J. R., Pearce, D E., Spencer, C., Leder, R., and Waldman, R. H.: Immunologic mechanisms in hypersensitivity pneumonitis. I: Evidence for cell-mediated immunity and complement fixation in pigeon breeders' disease. *J. Allergy Clin. Immunol. 52:* 225–230, 1973.
6. Emanuel, D. A., Wenzel, F. J., Bowerman, C. I., and Lawton, B. R.: Farmer's lung: Clinical, pathologic and immunologic study of twenty-four patients. *Am. J. Med. 37:* 392–401, 1964.
7. Fink, J. N., Banaszak, E. F., Barboriak, J. J., Hensley, G. T., Kurup, V. P., Scanlon, G. T., Schlueter, D. P., Sosman, A. J., Thiede, W. H., and Unger, G. F.: Interstitial lung disease due to contamination of forced air systems. *Ann. Intern. Med. 84:* 406–413, 1976.
8. Fink, J. N., Barboriak, J. J., Sosman, A. J., Bukosky, R. J., and Arkins, J. A.: Antibodies against pigeon serum proteins in pigeon breeders. *J. Lab Clin. Med. 71:* 20–24, 1968.
9. Fink, J. N., Moore, V. L., and Barboriak, J. J.: Cell-mediated hypersensitivity in pigeon breeders. *Int. Arch. Allergy Appl. Immunol. 49:* 831–836, 1975.
10. Flaherty, D. K., Iha, T., Chmelik, F., Dickie, H., and Reed, C. E.: HL-A8 in farmer's lung. *Lancet 2:* 507, 1975.
11. Ghose, T., Landrigan, P., Killeen, R., and Dill, J.: Immunopathological studies in patients with farmer's lung. *Clin. Allergy 4:* 119–129, 1974.
12. Hensley, G. T., Garancis, J. C., Cherayil, G. D., and Fink, J. N.: Lung biopsies of pigeon breeders' disease. *Arch. Pathol. 87:* 572–579, 1969.
13. Hensley, G. T., Fink, J. N., and Barboriak, J. J.: Hypersensitivity pneumonitis in the monkey. *Arch. Pathol. 97:* 33–38, 1974.
14. Johnson, K. J., and Ward, P. A.: Acute immunologic pulmonary alveolitis. *J. Clin. Invest. 54:* 349–357, 1974.
15. Moore, V. L., and Fink, J. N.: Immunologic studies in hypersensitivity pneumonitis—Quantitative precipitins and complement-fixing antibodies in symptomatic and asymptomatic pigeon breeders. *J. Lab. Clin. Med. 85:* 540–545, 1975.
16. Moore, V. L., Hensley, G. T., and Fink, J. N.: An animal model of hypersensitivity pneumonitis in the rabbit. *J. Clin. Invest. 56:* 937–944, 1975.

17. Pepys, J.: Immunopathology of allergic lung disease. *Clin. Allergy 3:* 1–22, 1973.
18. Pepys, J., and Jenkins, P. A.: Precipitin (F.L.H.) test in farmer's lung. *Thorax 20:* 21–35, 1965.
19. Reynolds, H. Y., Fulmer, J. D., Kazmierowski, J. A., Roberts, W. C., Frank, M. M., and Crystal, R. G.: Analysis of cellular and protein content of broncho-alveolar lavage fluid from patients with idiopathic pulmonary fibrosis and chronic hypersensitivity pneumonitis. *J. Clin. Invest. 59:* 165–175, 1977.
20. Richerson, H. B.: Acute experimental hypersensitivity pneumonitis in the guinea pig. *J. Lab. Clin. Med. 79:* 745–757, 1972.
21. Roska, K. B., Garancis, J. C., Moore, V. L., and Abramoff, P.: Immune complex disease in the lungs of guinea pigs. I: Elicitation by aerosol challenge, suppression with cobra venom factor, and passive transfer with serum. *Clin. Immunol. Immunopathol. 8:* 213–224, 1977.
22. Schlueter, D. P.: Response of the lung to inhaled antigens. *Am. J. Med. 57:* 476–492, 1974.
23. Seal, R. M., Hapke, E. J., Thomas, G. O., Meek, J. C., and Hayes, M.: The pathology of the acute and chronic stages of farmer's lung. *Thorax 23:* 469–489, 1968.
24. Ward, P. A., and Cochrane, C. G.: Bound complement and immunologic injury of blood vessels. *J. Exp. Med. 121:* 215–234, 1965.
25. Wenzel, F. J., Emanuel, D. A., and Gray, R. L.: Immunofluorescent studies in patients with farmer's lung. *J. Allergy 48:* 224–229, 1971.

Chapter 6

Recent Advances in Pneumoconiosis: The Pathologist's Role in Etiologic Diagnosis*

JERROLD L. ABRAHAM

The content of a review of "Recent Advances in Pneumoconiosis" depends a great deal on the definition of the term "pneumoconiosis." Pneumoconiosis (from the Greek roots meaning lung and dusty) is best defined rigidly as *the presence of dust in the lung and the lung's reaction to it.* While the word dust has a specific meaning that excludes fumes, vapors, and smoke,[144] it seems likely that when Zenker[204] coined the term in 1866, he did not intend to limit the scope to a particular kind of inhaled agent, and if the term were to be coined again today the more general term aerosol would probably be used instead of dust to refer to airborne particulate material. However, the term pneumoconiosis is so well entrenched in usage that its elimination is not realistic. Casual use of the term has resulted in considerable confusion and difficulty in comparing the work of various authors. One of the two recent texts on occupational lung problems uses the term repeatedly but nowhere can a definition be found.[129] The other text appropriately deals with this problem in its initial paragraphs.[144] To many, the term pneumoconiosis brings to mind aspects related to compensation litigation, and the phrase occupational disease also reminds many physicians of the unavoidable involvement in determining the presence, degree, and significance of the disease in question in a particular patient or group of patients. Some feel that the use of another term such as "environmental lung disease" is more acceptable as it is not linked with these previously mentioned connotations.[60] It is my contention that pathologists should not avoid this area, as it is their responsibility to be both the final and, in a sense, the initial sources of information on these diseases.

The years since the previous *International Academy of Pathology Monograph on the Lung*[113] have been ones of rapid expansion of the literature related to pneumoconiosis. A computer search of the literature for the past ten years yielded over four thousand articles related to this field. Articles continue to appear in the world's literature at the rate of approximately 50 to 100 per month. As this volume of material is beyond the scope of a brief review, I have limited this discussion to selected aspects of those problems related to the inhalation of

* Supported by Grant No. HL-19619 from the United States Public Health Service.

inorganic particulates. Organic dust disease[60, 93, 129, 144] and the oncogenic potential of these lesions[158] will only briefly be mentioned. Emphasis here will be on most recent results and on prospects for future developments. The reader is urged to consult the references for those aspects not adequately covered.

Two recent texts[129, 144] admirably collect and analyze most of the world's knowledge of occupational lung disease. Several international symposia and monographs on general and specific facets of the subject provide large collections of data.[19, 32, 47, 48, 79, 88, 96, 164, 167, 168, 188, 189, 203]

Review articles and state-of-the-art reports present additional data and opinions of workers in the field.[12, 25, 29, 30, 58, 60, 63, 69, 70, 80, 81, 83, 87, 93, 98, 101, 118, 128, 130, 133, 134, 137, 148, 150, 162, 163, 172, 174, 184, 194, 200, 205] However, neither in the previous *IAP Monograph*[113] nor in the references cited above has the role of the pathologist in etiologic diagnosis been specifically emphasized.

This is an area of many recent methodologic developments which are of increasing value to pathologists. Scanning electron microscopy (SEM) and X-ray microanalysis of inorganic materials in lung tissue were not routinely available a decade ago. The technical details of analytic lung pathology are beyond the scope of this chapter and have been reviewed elsewhere.[2, 6, 9, 193] Some basics of environmental and occupational (two terms which should be inseparable) inorganic dust diseases are essential for the understanding of these diseases.

TERMINOLOGY OF PARTICULATES

"Aerosol" includes both dispersed particles and droplets. Dust consists of solid particles dispersed in some medium such as air due to mechanical disintegration of solid materials or to agitation and dispersion of materials such as spores. Fumes consist of metal oxides ranging in size usually from 0.1–1 μ. Mists are liquid droplets formed by condensation of vapors or atomization of liquid around appropriate condensation nuclei. These may range from less than 0.1 μ up to 500 μ in diameter.[144] Since the division between types of aerosols is not sharp at the regions of overlap, the term particulate is used rather than dust.

PARTICULATE DEPOSITION AND CLEARANCE[14, 69, 116, 137, 144]

The structure of the respiratory tract is such that the larger particulates are filtered out or deposited in the more proximal portions, and only respirable particles penetrate deeply into the lung (*i.e.,* to the respiratory bronchioles and alveoli). Not only is the size of the particles important but also the shape and density interact to determine the final aerodynamic behavior. This is expressed for a given particle as its mass median aerodynamic diameter, which equates its behavior to that of a sphere of unit density. The shapes are defined as fibrous (length exceeding diameter by a factor of 3 to 1 or more) or compact (approximating a sphere). There are four mechanisms by which suspended particles are deposited.

Sedimentation is responsible for most of the deposition in larger airways of particles of aerodynamic diameter 2 μ or less. It is influenced less by the length and shape than by the falling speed of the particle which is determined by gravity and the density and cross-sectional area of the particle.

Inertial impaction is responsible for most of the deposition in the nose and larger airways of particles larger than 10 μ in diameter. Impaction is related to the density and cross-sectional area of the particles and to the diameter, change of direction, and rate of air flow in the airway.

Interception is responsible for deposition of irregular and fibrous particles. Long fibrous particles tend to orient with the air stream and avoid sedimentation and impaction in the larger airways until they are intercepted by collision with the walls of the terminal and respiratory bronchioles, particularly at bifurcations. With asbestos of different types for example, the deposition may vary, with the curled Chrysotile fibers being more likely to deposit on the walls of the narrow airways near their bifurcations and the very straight amphibole fibers such as Crocidolite being more likely to reach the periphery of the lung. This variation in penetration and deposition may be important in the resulting differences in patterns of disease associated with different kinds of particulates.

Diffusion affects only the very small particles (less than 0.1 μ in diameter). It influences the deposition of such particles independent of their density. There is some evidence[13, 14, 160] that the effect of cigarette smoking, whether it is due to a bronchoconstrictive effect of the smoke or to some other mechanism, tends to decrease the deposition of particles in the lung beyond the terminal bronchioles.

The pattern of respiration can greatly influence the deposition of particles. With a greater tidal volume there is deeper penetration of air into the lungs, and with increasing frequency of respiration the time for particles to become deposited decreases. With increasing effort both tidal volume and respiratory frequency are increased, thus the minute volume (the product of tidal volume and number of breaths per minute) increases, and persons engaged in heavy physical effort will have greater deposition of particles in a given environment than persons at rest.

As most of the calculations are based on theoretical models of aerodynamic behavior of particles in the branching system, the results may be considered as relative rather than absolute until confirmed by actual morphologic studies. Another factor to consider in interpreting the results of morphologic studies of dust particles examined *in situ* in tissues or recovered from tissues is the methodology involved. For example, a study using only light microscopy will almost always determine the average size of particles to be much larger than a study using transmission electron microscopy.

The distribution within the lungs of the air containing dust particles has been considered in relation to the zonal distributions of certain types of pneumoconiosis. During normal breathing all the zones are nearly uniformly ventilated. The lower zones are ventilated more than the upper when breathing from functional residual capacity, but this is reversed at lung volumes approaching residual volumes.[124] The combined effects of varying ventilation and perfusion ($\mathring{V}/\dot{Q}$ ratios)[193] related to pneumoconioses has not yet been well studied.

Figure 1 illustrates a fibrous glass filter from an environmental monitoring station in San Diego, as examined with the SEM. The filter exhibits nonselective deposition and no clearance, in contrast to the lung which is aerodynamically selective and has varying clearance mechanisms and rates.

The size of airborne particles plays a great role in determining their toxicity. In most urban aerosols analyzed, a large number of potentially toxic trace species have been detected, including lead, cadmium, antimony, selenium, nickel, vanadium, zinc, cobalt, bromine, manganese, sulfate, and benzo(a)pyrene.[110, 136, 140] The

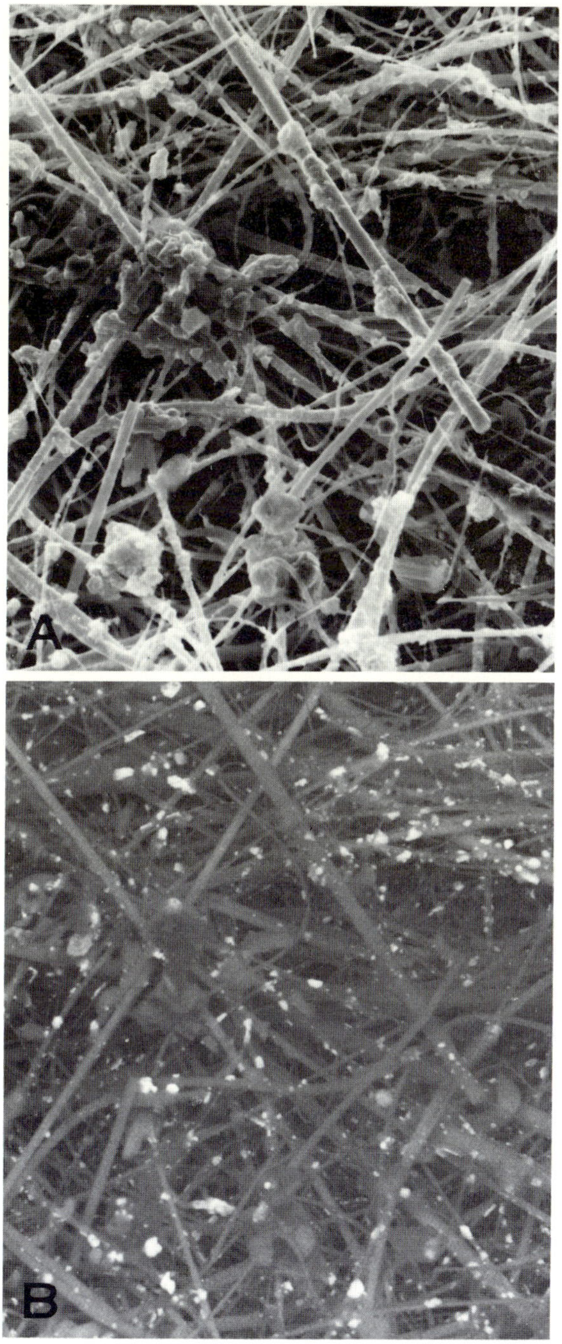

FIG. 1. Surface of fibrous glass ("Hi volume") filter with particles collected during 24 hours in San Diego County ambient air. Provided by San Diego Air Pollution Control District. Scanning electron micrograph, carbon-coated secondary electron image (*A*), and backscattered electron image (*B*). Larger particles with backscattered electron image brightness similar to fibrous glass filters are silicates. Note the numerous tiny brighter (higher atomic number) particles trapped on the filter. Most of these have been shown by X-ray microanalysis to contain lead and bromine, supporting their origin from automobile exhaust emissions. Others contain iron, copper, zinc, barium and gold. × 1400.

smallest particles emitted from high temperature combustion sources also contain many of these same species.[136] In general, the smaller the particle the more efficiently the body is able to extract trace components from it.

In addition to the particles, there may be volatile chemical species in the vapor phase of the atmosphere which by themselves might not deposit very efficiently in the lung. However, theoretical and experimental studies have shown that the vapor phase species can be adsorbed onto particle surfaces, greatly increasing their efficiency of deposition.[28]

Boren, in a review of the pathobiology of air pollutants, clearly documented that "the concept that one agent is responsible for one disease does not permit considerations of the full health impact of an environment polluted by continuously variable and ever increasing multiplicity of agents."[28] He presents the results of experiments showing that the combined effects of two agents together or in sequence is quite different from either agent alone and the order of exposure is also important in determining the effects. Thus conclusions drawn from exposure to single agents may not be complete in ruling out their toxic potential. "Such exposures may make the lung more susceptible to damage as indicated by subsequent challenge by NO_2." Also, "the failure to demonstrate morphologic change following exposure to a given agent does not necessarily mean that significant changes for the future have not been produced, just as the presence of an abnormality does not mean that a given agent is solely responsible for it."[28]

The extraction of toxic components from particles usually takes place at the site where they are retained. For example, large particles deposited in the nasal, pharyngeal and tracheobronchial regions do not remain there for long. They are usually cleared by ciliary action and swallowed within a matter of hours. Particles deposited in the pulmonary parenchyma may remain for weeks or years. Most toxic species are extracted more efficiently in the lung than in the stomach. For example, for lead it has been estimated that 60–80% is extracted from particles deposited in the lung, whereas only 5–15% is extracted from those in the stomach.[136] The influence of surface area for absorption as well as surface area of the particles can considerably influence extraction efficiency. For example, barium sulfate retained in the lung is extracted into the bloodstream within a matter of days, whereas ingested barium sulfate is not significantly absorbed at all.[115]

High temperature processes which may emit toxic trace elements into the atmosphere include internal combustion engines, power plants, blast furnaces, metallurgic smelters, cement kilns, municipal incinerators, etc. Urban aerosols contain 100- to 1,000-fold the natural abundance of elements such as lead, zinc, arsenic, cadmium, antimony, mercury, selenium, and sulphur. With decreasing particle size, the concentration of many of these increases markedly. These include lead, thallium, antimony, selenium, arsenic, nickel, chromium, zinc, and sulphur. Certain other elements show no strong dependence on particle size for their concentration. These include bismuth, tin, cobalt, iron, manganese, vanadium, titanium, calcium, potassium, magnesium, aluminum, beryllium, carbon, and silicon.[136]

It is thought that certain compounds become volatile at high temperatures and are then adsorbed onto the large surface area available on particulates.[136] This has been implicated in Los Angeles aerosols, where hydrocarbons seem to deposit on the surface of atmospheric particles.[136]

Recent work studying airborne particulates emitted from coal burning power plants has shown the spherical nature of many of the particles. The sphere-within-sphere microstructure was beautifully illustrated by Fisher, Chang, and Brummer[59] (Fig. 2). The smaller particles are potentially of toxicologic importance as it has been shown that the smaller particles are associated with higher concentrations of heavy metals.[140] Also, the surface predominance of trace elements (many of which are toxic) in fly ash has been demonstrated by Linton, Loh, Natusch, Evans, and Williams.[115] As it is the surface which is the interface between the particle and tissue, this is more than a scientific curiosity.

The automobile is probably the largest source of the smallest particulates. While the increasing use of lead-free gasoline has reduced the ambient lead air level significantly, there is some question about the catalytic devices designed to reduce higher oxides of nitrogen. Large numbers of metal containing particulates can be generated from these catalysts, which contain copper, chrome, nickel, platinum, aluminum oxide, barium, and possibly other metals. Up to and exceeding 1 million condensation nuclei per cc have been measured in testing some of these catalysts. The average size of the particulates is extremely small with an average on the order of 100–200 Å.[21] Also, one should be aware that the lead has been replaced by other non-inert agents such as manganese.

Until quite recently pulmonary clearance was thought by most to involve mucociliary clearance for particles deposited on the ciliated airways and macrophage mediated clearance for particles deposited more distally.[69, 97, 98, 118, 129, 130, 144] While these may be the major mechanisms, it is now known that the epithelial lining cells of large and small airways, as well as alveoli, are capable of phagocytosis of particles.[9, 11, 132, 171] The lymphatic and transairway passage of intracellular and extracellular particles is being actively investigated.[69, 109, 130, 131, 137, 184]

Sorokin and Brain[171] studied the clearance of submicronic particulate iron oxide in mice in great detail for up to fourteen months following single exposure. They found that the particles settled mostly on alveolar surfaces and that there were two clearance mechanisms, an extracellular mechanism fed by a fluid current sweeping across the surface, and a cellular mechanism principally involving macrophages. Early clearance by both mechanisms went through the airways. By twenty-four hours, uncleared residues had become ingested. Some uptake of particles by bronchial epithelial cells was demonstrated and may be more important in aerosols of particles deposited mostly in the bronchioles.

The route of delivery of particles is most important in designing and interpreting experimental exposures. A definitive study showing the differences in distribution of particles given by aerosol inhalation versus intratracheal instillation was done by Brain, Knudson, Sorokin, and Davis.[31] There is also variability in humans owing to respiratory rate, mouth versus nose breathing and use of respiratory protective equipment.[144] Tomenius[183] studied the deposition of radioactively tagged polystyrene particles in rabbits. He found that individual differences in deposition patterns could be repeatedly demonstrated using double labeling techniques and were not likely caused by differences in exposure technique or in the aerosols themselves. This relates to individual variability in humans as well.

The location of the primary damage by particulate material may be a reflection of its deposition behavior. Thus, large particles may damage large airways (*e.g.,*

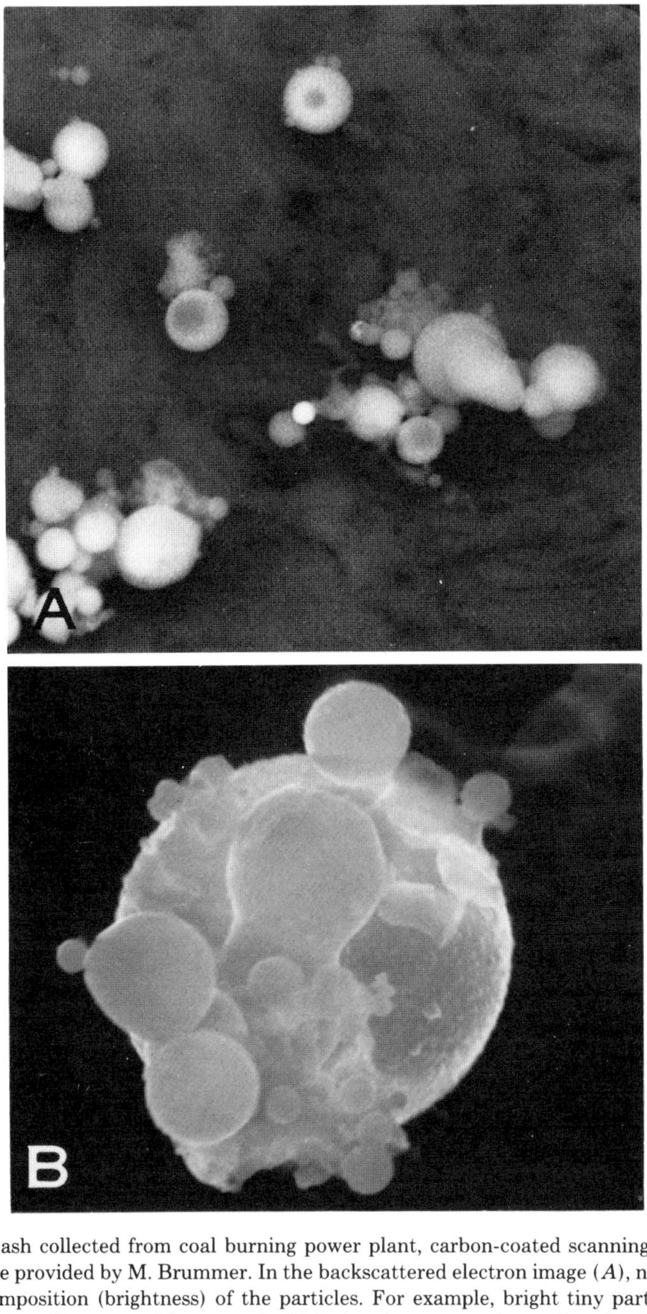

FIG. 2. Fly ash collected from coal burning power plant, carbon-coated scanning electron micrographs. Sample provided by M. Brummer. In the backscattered electron image (*A*), note the variation in size and composition (brightness) of the particles. For example, bright tiny particles amidst the common alumino-silicate particles contain high local concentrations of such elements as iron, strontium, vanadium, etc. Hollow nature of some particles is also revealed. × 1800. The complex surface is better seen in the secondary electron image of a group of particles (*B*). Note many adsorbed smaller particles on the larger ones. The surface predominance of many metals on fly ash particles reported by Linton, *et al.*[115] may be the result of such adsorption of discrete tiny particles rather than the more diffuse surface adsorption suggested by them.

industrial bronchitis[108]), respirable particles in the 1–5 μ range may damage respiratory bronchioles (*e.g.*, coal workers' pneumoconiosis),[52, 68, 86, 144] and submicron particles may damage the alveolar epithelium (*e.g.*, pulmonary alveolar proteinosis).[46, 72, 121, 153, 159, 175] The effective size probably increases rapidly with hydration of small particles, which might otherwise remain suspended in air.

The cellular events in conducting airways exposed to particles are being studied successfully with recently developed *in vitro* methods.[11, 132] Attention had not been focused on this area until recently despite the fact that the large airways are the site of origin for most neoplasms in the lungs.

The studies of Mossman, Kessler, Ley, and Craighead[132] show that asbestos fibers not only enter and cause damage and desquamation of tracheal epithelial cells but that small fibers can be found within the hyperplastic basal cells of the epithelium (Fig. 3). The relationship of particle size to the cells with which the particles interact has also been discussed by other workers.[136, 180–182]

While there is some variation in the degree of damage and proliferation caused

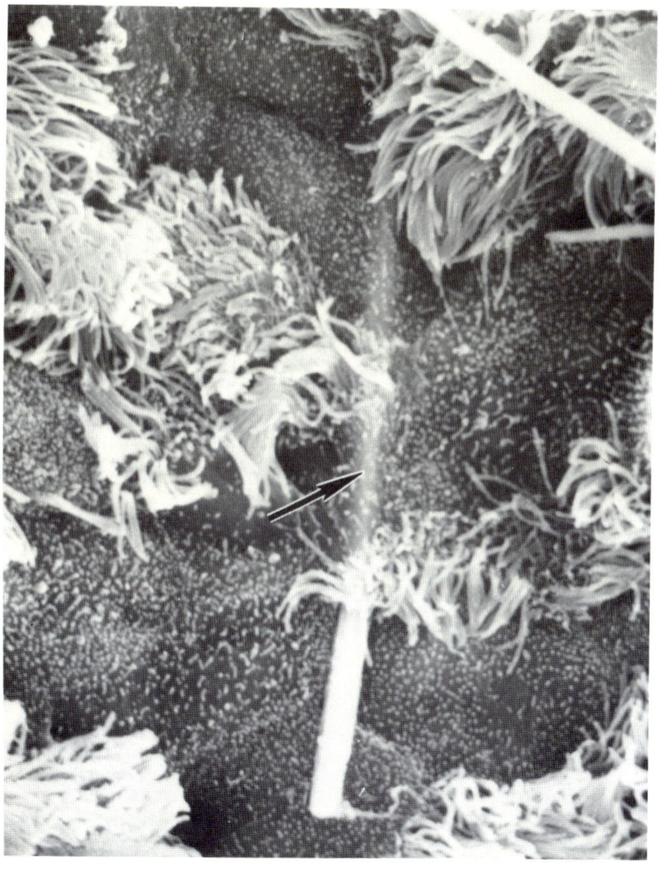

FIG. 3. Hamster tracheal epithelium *in vitro* exposed to Crocidolite asbestos fibers, metal coated. Micrograph provided through the courtesy of Dr. B. T. Mossman. Note the penetration of the epithelial cell by the asbestos fiber (*arrow*). Subsequent basal cell hyperplasia has been demonstrated.[132] Scanning electron micrograph, secondary electron imaging mode. × 3000.

by different particles,[11, 132] the same basic response to a variety of particles ranging from carbon, ferric oxide, and asbestos *in vitro,*[11, 132] and tantalum *in vivo*[9] suggests a nonspecific response to injury. Figure 4 shows some aspects of the response to tantalum.

The sequence of events in the response of tracheobronchial mucosa to nonparticulate injury has been studied using mechanical injury[103] and exposure to tobacco smoke[191] and is similar to that described for particles. There is a peak of mitotic activity as early as twenty-four hours after the injury.

In coal workers the response of the large airways to inhaled dusts has been shown indirectly by demonstrating a significant fall in expiratory flow rates during a single eight-hour work shift in the mine.[108] This is certainly consistent with the rapidity of the damage and desquamation of the epithelium shown in animal experimentation. One wonders why, if all this epithelial regeneration were taking place, there has not been demonstrated an increased risk of neoplasia in the coal mining population[45, 56, 143] comparable to that seen in asbestos workers.[158, 166] The answer is not available. One could speculate on the role of cigarette smoking, known to be an important co-carcinogen in asbestos workers.[166] Coal miners are not nonsmokers but are prohibited by fire hazards from smoking for one-third of each day spent underground. Asbestos particles would be more likely to come in contact with potential carcinogens from cigarettes than coal particles. One should not overlook the as yet undefined role of the particulate matter inhaled from cigarettes.[33]

It is not absolutely necessary that the particle damaging the epithelium be the same agent which induces change in the regenerating cells in the trachea or elsewhere. Presumably the stimulus of damage to the superficial epithelium is sufficient to cause proliferation of the basal cells. In the presence of suitable mutagens, these proliferating cells could become neoplastic, as was pointed out by Kotin in the previous *IAP Lung Monograph.*[100] Many of the trace elements associated with asbestos and in the environment can be shown to have mutagenic potential in an *in vitro* bacterial test system[61] similar to that used widely to screen organic compounds for mutagenicity and oncogenicity.[57]

ANALYTICAL LUNG PATHOLOGY

This term is used to emphasize the approach to lung disease known or suspected to be associated with some occupational or environmental exposure. While most pathologic diagnostic work is well performed with the light microscope, in these diseases there often is need for further analysis; pathologists may diagnose "pneumoconiosis" or "interstitial pneumonia." Valuable clinical, radiologic, and histologic patterns have been detailed which permit improved therapy and prognosis in some cases.[39] Approximately one-fourth of the interstitial lung disease studied by Carrington and Gaensler was related to known occupational exposure.[39] A large fraction of the remaining cases was of unknown etiology. It is possible that an analytical approach may allow the pathologist a chance to find the etiologic agents in those cases resulting from inorganic particulate exposure. Some factors to be considered are outlined in Table 1, page 110.

A wide variety of particles may be found in lungs in the absence of related disease, as the lungs are constantly sampling the air, over a much longer period of time than the filter shown in Figure 1. The importance of a careful and thorough occupational and environmental history in each case cannot be overemphasized.[144] In many cases the history will obviate the need for further analysis of the tissue.

The scanning electron microscope (SEM) has a resolution midway between the light microscope and transmission electron microscope (TEM). Most respirable particles are within the resolving power of the SEM. In addition, the SEM is able to provide information on the chemical composition of individual particles or regions of tissues. Currently the information is limited to elemental analysis, but within a few years the capability of organic compound microanalysis by ion beam etching and mass spectrometry may be commercially available.[104] The SEM is able to examine more varied samples than the TEM, ranging from pieces of tissues up to 3 cm^3 to ultrathin TEM sections. Easily accomodated are conventional 5-μ-thick paraffin sections as prepared for light microscopy, mounted on glass slides or other suitable substrates, such as carbon. For the study of respirable particles in pulmonary tissue, the thicker sections are desirable as the embedding paraffin is easily removed and the morphology of the intact particle can often be studied profitably. In ultrathin sections the particulate matter which is thicker than the section (usually less than 1000 Å or 0.1 μ) is often lost due to the difficulty of sectioning it, and if sectioned, only a cross-section rather than the important surface characteristics can be studied.

Analytical scanning electron microscopy. In the SEM, many different signals are generated simultaneously from the interaction of the electron beam and the specimen.[192] The familiar surface morphology results when the secondary electrons are collected and amplified to form an image. The X-rays generated provide information about the composition of the specimens. There are two types of analysis of X-rays: (1) wavelength dispersive spectrometry (WDXA) which uses a diffracting crystal to separate X-rays according to their wavelength; and (2) energy-dispersive X-ray spectrometry (EDXA) which uses a semiconductor device to separate the X-rays based on their energy. The former gives more precise separation of adjacent elements but only allows study of one element at a time, while EDXA facilitates much more rapid analysis of all elements from sodium through uranium simultaneously. EDXA is thus much better suited to searching for particulates of unknown composition in a minimum of time.[198]

Backscattered electrons (BSE) to date have been less utilized than secondary electrons and X-rays. They are especially useful for the detection of inorganic particulates in tissues, since the scattering of electrons is directly related to the atomic number of the specimen. Thus, any particulates of higher atomic number than carbon will scatter more electrons and give rise to a brighter image.[6, 8, 51] Particulates in tissues as small as 500 Å in diameter can be detected and analyzed with this system. Without BSE imaging one cannot locate *in situ* the particulates needing X-ray analysis.[53]

Much of the diagnostic use of the SEM to date has involved the analysis of inorganic materials retained in the lungs.[2, 3, 5, 6, 8, 9, 26, 33–35, 50–55, 76, 105, 106, 119, 121, 155, 156, 169]

The lung is constantly subjected to a barrage of particles which conveniently fall in the size ranges most suitable for SEM analysis.[130, 131] Only a few centers have yet developed the capability to do this work, although this is an area of rapid growth.[2, 26, 33, 52, 106, 119, 156, 169] Owing to the scarcity of both instrumentation and expertise, the scope of the analytical work has been rather limited to well-known disease entities such as asbestosis,[106] coal workers' pneumoconiosis,[52] and silicosis.[53, 169] The overwhelming majority of pulmonary diseases resulting from both recognized and unknown environmental (including occupational) exposures have either been analyzed only minimally or studied only by descriptive morphologic techniques.[60, 112, 163, 194] Identification of previously unrecognized toxic agents in the environment, as sampled by the most sophisticated dust sampler devised—the human lung—is possible. In some cases, findings may stimulate experimental studies in animals to investigate cause and effect relationships and to elucidate pathogenesis.

MAGNITUDE OF THE PROBLEM

The estimated number of persons at risk of developing occupational diseases of the lung, as well as other systems, is discussed in Ashford's[19] report. Several million workers are directly involved, and the numbers only increase when one adds the general population exposed at lower levels to the same industrial agents.

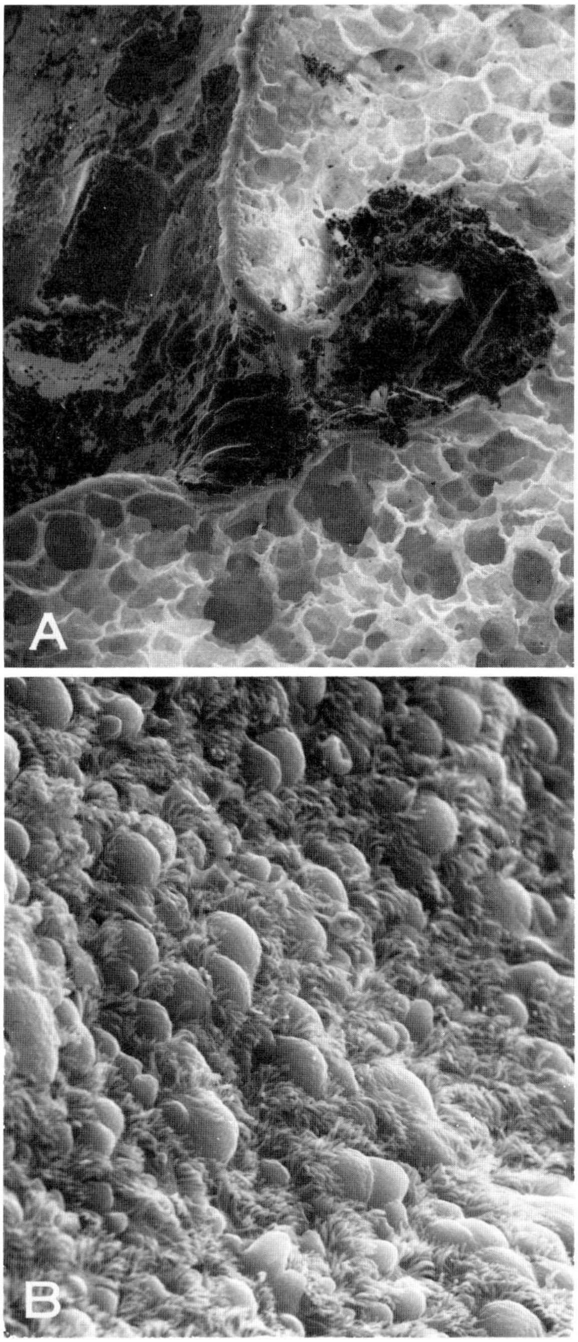

FIG. 4 A & B

These swollen cells are comprised of both Clara cells and mucous cells. × 1200. Six hours after instillation there is marked desquamation of cells (ciliated and nonciliated) in this comparable airway (*C*). The tiny bright areas are the tantalum particles in this secondary electron image. They are associated with the desquamated cells and cellular fragments. × 1200.

National Institute for Occupational Safety and Health (NIOSH) Survey. A survey letter to assess the national demand for analysis of lung tissues for inorganic particulates was mailed to over 10,000 pulmonary specialists and pathologists by NIOSH in May 1976. Through the courtesy of NIOSH[73] copies of the response to this survey were obtained. Of the 1600 respondents indicating they wished to participate in the study, 1200 had included in their response an estimate of the number of cases which they would submit per year. Based on the observed average of over 7 cases per year per respondent, one can calculate that the demand would be over 10,000 cases per year—well beyond the current capacity of any one laboratory, and most likely beyond the capacity of the entire nation.

SOME SPECIFIC EXAMPLES

Complete listings of pulmonary diseases related to occupational and environmental agents have taken two main organizational approaches. The first is a

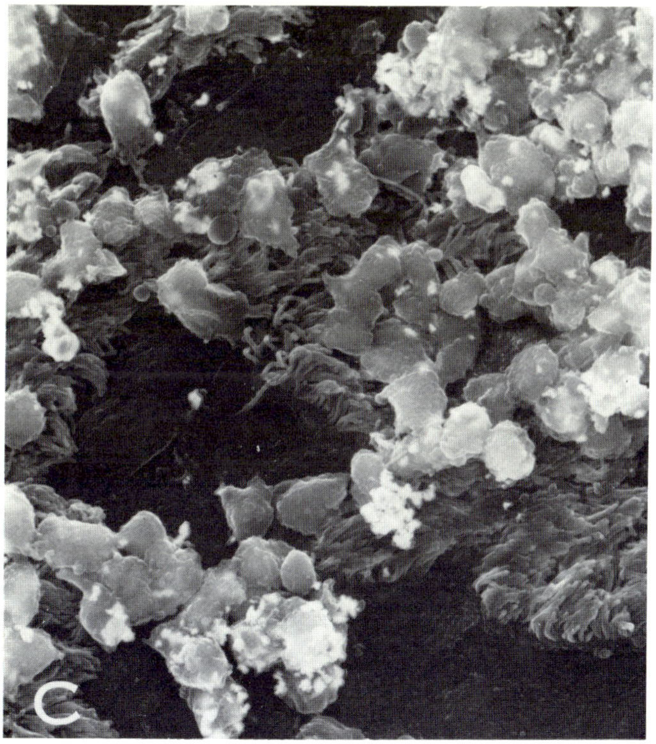

FIG. 4. Hamster lungs after intratracheal instillation of tantalum suspension,[9] scanning electron micrographs of glutaraldehyde fixed, critical point dried, carbon coated tissue. Two hours after instillation (*A and B*), large deposits of tantalum are seen on terminal bronchiolar surface and extending into a few alveoli of very short respiratory bronchiole. Tantalum appears dark in this combination of normal secondary electron image and negative backscattered electron image (*A*). × 120. Marked swelling of nonciliated cells, well above the cilated cells, is seen in the terminal bronchiole (*B*).

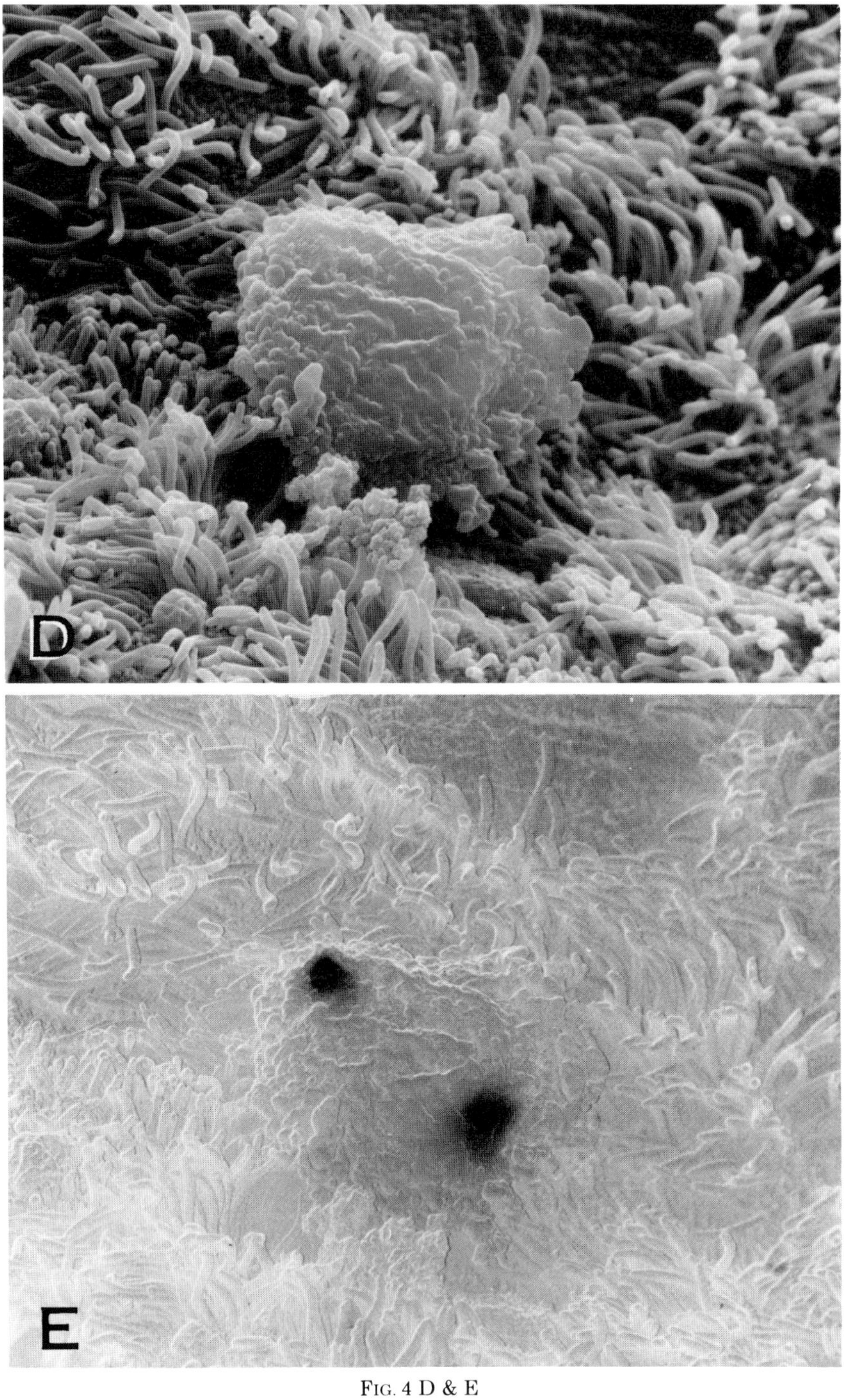

FIG. 4 D & E

Four days after instillation clearance of tantalum continues in macrophages travelling on the mucociliary escalator. The macrophage seen in the secondary electron image (*D*) is seen to contain two tantalum particles in the negative backscattered image (*E*). × 4000.

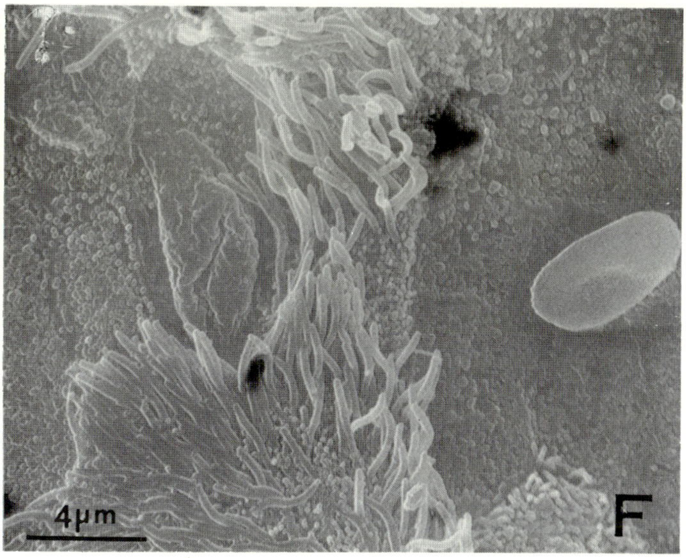

FIG. 4 F

The location of the tantalum particles within the bronchiolar epithelial cells can also be noted (*F*) owing to the ability of the backscattered electrons to penetrate a few micrometers of low density tissue (combination of secondary electron image and negative backscattered electron image). × 4000.

listing by agent such as in a toxicology text[67] and various others.[42, 65, 79, 129, 144, 172] The other is a grouping by type of host response to the agents.[39, 60, 129, 144, 194] While both types of reference are essential, the latter is of a more manageable size and likely to be of use to the pathologist confronted with a particular tissue reaction. Types of reaction should be characterized by light microscopy by their distribution, cell types, tissue pattern(s), connective tissue component(s), vascular components(s), and dust if present.

The reaction may be negligible (*e.g.,* NaCl dust) or may include interstitial fibrosis (*e.g.,* asbestosis[23, 164]), granulomatous reaction (*e.g.,* beryllium disease[62]), dense nodular fibrosis (*e.g.,* silicosis[205]), diffuse alveolar damage (*e.g.,* oxygen or metal fumes[95, 111, 112, 147]), bronchiolitis (*e.g.,* cigarette smoke[138, 139]), alveolar proteinosis (*e.g.,* acute silicosis),[22, 36, 121, 159, 175] and accumulation of dust with little associated reaction (*e.g.,* carbon, tin[120, 144, 190]). Most often exposures are to multiple agents varying in dose, size (deposition), and composition, and what is observed in the tissue is a combination of differing reactions.

The examination of the dust by light microscopy is commonly overlooked. Varying sizes and shapes of particles, their color, birefringence and index of refraction may all be usefully noted. However, none of these parameters permit chemical identification, which requires other analytical methods.[50, 92, 105, 174, 199] For instance, an opaque black, spherical 1-μ particle seen by light microscopy may contain carbon only or may contain many other elements, such as beryllium, iron, tungsten, or gold. The soot-like particles associated with smoking and urban living are usually spherical and fairly uniform in size. The presence of irregular, larger particles implies some exposure to a dust-generating process, either industrial (*e.g.,* mining) or environmental (*e.g.,* a wood-working hobby). Although

TABLE 1. ANALYTICAL LUNG PATHOLOGY

I. What are the indications for analysis of lung tissue?
  A. To identify toxic agents suspected to be present on the basis of history
    1) for verification of exposure
    2) for worker compensation
    3) for recognition of the relationship of the agent(s) with particular pathologic changes
    4) for quantitation of the agent in the tissue
    5) *Not* for any specific treatment, but for at least prevention of further exposure to the patient and other workers in similar jobs
  B. To identify agents suspected from the tissue findings
    1) unidentified particulates visible by light microscopy
    2) particles not visible by light microscopy owing to the nature of particle, its size, or its abundance
  C. To search for agents as a "fishing expedition"
  D. To document the "normal" condition for reference

II. What sorts of analyses can be done and what special preparation is needed?

Type of Analysis	Advantages	Disadvantages or Limitations
A. Bulk analysis (digestion of tissue and chemical analysis)	1. Best for quantitation of agent in the tissue 2. Can be most sensitive to very small traces of some agents 3. Fairly rapid (minutes to hours per case)	1. Requires large tissue sample (gms) 2. Sacrifices histology 3. Does not allow correlation of analysis with specific lesions except on a gross scale
B. *In situ* microanalysis [Scanning EM (SEM) + X-ray microanalysis (EDXA and WDXA); Transmission EM (TEM) with electron diffraction (SAED); Ion microprobe mass analysis (IMMA)]	1. Best for identification of specifilc associations of agents with pathology 2. Requires only a conventional formalin-fixed tissue block or paraffin block for preparation of section to be analyzed 3. Allows detection and analysis of individual respirable particles with better resolution than light microscope 4. Documents associations of elements in single particles, which may suggest a specific source	1. Very time consuming (hours to days per case) 2. Requires skilled microanalyst 3. Difficult to quantitate 4. Usually identifies single elements rather than compounds 5. Limited to inorganic analysis at present 6. Not generally as sensitive to trace elements as wet chemical techniques, unless trace elements occur as discrete particles

finding a specific particle in a diseased lung sampled at one point in time does not prove an etiologic relationship the association of particulate material with a specific lesion should stimulate further study. The location of the dust may in some cases be helpful in suggesting a relationship. Knowledge of the predominant dust clearance pathways enables one to search more efficiently for dust, using the omnipresent opaque dust from smoke as a marker. In very acute exposures there may be retention of the inciting particulate at the site of damage, having had little or no time for clearance to the usual peribronchial and perivascular lymphatics, where materials from both remote and recent exposure are intermingled. It should be possible to exclude incidental passage of macrophages through areas of specific particulate damage, as the content of the macrophages would be similar to that of those elsewhere if there were no relationship to the toxic particulate.[121] This phenomenon of macrophages carrying with them the undigestible remains of previous meals has complicated the interpretation of scars in the lung, in which macrophages accumulate. It becomes difficult to unravel the relationship of dust to scar to neoplasia.[123]

Coal Workers' Pneumoconiosis (CWP)

This entity, recognized as separate from silicosis in the United States long after the remainder of the world, has been studied extensively for over 3 decades.[128, 129, 144, 167] Nevertheless, there is still considerable debate over its definition, its significance and its pathology.[128, 129, 133, 134, 144, 167] Most of the work done in the United States has been epidemiologic, utilizing questionnaires, spirometry, and chest roentgenography.[128] Although a detailed classification of the radiology of pneumoconioses has been internationally promoted and tested,[128, 129, 144, 186] such a system for pathology is only in its early developmental stages.[4] Morgan[127] is of the opinion that CWP does not exist in the absence of a positive chest X-ray! The interpretation of this must be based on his broad epidemiologic experience,[128, 129] showing that demonstrable physiologic impairment due to inhalation of coal dust is unlikely with a negative chest X-ray. From the morphologic standpoint, the basic lesion of CWP is the dust macule containing dust compatible with that generated in mining coal (coal mine dust is the term preferred over coal dust).[68, 86] Often coexisting with the macule is a varying degree of centrilobular emphysema, so-called focal dust emphysema by Gough.[68] Neither the dust macule nor the dilatation of the respiratory bronchioles is specific for CWP, but both represent responses of the lung to inhalation of dust (Fig. 5). In an analytical study of CWP, DeNee, Abraham, and Gelderman[52] illustrated the types of particles present in macules and more nodular lesions as seen in silicosis. There is a gradation of lesions and in my experience a mixture of carbon, silicates and silica (SiO_2) are found in all cases. The more silica particles the more chance for a fibrotic reaction. The critical dose of silica is not defined and it is likely that different forms of silica[203] and differing silicates may modify the fibrogenicity of silica.

Silicon, the pure element, is not naturally occurring. *Silica,* SiO_2, is common, as are various *silicates* (silica combined with many other cations such as Mg, Al, K, Ca, and Fe). These three terms should not be used interchangeably if one wishes to avoid unnecessary confusion.

An attempt to solve the problem of CWP pathology was initiated with the 1971 implementation of the United States National Coal Workers' Autopsy Study (NCWAS).[40] This represents the first national occupational autopsy program of its kind. Other coal mining nations[167] have laws mandating necropsies on all miners who had been awarded compensation. The NCWAS was designed to provide a broader coverage; although voluntary, any person who had worked one day or more at an underground coal mine was eligible for inclusion. While the NCWAS has limitations both epidemiologically (uncontrolled sampling) and pathologically (limited examination of the lungs and heart rather than whole organ studies) it has yielded some data of interest. In its first three and one-half

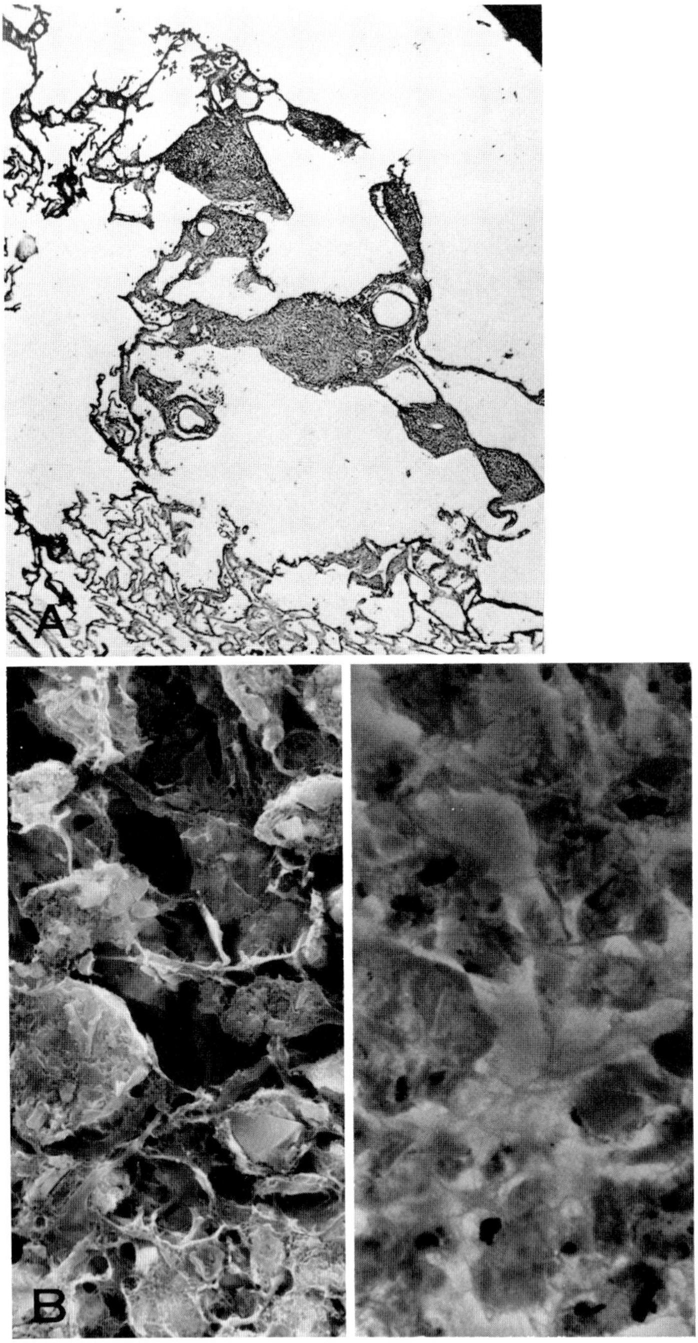

FIG. 5. Coal Worker's Pneumoconiosis (CWP), SEM of standard 5-μ paraffin section on carbon disc, deparaffinized. (*A*), Typical macule of CWP showing collections of dust-filled macrophages surrounding dilated respiratory bronchioles and enveloping small arterioles (negative secondary electron image). × 30. (*B*), Higher magnification of macule showing variety of sizes and shapes of particles (secondary electron image, *left*) and varying composition (negative backscattered electron image, *right*). Light gray particles are coal, black or dark gray particles are silica or silicates, some also containing iron. × 1400.

years 1300 cases were accessioned, being submitted by over 150 pathologists in 26 states. Of these, less than 10% showed no macules of CWP. Thus the prevalence of the basic CWP lesion was greater than 90% at death. These data are not an index of severity or profusion of lesions, nor by any means related to disability from CWP. They, however, emphasize the important difference between CWP as defined pathologically and as used clinically. The frequency of positive chest X-rays for CWP was below 30% in the NCWAS cases. Basic data on the characteristics of the NCWAS population are shown in Tables 2 through 5. It seems likely that the NCWAS population is more nearly representative of the older coal miners than the usual hospital-based autopsy study. Comparison of autopsy diagnoses with death certificate diagnoses showed the expected inaccuracy of the latter.[142]

Lung cancer in coal miners has been a subject of controversy. James'[91] large series from Britain showed no increased prevalence of lung cancer in miners with increasing severity of pneumoconiosis. However, this sampling included only those who had pneumoconiosis by X-ray, and smoking history was not examined. Most,[45, 91, 143] but not all[56, 126, 161] studies either from death certificates or from autopsies have shown no increased risk of lung cancer associated with coal

TABLE 2. DISTRIBUTION OF AUTOPSIES IN U.S. NATIONAL COAL WORKERS' AUTOPSY STUDY (1296 CASES)

Type of death	Type of autopsy		
	Complete 254 (19.60%)	Brain excluded 871 (67.21%)	Heart and lungs only 171 (13.19%)
Hospital 297 (22.92%)	131 (10.11%)	143 (11.03%)	*23 (1.77%)*
Dead on arrival 103 (7.94%)	21 (1.62%)	35 (2.70%)	*47 (3.63%)*
Embalmed 896 (69.14%)	*102 (7.87%)*	*693 (53.47%)*	*101 (7.79%)*

Italicized data indicate minimum estimate of autopsies assumed performed for NCWAS, 969 or 74.54%.

TABLE 3. U.S. NATIONAL COAL WORKERS' AUTOPSY STUDY CASES BY STATE OF DEATH

State of death	Number	Percent
Pennsylvania	594	47
West Virginia	350	28
Illinois	71	6
Ohio	50	4
Kentucky	49	4
Virginia	41	3
Wyoming	26	2
Colorado	23	2
Utah	9	1
New Mexico	7	1
Kansas, Michigan	6	0.5
Tennessee	5	0.4
Oklahoma, Missouri	4	0.3
Indiana, New Jersey	3	0.23
New York, Washington, Washington, D.C.	2	0.16
Arizona, Connecticut, Florida, Georgia, Oregon, Texas	1	0.08

TABLE 4. FREQUENCY OF SELECTED DIAGNOSES IN THE U.S. NATIONAL COAL WORKERS' AUTOPSY STUDY

Cause of death	Number	Percent
All lung cancer	104	8.0
All gastrointestinal cancer	85	6.5
All cancer	315	24.3
Ischemic heart disease (as primary cause of death)	455	35.0
Accidents, suicides, homicides	100	7.7

TABLE 5. SMOKING HISTORY IN THE U.S. NATIONAL COAL WORKERS' AUTOPSY STUDY

Smoking status	Number	Percent
Never smoker	334	25.7
Cigar or pipe only	31	2.4
Ex-smoker	509	39.2
Current smoker	394	30.3
Unknown status	31	2.2
Total	1299	100

mining. The data presented in Table 6 suggest there may be some increased risk related to inhalation of coal mine dust, although cigarette smoking is the predominant factor. The collection of enough cases of lung cancer in nonsmokers has made such analyses difficult in smaller series.[157, 161] A large number of cases is necessary to pick up minor effects so overshadowed by cigarette smoking.

The form of CWP discussed above, with macules and/or nodules less than 1 cm in size (defined radiologically[186]) is called simple CWP. *Complicated CWP,* or progressive massive fibrosis (PMF), is another entity in that it is definitely disabling. Its etiology and pathogenesis are not well understood. Evidence for mycobacterial infection[90, 129, 144] is supported by experimental studies.[203] Immune mechanisms[38, 144] also have some support. There is not conclusive evidence for a direct dust dose-response relationship in PMF,[135, 188] but Pratt[146] reanalyzed the data of Nagleschmidt et al.,[135] showing increased silica concentration in the PMF lesions. PMF is not restricted to CWP. It can occur in most any other pneumoconiosis such as silicosis, talcosis, and asbestosis.[129, 144, 185]

Caplan's syndrome[38, 144] is the development of complicated pneumoconiosis in a patient with rheumatoid arthritis. These lesions usually do not appear on a background of simple pneumoconiosis but appear to represent an altered response to the dust injury. The nodules may show features similar to a rheumatoid nodule.[144] Whether the rheumatoid arthritis occurs before the pneumoconiosis or as a result of it has not been resolved. This caveat may be extended to many of the associations shown between pneumoconiosis (and other lung diseases) and collagen vascular disease such as lupus erythematosus, progressive systemic sclerosis (scleroderma), rheumatoid disease and glomerulonephritis.[37, 39, 144, 152, 175]

One may develop a rather general, simple hypothesis that particulate matter which damages the lung (or for that matter, lung damage of almost any etiology) will result in loss of some normal components of lung tissue. These may be both cellular and extracellular components. Some may be released as soluble or bound

TABLE 6. LUNG CANCER IN U.S. NATIONAL COAL WORKERS' AUTOPSY STUDY

Case parameters	Smokers				Ex-smokers				Never smokers		
	Lung cancer		Others		Lung cancer		Others		Lung cancer		Others
Number	30		380	↔ [b]	64		444	↔ [b]	10		352
Age at death[a]	65.7 ± 10.1	↔ [b]	58.8 ± 10.1		64.1 ± 9.4		64.2 ± 9.9		71.2 ± 8.05		69.7 ± 11.63
Smoking history,[a] (pack-years)	36.8 ± 24.1	↔ [c]	27.5 ± 19.7		24.9 ± 15.4	↔ [c]	19.9 ± 16.9		0		0
Years in underground job[a]	30.4 ± 15.6		26.8 ± 12.1		29.2 ± 14.4		28.5 ± 13.2		40.0 ± 8.98	↔ [c]	29.7 ± 13.31

[a] Mean ± SD
[b] $P < 0.01$
[c] $0.01 < P < 0.05$

to certain macromolecules and others may be only removed from the lung by cellular transport. Any of these materials leaving the lung will reach the general circulation directly if they enter the pulmonary venous circulation or via the lymphatic drainage of the lung, in which case a large proportion will be recycled through the lung before entering the systemic circulation. It does not seem unreasonable to expect that these materials may in some cases stimulate the formation of humoral or cellular immune responses. Those sites in the body where filtration of the blood occurs may show the accumulation of these products and in some cases may be the site of a localized response. Such sites would include renal glomeruli and tubular epithelial cells, the synovial lining cells of joints and the choroid plexus. There is no question that there is some loss of lung parenchyma with age.[179] This tissue lost must be removed either through bronchial clearance mechanisms or by way of the circulation. The tendency to react to these hypothetical breakdown products may be at least partially genetically determined. An association has been shown between rheumatoid arthritis and interstitial lung disease, but it is not yet known which is the chicken and which is the egg, assuming that one or the other is the primary site of damage.

Some of the vasculitides, by extension, might be thought of as induced by transport of cleared materials to the perivascular areas, at which point antibodies and antigens might diffuse through the vascular wall, the reaction conceptually resembling a modified Ouchterlony plate.

With the projected increasing demand for coal as an alternate energy source the prevention of CWP will shortly take on new magnitude. The pathologist of the next generation will be the judge of this generation's success or failure.

Silicosis

This is the classic model of pneumoconiosis, existant in any civilization breathing silica from the environment (*e.g.,* desert sand[22, 178]) or industry.[129, 144, 175, 205] The exact mechanism of interaction of silica with biological tissue, despite decades of research, is unresolved.[15-17, 47, 48, 99, 129, 144, 188, 189, 203, 205] Hypotheses dealing with solubilization of silicic acid, surface charge and availability of electrons are the strongest contenders. The cellular biology of particulate interaction has been meticulously studied by Allison.[15-17] Observed progression of silicotic lesions in the absence of further exposure can be understood by knowledge of the continued cycle of phagocytosis → formation of phagolysosomes → lysis of phagolysosomes and cells → release of particle → phagocytosis, etc. Some evidence that particles recovered from the lungs are smaller than those inhaled[77] might be interpreted as indicating partial dissolution of the particles. However, when the normal deposition and clearance mechanisms are considered, it must be recognized that particles retained in and recovered from the lung are not necessarily the same total population of particles deposited.

Classic nodular silicosis has been well reproduced in animals.[203] Under certain conditions of large doses and small particle size, a lesion is produced in animals called acute silicosis or acute silico-proteinosis. This may resemble pulmonary alveolar proteinosis as seen in man,[153] but often shows more interstitial reaction than the latter, which is usually devoid of interstitial change. Acute silicosis has been noted in sandblasters working with fine sand or high-pressure sandblasting of steel, as in a shipyard.[20, 36, 159, 175] Acute in this case means development of the disease in months or a very few years as opposed to the decades usually preceding the onset of classic nodular silicosis. These cases show some areas resembling pulmonary alveolar proteinosis (PAP). In reviewing human cases of PAP, McEuen and I have used polarized light microscopy plus SEM and X-ray microanalysis to search for particulates in areas of PAP.[121, 122] We found that 29 of 37 cases (78%) of PAP contained significantly higher concentrations of birefringent particles (most of which were less than 1 μ in diameter) than controls. SEM and X-ray microanalysis identified many of these particles as silica, others were silicates. Particles which were not birefringent and/or too small to resolve by light microscopy are detectable with SEM imaging.[2]

Another reaction to particulate matter or irritant gases may be bronchiolitis obliterans.[66] De Nee, Abraham, Gelderman, and Shaw[53] presented a case in which this reaction developed after exposure to burning jute. In addition to the soot particles in many bronchioles, birefringent crystals were noted (Fig. 6). SEM and X-ray analysis identified some of these as silica. The origin may have been the naturally occurring silica in the jute. These biogenic silica particles, or phytoliths,

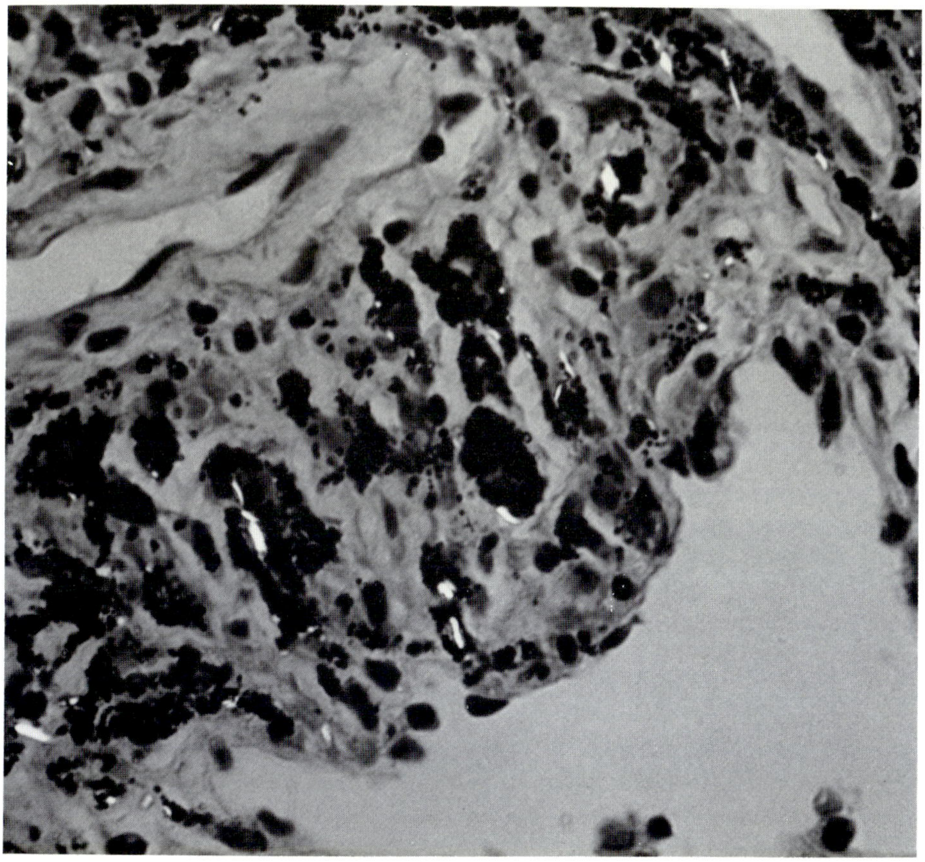

FIG. 6. Bronchiolitis obliterans. Polarized light micrograph illustrating association of soot particles and birefringent particles in bronchiolar epithelium. × 900.

are common in most plants.[197] Many are in the respirable size range. The medical significance of these particles in other plant or plant product exposures (*e.g.*, cotton workers, tobacco smokers) remains unknown.

While the use of SEM and X-ray microanalysis allows identification of inorganic materials in tissues to proceed further than is possible with light microscopy, certain limitations must be recognized. Some of these are in the instrumentation, allowing detection of only certain elements (for example, in energy dispersive X-ray analysis those elements of atomic number less than eleven, sodium, are not detectable). Elements must be present in sufficient concentration to be detected by this method, usually 0.1–1% weight concentration in the volume analyzed. Examination of tissues at relatively low magnification, with the electron beam scanning over a larger area, may result in failure to detect certain elements present in high concentration within individual particles.[2] It is usually necessary to analyze individual particles, and to analyze sufficient numbers to ensure representative sampling of those present in the tissue. A recent report by Pintar, Funahashi, and Siegesmund[145] illustrates this problem. The diagnosis of silicosis was made (even though the reaction was atypical) based on the finding of significant X-ray counts for the element silicon in the thickened but non-nodular tissue in three foundry workers. This analysis was done at low magnification rather than analyzing individual particles. I have found similar lesions in a foundry worker (Fig. 7). The analysis at low magnification again revealed silicon, but analysis of individual particles revealed several kinds of particles, the most common being zircon ($ZrSiO_4$) and silica (SiO_2). Perhaps similar materials were present in the tissues examined by Pintar *et al.*[145] but were not detected owing to the method of analysis.

ASBESTOSIS

Asbestos has been a subject of exhaustive research and profuse publications in recent years.[23, 32, 83, 129, 144, 158, 164, 168, 189, 203] Harington[83] has recently reviewed the geology and cellular biochemistry. To the geologist, asbestos defines a large group of minerals with some properties in common. The differences in composition and structure of the minerals may be importantly related to the biologic effects in the exposed subject. Chrysotile (white asbestos) accounts for over ninety percent of the current world use. Crocidolite (blue asbestos) and Amosite (brown asbestos) each account for approximately 3% of the world's consumption. Anthophyllite, Tremolite, and Actinolite each account for less than 1% of use.

The most soluble type of asbestos is the most common, Chrysotile. It is likely that much of the Chrysotile deposited in the lung may lose considerable magnesium, complicating its identification in tissue. Also, different kinds of asbestos have different flexibility, and tend to fragment into shorter and thinner particles during processing and perhaps also during residence in tissues. As the size of the particle may be as important as its composition in determining the response of the tissue[83, 181] these factors must be considered in any evaluation of the biologic effects of asbestos.

Electron microscopic examination of tissue as well as of environmental samples reveals that for every fiber visible by light microscopy there are likely to be hundreds or thousands of particles visible only by electron microscopy.[125] This raises obvious questions of the merits of the monitoring criteria which are based on light microscopy alone.[141] Furthermore such examination of tissues has revealed that the large majority of fibers remain uncoated.[125] Thus the absence of asbestos bodies does not rule out the presence of asbestos in the tissues.

The finding that pulmonary interstitial fibrosis in asbestosis affects the peripheral regions of the lower zones more than the upper zones has not been sufficiently well explained. Explanations based on posture and gravity have been advanced.[129, 144] It is not unreasonable to expect that there might be some preferential deposition in the lower lobes of the long fibers which might have difficulty "turning the corner" in the bronchial tree to allow their distribution to the upper zones.

The underlying physiologic differences in upper versus lower lung zones[193] may be somehow related to the differences in reaction to different toxic particulates. Most respirable particulates such as silica or coal tend to involve the upper zones earlier or to a greater degree than the lower.[129, 144] The distribution of ventilation at rest, during exercises, and with changes in posture influences the deposition patterns of inhaled materials. Changes in perfusion distributions do not likely affect the deposition of particles but may produce different chemical and cellular milieu for the reaction to the particles. For example, the common distribution of centrilobular emphysema shows predominance in the upper lobes. This emphysema is usually thought to be related to exogenous pulmonary insult, such as cigarette smoking. The emphysema occurring in α_1-antitrypsin deficiency, in contrast, seems to be predominantly lower lobe.[179] Whether this represents a fundamental difference in response to purely exogenous versus at least partially endogenous factors has not been proven. However, it seems likely that the differences in perfusion, and possibly in degree of aerobic *versus* anaerobic metabolism, in different zones of the lung may result in varying cell populations with varying metabolic (including hydrolytic enzymes) activity. The metabolic state of the cells involved in the reaction certainly might determine the probability of cellular damage leading to fibrosis.

The recent findings of phagocytic activity by ciliated and nonciliated bronchial and bronchiolar lining cells[9, 11, 31, 132, 171] raises new questions about the route of inhaled particles to the parenchyma. The peribronchiolar fibrosis associated with asbestos exposure may be largely the consequence of direct penetration of the bronchiolar epithelium rather than of clearance of more peripherally deposited particles to the peribronchiolar regions. The same considerations may apply to the location of dust deposits seen in coal workers' lungs. These also resemble the distribution of lesions seen in smokers' peripheral airways.[138, 139] It is quite possible that the fibers of asbestos greater than the size expected to be found in alveoli got there by penetration through the adjacent bronchioles upon which they impacted rather than by peculiar aerodynamic behavior.

The mechanism or mechanisms whereby asbestos fibers reach the pleura and other organs remain unclear. It is the parietal rather than the visceral pleura which is the site of development of fibrous plaques. The uncoated fibers visible only by electron microscopy may be found associated with mesotheliomas or in the parietal pleura even in the absence of coated fibers in the lung itself. The pathogenesis of mesothelioma appears to be unrelated to co-factors such as the association of asbestos exposure, smoking and lung cancer.[158, 166]

Asbestos bodies (Fig. 8) are more properly referred to as ferruginous bodies

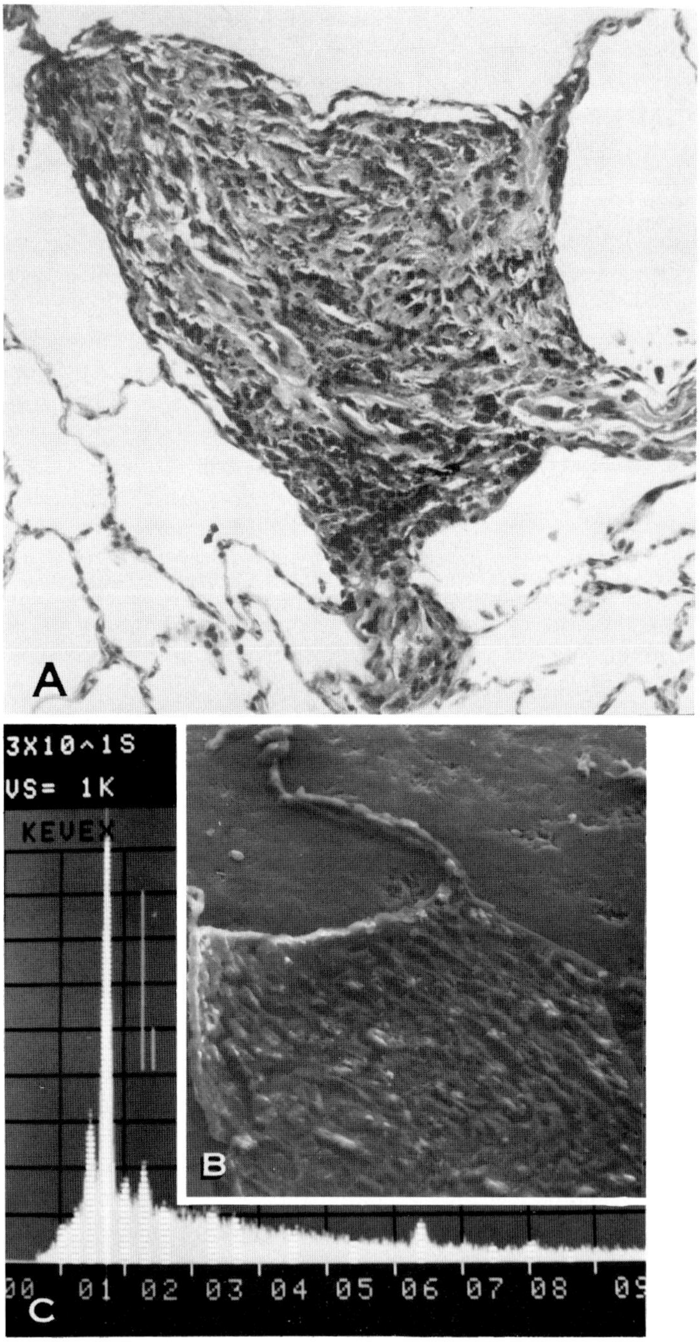

FIG. 7. Foundry worker. Tissue provided by Dr. F. B. Askin. (*A*), Macules of dust with minimal fibrosis noted by light microscopy. × 400. (*B*), Similar macule as seen by SEM, secondary electron image. × 450. *Inset* in *C*, EDXA spectrum from analysis of entire macule seen in *B*, showing presence of silicon and sulfur as the major elements. Aluminum, phosphorous, potassium and iron are also present. (*D*), Higher magnification of same area, SEM, negative backscattered electron image,

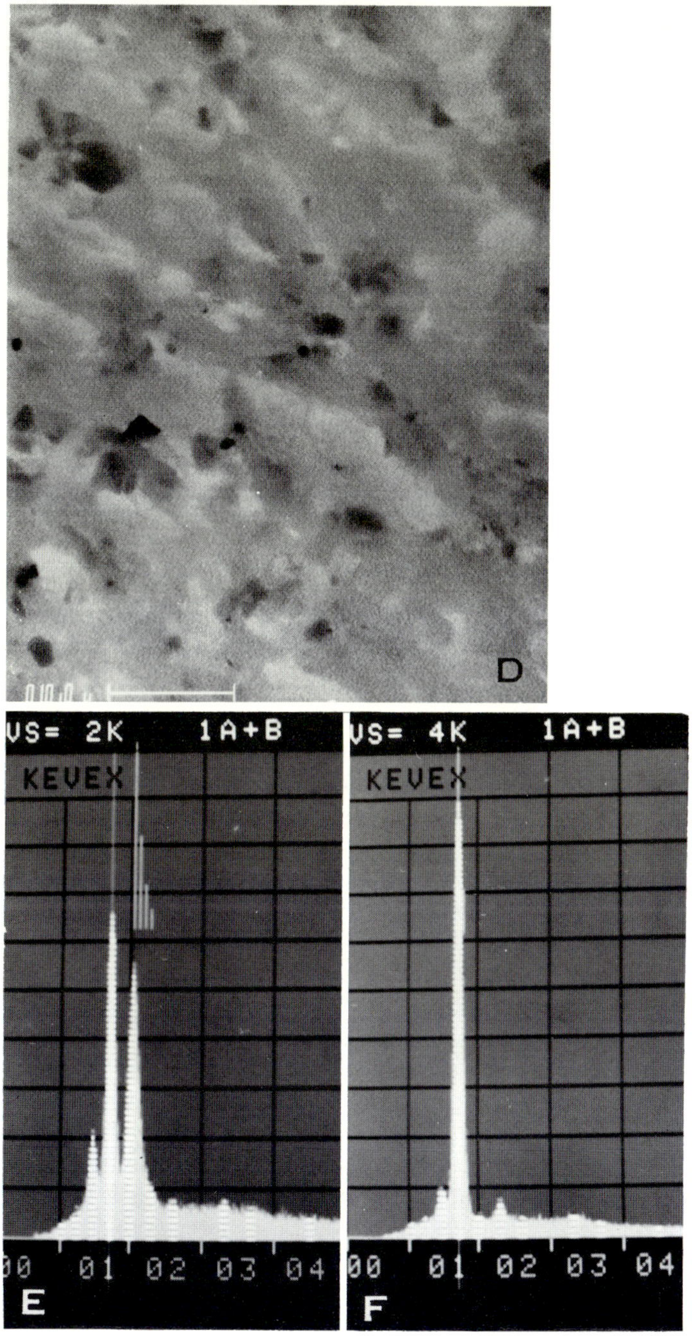

showing numerous individual particles of varying atomic number (highest atomic number particles are darkest). × 2000. (*E*), EDXA spectrum from a single very dark particle showing zirconium and silicon, allowing identification of particle as zircon ($ZrSiO_4$). (*F*), EDXA spectrum from a gray particle in *D*, showing Si only, identifying particle as silica (SiO_2).

since they are not specific for the presence of asbestos.[43, 64] These are rod-shaped structures with clubbed ends, often appearing beaded along their length. The length ranges from 10–30 μ and the thickness from 1–6 μ. Sometimes one can see a central paler core which may be mildly birefringent. The coating consists of ferritin and proteinaceous material deposited around the fibers by macrophages which ingest all or a portion of the particles. Several macrophages may be needed to engulf the larger fibers. The coating is not a rapid process and seems to continue to occur for months or years after inhalation.[176] Also some dissolution of the coating and of the fibers occurs with time. The coating is more evident on larger fibers which cannot be completely engulfed by one macrophage.[49]

Other materials which may become coated and give rise to ferruginous bodies or pseudoasbestos bodies include glass and cotton fibers, talc, graphite, carborundum and other particles. It is possible to identify the materials in the core of the ferruginous body using electron beam techniques. Using these techniques it has been shown that all types of asbestos may produce ferruginous bodies, but in man the kind found most frequently as the core of a ferruginous body is the amphibole fiber, even though exposure to Chrysotile fibers is more common. Possibly this occurs because of fibril size of the Chrysotile or of its tendency to break down into shorter lengths, thus being too small to be observed by light microscopy or too small to elicit a coating response. It may be possible not only to identify the type of mineral present but its specific geographic region of origin since each mineral apparently has unique combinations of trace elements associated with the major mineral.[107]

The prevalence of asbestos bodies at different periods in time has been reported by several observers. The results seem quite dependent on the technique used for collecting and quantitating the number. Selikoff and Hammond[165] studied the yield of asbestos bodies by light microscopy in ashed sections of tissue from 1934 to 1967. The tissue sampling was limited to sections 175 μ in thickness. They found 53% of cases positive in 1934 and 60% in 1967. In contrast, Bhagavan and Koss[27] studied wet formalin-fixed tissue (approximately 5–10 gm of lung tissue per case, compared with a few mg at most in the study reported by Selikoff and Hammond). This later study found that in the period of 1940–1949, 41% of cases had asbestos bodies and in the 1970–1972 period, 91% of cases had asbestos bodies. Also the mean number of asbestos bodies per 5 gm of lung tissue increased from 4.0 in the 1940's to 28.6 in the 1970's. The median number increased from zero in the 1940's to 3.8 in the 1950's to 14.0 in the 1970's. The number per 5 gm of lung also increased with age in each period studied. Neither of these reports actually involved identification of the fibrous core of the asbestos bodies but it is likely that the concentration of asbestos bodies or ferruginous bodies in the lungs is related to the amount of asbestos in the lungs. Recent work by Churg and Warnock[43] suggests that over 90% of ferruginous bodies in non-occupationally exposed individuals have, in fact, asbestos cores.

There seems to be a strong correlation between the hemolytic and cytotoxic activities of a wide range of mineral fibers *in vitro*.[83] This applies to asbestos as well as to silica and other silicates. In the direct hemolysis tests involving incubation of minerals with a suspension of erythrocytes and measuring the free

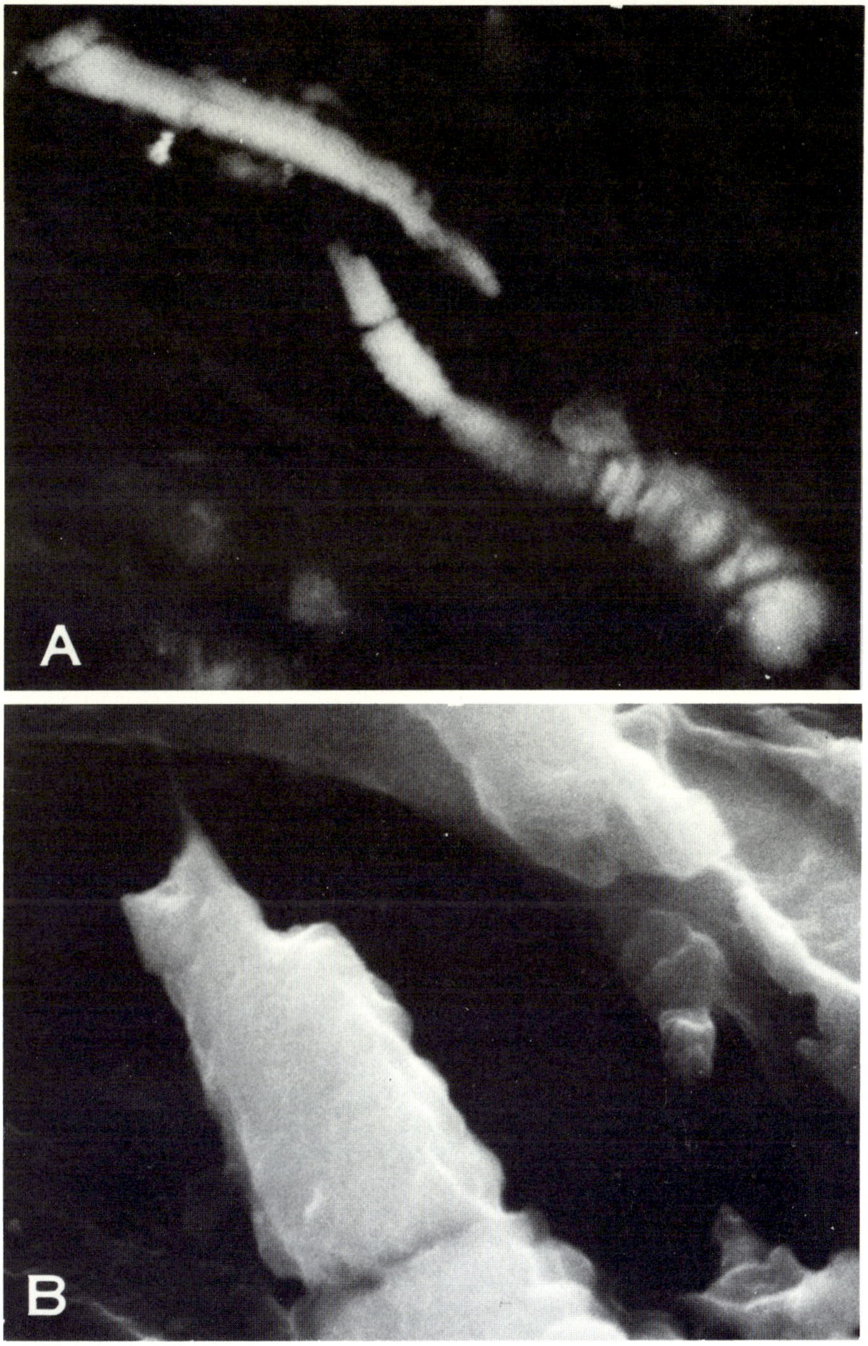

FIG. 8. SEM illustration of asbestos body easily found in standard 5 μ paraffin section of welder's lung, mounted on carbon, deparaffinized. (*A*), Backscattered electron image. × 2500. (*B*), Fibers in center of broken asbestos body seen in secondary electron image. × 16,000.

hemoglobin resulting, Chrysotile asbestos shows high activity and other forms such as Crocidolite and Amosite show little activity. This hemolytic effect is evidently directly related to the solubility of divalent magnesium from the Chrysotile fiber surface. Specific inhibitors of the hemolytic activity of Chrysotile are specific chelators for magnesium. Also the ratio of the magnesium to silicon of different varieties of asbestos seems to be directly related to the hemolytic activity of the mineral. The mechanism of hemolysis caused by silica does not involve magnesium but seems to involve hydrogen bonding. This is apparently the mechanism of inhibition of hemolysis of silica by polyvinylpyridine oxide (PVPNO). The hemolytic activity of Chrysotile is also inhibited by some acidic water soluble polymers such as sodium carboxymethylcellulose (CMC). The polymer presumably binds firmly to the Chrysotile surface.

The role of sialic acid in the interaction between erythrocyte surface membranes and Chrysotile was investigated by Harington, Gilson and Wagner[84] who found that sialic acid was an inhibitor of Chrysotile hemolysis. The interaction of sialic acid and magnesium containing compounds such as asbestos may be of general interest in cell biology. Asbestos may strongly absorb sialic acid or substances containing sialic acid from the surfaces of cells. The role of cell surface macromolecules in the regulation of cellular interactions, cellular division and growth may be speculatively related to asbestos carcinogenesis in light of the findings that the surface glycoproteins necessary for cellular communication and recognition may be altered or lost in malignant cells.[117]

Asbestos-related tissue changes range from a reaction resembling desquamative interstitial pneumonia (DIP)[44, 114] through the more common, nonspecific, characteristically peribronchiolar, interstitial inflammation with fibrosis to a progressive massive fibrosis type of lesion. The latter is not common and differs from the PMF seen in coal workers and silicotics in that it is more likely to occur in the lower lobes. Also the question of mixed exposures to silica or talc has been raised in some of these cases.[170, 185]

Although this review largely excludes the neoplastic aspects of pneumoconiosis, the association between exposure to asbestos and subsequent development of pleural and peritoneal mesothelioma and to the development of carcinoma of the lung merits mention. The histologic types of these neoplasms have been thoroughly discussed in several reviews, and the relationship between dose, latency, and other factors such as cigarette exposure has been well studied.[23, 89, 158, 166, 195] The relationships between specific particle types and sizes and the response of the organism are still being investigated because human exposures to pure fiber types are rare. Mixed exposures to various types of asbestos, as well as to other dusts, are the rule.

There is no question that the risk of carcinoma of the lung associated with exposure to asbestos in persons smoking cigarettes is increased several fold over the risk in smokers not exposed to asbestos. The nonsmoker exposed to asbestos has not yet been conclusively shown to be at increased risk for carcinoma of the lung (although smoking does not seem to be involved in the pathogenesis of mesothelioma).[158, 166] The difficulty in collecting a large enough series of nonsmokers, especially of finding nonsmokers with lung cancer, regardless of asbestos exposure, probably accounts for most of the remaining dispute among epidemiologists.

The association of lung cancer with asbestos exposure is also supported pathologically by differences from such cancer in the general population. The tumors are commonly located in the lower lobes where the fibrosis of asbestos tends to be most marked.[89] The distribution of histologic types seems different from that in the non asbestos-exposed population,[24, 202] with a greater proportion of adenocarcinoma.[195] Not all series show this histologic distribution.[94] The problem of interpretation of histologic type of lung cancer by different observers using different criteria is a major one in any such geographic studies.[202] With new criteria or classification systems frequently being adopted, it seems unlikely that this problem of comparison between different centers and nations will be resolved in the next few years. This should reemphasize the need for morphologic standards for pneumoconiosis as have been adopted by the radiologists for chest X-rays.[186]

The hypothesis that carcinogens in cigarette smoke may be bound to the particles and fibers and thus delivered to the more peripheral regions of the bronchial tree has been advanced by Whitwell and Rawcliffe.[195, 196] It seems equally likely that the nonspecific damage caused by asbestos and other dusts increases the susceptibility of the epithelium to carcinogens from cigarette smoke, etc. by damage to, and subsequent increased regenerative proliferation of the epithelium. Common sites of neoplasia are sites of rapid cell turnover such as the skin, the reticuloendothelial system and the gastrointestinal tract. The lung has only become a major site of carcinoma since the advent of widespread cigarette smoking.

Asbestos has been associated with increased risk of laryngeal as well as pulmonary cancer.[75] It is worth noting that one coal miner in the lung cancer series of the U.S. National Coal Workers' Autopsy Study (with adenocarcinoma of the lung) underwent a previous resection for epidermoid cancer of the larynx. The lung contained numerous ferruginous bodies. Similar cases are not uncommon.[102, 201]

Although use of asbestos is being curtailed and better safety precautions taken in its use, it remains in many buildings and ships which may someday be demolished. This, coupled with the latency of decades for development of a disease such as mesothelioma implies that pathologists will be seeing much more of this now ubiquitous material and its sequelae before they see less. The fibrous materials such as fibrous glass[41, 71] currently being used in place of asbestos have not been shown to be carcinogenic, but the human experiment of exposure for several decades is well underway, and the final answer should be available in the next decade or two.

Beryllium Disease

The recognition of beryllium as the cause of acute and chronic pulmonary and systemic disease in workers in the fluorescent lamp industry in the late 1930's and early 1940's led to the discontinuance of its use in that industry in 1949. Nevertheless, the consumption of beryllium, as beryl, its principle ore, steadily increased from 1200 tons in 1941 to nearly 9000 tons in 1968. It is used in industry predominantly in three forms—as the metal, as alloys, and as the oxide. Beryllium metal is used in many applications because of its light weight, rigidity, and stability. It is used increasingly in aerospace applications, in structural materials, guidance systems, optical devices, rocket motor parts, heat shields, and airplane brakes. As an alloying agent it improves the quality and performance of several metals. Beryllium copper alloys have high tensile strength, high electrical and thermal conductivity, resistance to corrosion and fatigue, and antisparking and antimagnetic qualities. Beryllium copper alloys are used in springs, electrical contacts, connectors in electrical equipment, bearings, gears, antispark tools, welding electrodes, and many other items. Beryllium nickel alloys, which are comparable or superior to heat treated stainless steel in some ways, are used in high temperature springs, diamond drill bits, fuel pumps, and business machines. Beryllium oxide has the unusual property of being both a good conductor of heat and an electrical insulator. It is used in ceramic parts for the electronics industry, for thermal coatings and crucibles, and in nuclear reactors.[80, 173, 177]

The sources of exposure to beryllium in industry are extremely broad, involving melting, sawing, grinding, welding, milling, machining, etc. In addition to direct industrial exposure beryllium is easily dispersed into the air and the scrap material can be subsequently used without knowledge of its beryllium content.

Neighborhood cases in the region around industrial sources have been recorded in individuals exposed to beryllium compounds within half a mile of industrial source or by handling contaminated clothing of workers. The occupational history alone may not elicit beryllium exposure, as illustrated by a case recently acces-

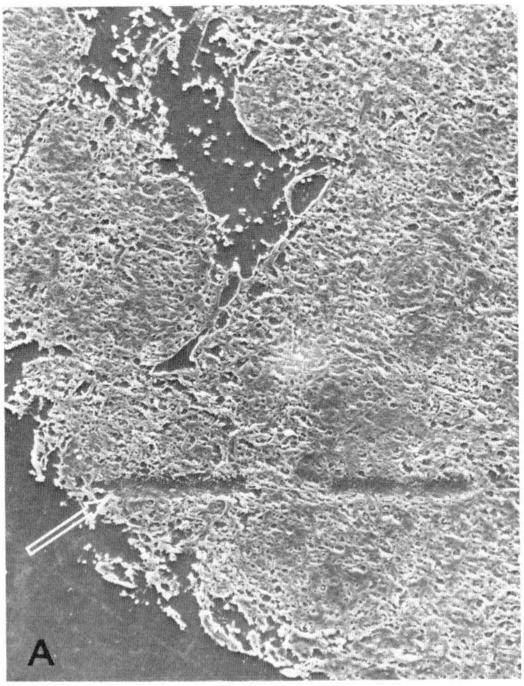

FIG. 9. Beryllium disease. Standard 5 μ paraffin section on carbon deparaffinized. (*A*), SEM illustration of noncaseating granulomas in intrapulmonary lymph node. Lines (*arrow*) indicate 150 μ wide regions analyzed with ion microprobe (IMMA). Smooth regions represent epithelioid cells. Rougher areas contain lymphoid cells and macrophages. × 160.

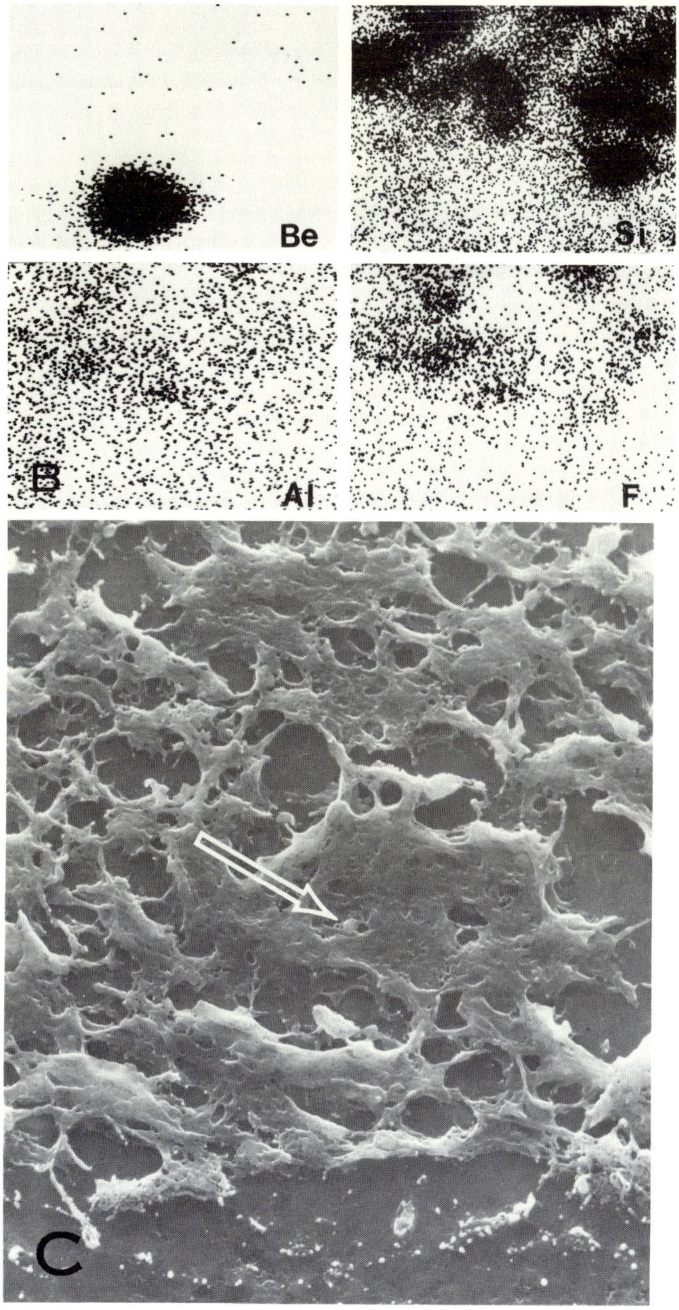

FIG. 9 B & C

(*B*), IMMA distribution maps of the indicated line at left in 9*A* are shown for Be, Si, Al, and F. Absence of elements other than Be from single focus rules out compounds of Be other than BeO. (*C*), SEM reveals a 1 μ hexagonal BeO particle detected in IMMA maps (*arrow*) is located within the epithelioid granuloma. $\times$ 1500.

sioned by the Beryllium Case Registry.[82, 85] The patient was a secretary working in a nonindustrial office. Only after repeated questioning was it learned that she worked in a building shared with a beryllium processing industry, and to get to and from her office she had to walk through the beryllium plant at least twice a day.

The morphologic reaction in beryllium disease is classically the formation of noncaseating granulomas as in sarcoidosis. There may also be lymphocytic infiltration and some necrosis. Asteroid bodies, Schaumann's bodies and hyalinization of granulomata are present in some cases. Blebs and bullae may form and may be the cause of pneumothorax. The critical difference between sarcoidosis and beryllium disease is the documentation of beryllium exposure either by finding beryllium in the urine or tissues, or by strong epidemiologic evidence of exposure. Freiman and Hardy[62] reported a better prognosis associated with lesions showing less interstitial reaction.

Analysis of tissue or fluids for beryllium is a nonroutine procedure, best performed by experienced laboratories. Lungs of coal miners and urban dwellers where soft coal is burned may also contain beryllium. The detection of beryllium in the tissue gives evidence of past or recent exposure to beryllium, but does not, by itself, document beryllium disease. A large sample of tissue is necessary for the chemical methods used, which involve extraction and treatment to separate beryllium oxide and other compounds from naturally occurring beryl prior to spectroscopic analysis. These techniques, of course, do not allow localization of beryllium in specific lesions and do not allow identification of specific beryllium compounds. Recent work using microprobe techniques has allowed the demonstration of beryllium in the granulomas using a laser microprobe,[149, 151] and most recently, using the ion microprobe mass analyzer in conjunction with electron beam microanalysis, it has been possible to identify beryllium oxide within the epithelioid cells of granulomas and to characterize the individual particles using scanning electron microscopy[3, 8, 10, 18] (Fig. 9).

The mechanism of beryllium toxicity is not well understood despite much work. Biochemical studies in animals have shown that beryllium becomes associated with the lysosomal fraction and the nucleus of the cells. The role of steroid hormones (sometimes effective in humans) in regulating beryllium disease has also been studied in animals. Those whose adrenal cortical function was markedly reduced rapidly showed pronounced beryllium toxicity which was reduced by steroid treatment.[173] In animals, beryllium compounds were able to induce pulmonary adenomatous tumors and osteosarcoma.[173] The counterparts in the human have not been seen despite careful scrutiny of cases in the Beryllium Registry to date.[82] This toxic material is being used increasingly and no doubt an increase in cases of beryllium disease will be seen over the next decades.

Other Pneumoconioses

One has only to examine the lists of texts and monographs cited at the outset of this chapter to appreciate the need for great selectivity in choosing topics for discussion. In addition to the well described, more common pneumoconioses that have been discussed, there are numerous others as well as yet undetected reactions to particulate toxic agents. In any lung disease of unknown etiology, ranging from acute diffuse alveolar damage, as with exposure to nickel fumes,[2, 78] to interstitial fibrosis,[39, 156] to granulomatous "sarcoid" reactions as with exposure to aluminum, beryllium, etc.,[4, 74, 144] such environmental or occupational exposure must be considered.

It is fortunate for pathologists that many inorganic particulates are retained in the lung to provide clues in the study of lung diseases. Only by thorough correlation of pathology with clinical and occupational/environmental history, physiology, radiology, and chemical analysis[7, 120, 154, 174] will we derive adequate information for patient diagnosis. Identification of causal agents will be important, especially for prevention of disease.

SUMMARY

Pneumoconiosis is broadly defined as dust in the lung. The reaction to the dust may range from none to severe. Hundreds of thousands of active people annually are partially or totally disabled by inorganic dust induced lung disease (IDILD). The rather unusual aspect of IDILD is that if one can search by appropriate methods, the etiologic agent may often be detected in tissue obtained at biopsy or necropsy. Perhaps in no other area of pathology does the identification in tissue of the etiologic agent of a patient's disease offer as little help in directing corrective therapy as in IDILD. However, in few other diseases is such identification of greater importance to the current and future health of large numbers of persons.

It is sobering to consider that many known occupational and environmental diseases have a latency of, or require a cumulative exposure for, many years or decades. How many discoveries like vinyl chloride and angiosarcoma of the liver, or asbestos and mesothelioma lie ahead? I believe that pathologists are in a position to hasten these discoveries; they have the means and the responsibility to provide a special service to both the patient and society.

A recent survey by the U.S. National Institute for Occupational Safety and Health suggests that IDILD is suspected in over 10,000 lung biopsies or necropsies per year. Pathologists will receive increasing requests for analysis of tissues for evidence of exposure to occupational and environmental agents. Clinicians and patients will seek their opinion as to the relationship between exposure and disease, including neoplasia.

It is not enough to stop at a diagnosis of dust disease, any more than it is enough to diagnose caseating granuloma, and not perform special stains for infectious agents. The responsible agents are most often retained in the tissues and are available for analysis, even after the usual tissue processing through fixatives, solvents, and embedding media. Recent additions to the pathologist's armamentarium of research and diagnostic instrumentation allow fairly rapid analysis of inorganic respirable particulate materials in routinely prepared tissue sections. A most essential aspect of any such study is the correlation of such analyses with the environmental and occupational history of the patient. Development of interest and skill in obtaining the latter is equally important to mastering the techniques of microanalysis.

The added topographic information resulting from *in situ* microanalysis may be of value in separating recent dust exposure related to specific tissue changes from remote or chronic dust exposure, which may complicate the interpretation of bulk tissue analyses or analyses of particles isolated from tissue. Major unsolved problems facing all pathologists dealing with environmental/occupational diseases include: the need for standardization of morphologic evaluation and reporting, quantitation of the findings, the relationship to lung (and other) cancer, and the need for some coordinated effort to facilitate early recognition of the many as yet unrecognized effects of multitudes of inhaled materials.

REFERENCES

1. Abraham, J. L.: Lung cancer in the U.S. National Coal Workers' Autopsy Study: Analysis of 1300 necropsies. *Am. Rev. Resp. Dis. 113:* 104, 1976. (abstr.)
2. Abraham, J. L.: SEM as an aid in diagnosis—An overview. In *Scanning Electron Microscopy,* edited by Johari, O., Vol. 2, pp. 119–128. Chicago, IIT Research Institute, 1977.
3. Abraham, J. L.: Multiple imaging and microanalytical modes for biological specimens—Electron and ion beam studies. *Proc. Microbeam Anal. Soc.,* Boston, August, 1977.
4. Abraham, J. L. Unpublished results.
5. Abraham, J. L., and DeNee, P. B.: Scanning-electron-microscope histochemistry using backscatter electrons and metal stains. *Lancet 1:* 1125, 1973.
6. Abraham, J. L., and DeNee, P. B.: Biomedical applications of backscattered electron imaging—One year's experience with SEM histochemistry. In *Scanning Electron Microscopy,* edited by Johari, O., and Corvin, I., pp. 251–258. Chicago, IIT Research Institute, 1974.
7. Abraham, J. L., and DeNee, P. B.: Roentgenologic-pathologic-microanalytic correlative study of coal workers' pneumoconiosis. *Lab. Invest. 32:* 462, 1975. (abstr.)
8. Abraham, J. L., Rossi, R. Marquez, N., and Wagner, R. M.: Ion microprobe mass analysis of beryllium *in situ* in human lung: Preliminary results. In *Scanning Electron Microscopy,* edited by Johari, O., Vol. 2, pp. 501–506. Chicago, IIT Research Institute, 1976.
9. Abraham, J. L., Wagner, R. M., Miyai, K., Bullock, R., and Friedman, P. J.: Choice of imaging modes in SEM study of respirable radiographic contrast medium: Tantalum particles in the lung. In *Scanning Electron Microscopy,* edited by Johari, O., Vol. 2, pp. 691–698. Chicago, IIT Research Institute, 1976.
10. Abraham, J. L., and Whatley, T. A.: Ion microprobe analysis of beryllium-containing particles *in situ* in human lungs. *Fed. Proc. 36:* 1090, 1977 (abstr.)
11. Adler, K. B., Mossman, B. T., and Craighead, J. E.: Personal communication.
12. The Eighth Annual air pollution medical research conference. *Arch. Environ. Health 14:* 1–233, 1967.
13. Albert, R. E., Lippmann, M., and Briscoe, W.: The characteristics of bronchial clearance in humans and the effects of cigarette smoking. *Arch. Environ. Health 18:* 738–755, 1969.
14. Albert, R. E., Lippmann, M., Peterson, H. T., Jr., Berger, J., Sanborn, K., and Bohning, D.: Bronchial deposition and clearance of aerosols. *Arch. Intern. Med. 131:* 115–127, 1973.
15. Allison, A. C. Lysosomes and the responses of cells to toxic materials. *Sci. Basis Med. Ann. Rev. 2:* 18–30, 1968.
16. Allison, A. C. Effects of silica and asbestos on cells in culture. *Inhaled Part. Vap. 3:* 437–445, 1970.
17. Allison, A. C., Harington, J. S., and Birbeck, M.: An examination of the cytotoxic effects of silica on macrophages. *J. Exp. Med. 124:* 141–154, 1966.
18. Andersen, C. A., and Hinthorne, J. R.: Ion microprobe mass analyzer. *Science 175:* 853–860, 1972.
19. Ashford, N. A.: *Crisis in the Workplace.* Cambridge, Mass., M.I.T. Press, 1976.
20. Bailey, W. C., Brown, M., Buechner, H. A., Weill, H., Ichinose, H., and Ziskind, M.: Silico-mycobacterial disease in sandblasters. *Am. Rev. Resp. Dis. 110:* 115–125, 1974.
21. Balgord, W. D. Fine particles produced from automotive emissions-control catalysts. *Science 180:* 1168–1169, 1973.

22. Bar-Ziv, J., and Goldberg, G. M.: Simple siliceous pneumoconiosis in Negev Bedouins. *Arch. Environ. Health 29:* 121–126, 1974.
23. Becklake, M. R.: Asbestos-related diseases of the lung and other organs: Their epidemiology and implications for clinical practice. *Am. Rev. Resp. Dis. 114:* 187–227, 1976.
24. Berge, T., and Toremalm, N. G.: Bronchial Cancer—A clinical and pathological study. I. Histopathology and metastases. *Scand. J. Resp. Dis. 56:* 109–119, 1975.
25. Berman, D. M. Why work kills—A brief history of occupational safety and health in the U.S. *Inter. J. Health Serv. 7:* 63–87, 1977.
26. Berry, J. P., Henoc, P., Galle, P., and Pariente, R.: Pulmonary mineral dust. A study of ninety patients by electron microscopy, electron microanalysis, and electron microdiffraction. *Am. J. Pathol. 83:* 427–456, 1976.
27. Bhagavan, B. S., and Koss, L. G. Secular trends in prevalence and concentration of pulmonary asbestos bodies—1940 to 1972. A necropsy study. *Arch. Pathol. Lab. Med. 100:* 539–541, 1976.
28. Boren, H. G.: Pathobiology of air pollutants. *Environ. Res. 1:* 178–197, 1967.
29. Bouhuys, A.: Respiratory disease: Etiologic role of industrial agents—Prepared for the *NIEHS Task Force on Research Planning in Environmental Health Science.* On deposit at the National Library of Medicine, Bethesda, Maryland, 1969.
30. Bouhuys, A., and Peters, M. J.: Control of environmental lung disease. *N. Engl. J. Med. 283:* 573–582, 1970.
31. Brain, J. D., Knudson, D. E., Sorokin, S. P., and Davis, M. A.: Pulmonary distribution of particles given by intratracheal instillation or by aerosol inhalation. *Environ. Res. 11:* 13–33, 1976.
32. Brodeur, P.: *Expendable Americans.* New York, Viking Press, 1974.
33. Brody, A. R., and Craighead, J. E.: Cytoplasmic inclusions in pulmonary macrophages of cigarette smokers. *Lab. Invest. 32:* 125–132, 1975.
34. Brody, A. R., Dwyer, D. M., Vallyathan, N. V., Visco, G. P., and Craighead, J. E.: The elemental content of granulomata: Preliminary studies of pulmonary sarcoidosis and hypersensitivity pneumonitis. In *Scanning Electron Microscopy,* edited by Johari, O., Vol. 2, pp. 129–136. Chicago, IIT Research Institute, 1977.
35. Brody, A. R., Vallyathan, N. V., and Craighead, J. E.: Distribution and elemental analysis of inorganic particles in pulmonary tissue. In *Scanning Electron Microscopy,* edited by Johari, O., Vol. 1, pp. 477–484. Chicago, IIT Research Institute, 1976.
36. Buechner, H. A., and Ansari, A.: Acute silico-proteinosis. A new pathologic variant of acute silicosis in sandblasters, characterized by histologic features resembling alveolar proteinosis. *Dis. Chest 55:* 274–284, 1969.
37. Burrell, R.: Immunology of occupational lung diseases. In *Occupational Lung Diseases,* edited by Morgan, W. K. C., and Seaton, A. Chapter 6, pp. 65–79. London, W. B. Saunders Co., 1975.
38. Caplan, A.: Certain unusual radiological appearances in the chest of coal-miners suffering from rheumatoid arthritis. *Thorax 8:* 29–37, 1953.
39. Carrington, C. B., and Gaensler, E.: See Chapter 4 of this volume.
40. Cassidy, E. P. The National Coal Workers' Autopsy Study. The development and implementation of an occupational necropsy study. *Arch. Pathol. 94:* 133–136, 1972.
41. Chapman, J. S. Oncogenicity of fiber glass (editorial). *Arch. Environ. Health 31:* 107, 1976.
42. Christensen, H. E., and Luginbyhl, T. T. (eds.): *The Toxic Substances List.* U.S. Dept. Health, Education and Welfare Public Health Service, Center for Disease Control. National Institute for Occupational Safety and Health. Rockville, Maryland, 1974.
43. Churg, A., and Warnock, M. L.: Analysis of the cores of ferruginous (asbestos) bodies from the general population. I. Patients with and without lung cancer. *Lab. Invest. 37:* 280–286, 1977.
44. Corrin, B., and Price, A. B.: Electron microscopic studies in desquamative interstitial pneumonia associated with asbestos. *Thorax 27:* 324–331, 1972.
45. Costello, J., Ortmeyer, C. E., and Morgan, W. K. C.: Mortality from lung cancer in U.S. coal miners. *Am. J. Pub. Health 64:* 222–224, 1974.
46. Davidson, J. M., and Macleod, W. M. Pulmonary alveolar proteinosis. *Br. J. Dis. Chest 63:* 13–28, 1969.
47. Davies, C. N.: *Inhaled Particles and Vapours I.* Proceedings of an International Symposium organized by the British Occupational Hygiene Society, Oxford, 29 March–1 April, 1960. Oxford, Pergamon Press, 1961.
48. Davies, C. N.: *Inhaled Particles and Vapours II.* Cambridge, Pergamon Press, 1965.

49. Davis, J. M. G., Gross, P., and de Treville, R. T. P.: "Ferruginous bodies" in guinea pigs. Fine structure produced experimentally from minerals other than asbestos. *Arch. Pathol. 89:* 364–373, 1970.
50. DeNee, P. B.: Identification and analysis of particles in biological tissue using SEM and related techniques. In *Scanning Electron Microscopy,* edited by Johari, O., and Corvin, I., Vol. 2, pp. 461–468. Chicago, IIT Research Institute, 1976.
51. DeNee, P. B., and Abraham, J. L.: Backscattered electron imaging: Application of atomic number contrast. In *Principles and Techniques of Scanning Electron Microscopy,* edited by Hayat, M. A., pp. 144–180. New York, Van Nostrand Reinhold Co., 1976.
52. DeNee, P. B., Abraham, J. L., and Gelderman, A. H.: Methods for a scanning electron microscope study of coal workers' pneumoconiosis. In *Scanning Electron Microscopy,* edited by Johari, O., and Corvin, I., pp. 411–418. Chicago, IIT Research Institute, 1973.
53. DeNee, P. B., Abraham, J. L., Gelderman, A. H., and Shaw, G. B.: SEM identification of biogenic silica in jute: Silica in human lung following exposure to burning jute. *Proc. Microbeam Anal. Soc.* Ottawa, Article 10, July, 1974.
54. DeNee, P. B., Abraham, J. L., and Willard, P. A.: Histochemical stains for the scanning electron microscope—Qualitative and semiquantitative aspects of specific silver stains. In *Scanning Electron Microscopy,* edited by Johari, O., and Corvin, I., pp. 259–266. Chicago, IIT Research Institute, 1974.
55. DeNee, P. B., Walker, E. R., and Abraham, J. L.: SEM characterization of respirable dust in lung tissue using ashing and digestion techniques. *Proc. Microbeam Anal. Soc.* Las Vegas, Article 51, August, 1975.
56. Enterline, P. E.: Mortality rates among coal miners. *Am. J. Pub. Health 54:* 758–768, 1964.
57. Environmental mutagenic hazards. *Science 187:* 503–514, 1975.
58. Epstein, S. S.: Environmental pathology. A review. *Am. J. Pathol. 66:* 352–374, 1972.
59. Fisher, G. L., Chang, D. P. Y., and Brummer, M.: Fly ash collected from electrostatic precipitators: Microcrystalline structures and the mystery of the spheres. *Science 192:* 553–555, 1976.
60. FitzGerald, M. X., Carrington, C. B., and Gaensler, E. A.: Environmental lung disease. *Med. Clin. N. Am. 57:* 593–622, 1973.
61. Flessel, P.: Metals as mutagens. In *Inorganic and Nutritional Aspects of Cancer,* edited by Schrauzer, G. N., Plenum Press, 1978.
62. Freiman, D. G., and Hardy, H. L.: Beryllium disease. The relation of pulmonary pathology to clinical course and prognosis based on a study of 130 cases from the U.S. Beryllium Case Registry. *Hum. Pathol. 1:* 25–44, 1970.
63. Frost, J. K., Gupta, P. K., Erozan, Y. S., Carter, D., Hollander, D. H., Levin, M. L., and Ball, W. C., Jr.: Pulmonary cytologic alterations in toxic environmental inhalation. *Hum. Pathol. 4:* 521–536, 1973.
64. Gaensler, E. A., and Addington, W. W.: Asbestos or ferruginous bodies. *N. Engl. J. Med. 280:* 488–492, 1969.
65. Gafafer, W. M.: *Occupational diseases. A guide to their recognition.* U.S. Department of HEW, PHS, Division of Occupational Health, U.S. Government Printing Office, Public Health Service publication No. 1097, 1964.
66. Gosink, B. B., Friedman, P. J., and Liebow, A. A.: Bronchiolitis obliterans: Roentgenologic-pathologic correlation. *Am. J. Roentgenol. Rad. Ther. Nucl. Med. 117:* 816–832, 1973.
67. Gosselin, R. E., Hodge, H. C., Smith, R. P., and Gleason, M. N.: *Clinical Toxicology of Commercial Products.* Acute Poisoning. 4th ed. Baltimore, The Williams & Wilkins Co., 1976.
68. Gough, J.: Pneumoconiosis in coal trimmers. *J. Pathol. Bacteriol. 51:* 277–285, 1940.
69. Green, G. M., Jakab, G. J., Low, R. B., and Davis, G. S.: Defense mechanisms of the respiratory membrane. *Am. Rev. Resp. Dis. 115:* 479–514, 1977.
70. Gross, P.: Some aspects of pneumoconiosis. *Pathol. Annu. 6:* 61–79, 1971.
71. Gross, P.: The biologic categorization of inhaled fiber glass dust: A critical review of pertinent studies and reports. *Arch. Environ. Health 31:* 101–107, 1976.
72. Gross, P., and deTreville, R. T. P.: Alveolar proteinosis. Its experimental production in rodents. *Arch. Pathol. 86:* 255–261, 1968.
73. Groth, D., and Finklea, J.: Personal communication.
74. Guidotti, T. L.: Pulmonary aluminosis. A review. *Bull. Soc. Pharmacol. Environ. Pathol. 3:* 16–18, 1975.

75. Guidotti, T. L., Abraham, J. L., and DeNee, P. B.: Asbestos exposure and cancer of the larynx. *West. J. Med. 122:* 75, 1975.
76. Guidotti, T. L., Abraham, J. L., DeNee, P. B., and Smith, J. R.: Arc welders' pneumoconiosis: Application of advanced SEM. *Arch. Environ. Health* 1978 (in press).
77. György, U., Pal, H., Zsuzsa, B., et al.: Electron microscopic study of natural SiO_2 particles and SiO_2 particles isolated from rat lung. *Morphol. Igazsagugyi Orv Sz 16:* 225-232, 1976.
78. Hackett, R. L., and Sunderman, F. W., Jr.: Pulmonary alveolar reaction to nickel carbonyl. Ultrastructural and histochemical studies. *Arch. Environ. Health 16:* 349-362, 1968.
79. Hamilton, A., and Hardy, H. L.: *Industrial Toxicology.* 3rd ed. Acton, Mass., Publishing Sciences Group, Inc., 1974.
80. Hardy, H. L.: Beryllium poisoning-lessons in control of man-made disease. *N. Engl. J. Med. 273:* 1188-1199, 1965.
81. Hardy, H. L.: Annual discourse—Risk and responsibility. A physician's viewpoint. *N. Engl. J. Med. 293:* 801-806, 1975.
82. Hardy, H. L.: Personal communication.
83. Harington, J. S.: The biological effects of mineral fibres, especially asbestos, as seen from *in vitro* and *in vivo* studies. *Ann. d'Anat. Pathol. (Paris), 21:* 155-198, 1976.
84. Harington, J. S., Gilson, J. C., and Wagner, J. C.: Asbestos and mesothelioma in man. *Nature 232:* 54-55, 1971.
85. Hasan, F. M., and Kazemi, H.: Progress Report—U.S. Beryllium Case Registry, 1972. *Am. Rev. Resp. Dis. 108:* 1252-1253, 1973.
86. Heppleston, A. G.: The pathological anatomy of simple pneumokoniosis in coal workers. *J. Pathol. Bacteriol. 66:* 235-246, 1953.
87. Higginson, J.: The role of the pathologist in environmental medicine and public health. *Am. J. Pathol. 86:* 460-484, 1977.
88. Hunter, D.: *The Diseases of Occupations.* 5th Ed. London, English University Press, 1975.
89. Jacob, G., and Anspach, M.: Pulmonary neoplasia among Dresden asbestos workers. *Ann. N.Y. Acad. Sci. 132:* 536-548, 1965.
90. James, W. R. L.: The relationship of tuberculosis to the development of massive pneumokoniosis in coal workers. *Br. J. Tuberc. 48:* 89-101, 1954.
91. James, W. R. L.: Primary lung cancer in South Wales coal-workers with pneumoconiosis. *Br. J. Ind. Med. 12:* 87-91, 1955.
92. Johnson, F. B.: Crystals in pathologic specimens. In *Pathology Annual,* edited by Sommers, S. C., Vol. 7, pp. 321-344. New York, Appleton-Century-Crofts, 1972.
93. Kaltreider, H. B.: Expression of immune mechanisms in the lung. *Am. Rev. Resp. Dis. 113:* 347-379, 1976.
94. Kannerstein, M., and Churg, J.: Pathology of carcinoma of the lung associated with asbestos exposure. *Cancer 30:* 14-21, 1972.
95. Katzenstein, A-L. A., Bloor, C. M., and Liebow, A. A.: Diffuse alveolar damage—The role of oxygen, shock and related factors. A review. *Am. J. Pathol. 85:* 210-228, 1976.
96. Key, M. M., Kerr, L. E., and Bundy, M. (eds.): *Pulmonary Reactions to Coal Dust. A Review of U.S. Experience.* New York, Academic Press, 1971.
97. Kilburn, K. H.: A hypothesis for pulmonary clearance and its implications. *Am. Rev. Resp. Dis. 98:* 449-463, 1968.
98. Kilburn, K. H. (Guest Editor): Symposium on pulmonary responses to inhaled materials: An evaluation of model systems. *Arch. Intern. Med. 126:* 415-511, 1970.
99. Klosterkötter, W., and Robock, K.: 1975 Yant Memorial Lecture. New aspects on dust and pneumoconiosis research. *Am. Ind. Hyg. Assoc. J. 36:* 659-668, 1975.
100. Kotin, P.: Carcinogenesis of the lung: Environmental and host factors. In *The Lung,* edited by Liebow, A. A., and Smith, D. E., Chapter 14, pp. 203-225. Baltimore, The Williams & Wilkins Co., 1968.
101. Kotin, P.: Environmental diseases—A pathologist's overview and public health responsibility. *Am. J. Pathol. 64:* 225-234, 1971.
102. Lane, B. P.: Personal communication.
103. Lane, B. P., and Gordon, R.: Regeneration of rat tracheal epithelium after mechanical injury. I: The relationship between mitotic activity and cellular differentiation. *Proc. Soc. Exp. Biol. Med. 145:* 1139-1144, 1974.

104. Lane, W. C., and Yew, N. C.: Ion analysis in the SEM. In *Scanning Electron Microscopy,* edited by Johari, O., and Corvin, I., p. 81. Chicago, IIT Research Institute, 1973.
105. Langer, A. M.: Inorganic particles in human tissues and their association with neoplastic disease. *Environ. Health Persp. 9:* 229–233, 1974.
106. Langer, A. M., Rubin, I. B., and Selikoff, I. J.: Chemical characterization of asbestos body cores by electron microprobe analysis. *J. Histochem. Cytochem. 20:* 723–734, 1972.
107. Langer, A. M., and Wolff, M. S.: Asbestos carcinogenesis. In *Inorganic and Nutritional Aspects of Cancer,* edited by Schrauzer, G. N. Plenum Press, 1978.
108. Lapp, N. L.: Industrial bronchitis. In *Occupational Lung Diseases,* edited by Morgan, W. K. C., and Seaton, A., Chapter 13, pp. 265–273. Philadelphia, W. B. Saunders Co., 1974.
109. Lauweryns, J. M., and Baert, J. H.: Alveolar clearance and the role of the pulmonary lymphatics. *Am. Rev. Resp. Dis. 115:* 625–683, 1977.
110. Lee, R. E., Jr.: The size of suspended particulate matter in air. *Science 178:* 567–575, 1972.
111. Liebow, A. A.: New concepts and entities in pulmonary disease. In *The Lung,* edited by Liebow, A. A., and Smith, D. E., Chapter 24, pp. 332–365. Baltimore, The Williams & Wilkins Co., 1968.
112. Liebow, A. A.: Definition and classification of interstitial pneumonias in human pathology. *Prog. Resp. Res. 8:* 1–33, 1975.
113. Liebow, A. A., and Smith, D. E. (eds.): *The Lung.* The Williams & Wilkins Co., Baltimore, Maryland 1968.
114. Liebow, A. A., Steer, A., and Billingsley, J. G.: Desquamative interstitial pneumonia. *Am. J. Med. 39:* 369–404, 1965.
115. Linton, R. W., Loh, A., Natusch, D. F. S., Evans, C. A., and Williams, P.: Surface predominance of trace elements in airborne particles. *Science 191:* 852–854, 1976.
116. Lippmann, M., Albert, R. E., and Peterson, H. T.: The regional deposition of inhaled aerosols in man. *Inhaled Part. Vap. 3:* 105–122, 1970.
117. Loewenstein, W. R.: On the genesis of cellular communication. *Develop. Biol. 15:* 503–520, 1967.
118. Lourenco, R. V. (ed): Inhaled aerosol symposium. *Arch. Int. Med. 131:* 21–166, 1973.
119. Määttä, K., and Arstila, A. U.: Pulmonary deposits of titanium dioxide in cytologic and lung biopsy specimens. Light and electron microscopic X-ray analysis. *Lab. Invest. 33:* 342–346, 1975.
120. McCallum, R. I., Underhill, J., and Aird, E. G. A.: Measurement of antimony oxide dust in human lungs *in vivo* by X-ray spectrophotometry. *Inhaled Part. Vap. 2:* 611–618, 1970.
121. McEuen, D. D., and Abraham, J. L.: Particulate concentrations in pulmonary alveolar proteinosis. *Am. J. Pathol.,* (submitted for publication).
122. McEuen, D. D., and Abraham, J. L.: Unpublished results.
123. Meyer, E. C., and Liebow, A. A.: Relationship of interstitial pneumonia, honeycombing and atypical epithelial proliferation to cancer of the lung. *Cancer 18:* 322–351, 1965.
124. Milic-Emili, J., Henderson, J. A. M., and Kaneko, H.: Regional distribution of pulmonary ventilation. In *Form and Function in the Human Lung,* edited by Cumming, G., and Hunt, L. B., pp. 66–75. London, E. & S. Livingstone Ltd., 1968.
125. Miller, A., Langer, A. M., Tierstein, A. S., and Selikoff, I. J.: "Nonpsecific" interstitial pulmonary fibrosis. Association with asbestos fibers detected by electron microscopy. *N. Engl. J. Med. 292:* 91–93, 1975.
126. Mooney, F.: Coal worker's pneumoconiosis and carcinoma of the lung. *Lancet 1:* 43, 490, 1975.
127. Morgan, W. K. C.: Personal communication.
128. Morgan, W. K. C., and Lapp, N. L.: Respiratory disease in coal miners. *Am. Rev. Resp. Dis. 113:* 531–559, 1976.
129. Morgan, W. K. C., and Seaton, A.: *Occupational Lung Diseases.* Philadelphia, W. B. Saunders Co., 1975.
130. Morrow, P. E.: Experimental studies of inhaled materials. A basis for respiratory models. *Arch. Intern. Med. 126:* 466–470, 1970.
131. Morrow, P. E.: Lymphatic drainage of the lung in dust clearance. *Ann. N.Y. Acad. Sci. 200:* 46–65, 1972.
132. Mossman, B. T., Kessler, J. B., Ley, B. W., and Craighead, J. E.: Interaction of Crocidolite asbestos with hamster respiratory mucosa in organ culture. *Lab. Invest. 36:* 131–139, 1977.

133. Naeye, R. L.: The anthracotic pneumoconioses. *Curr. Top. Pathol. 55:* 37–68, 1971.
134. Naeye, R. L.: Black lung disease, the anthracotic pneumoconioses. *Pathol. Annu. 8:* 349–377, 1973.
135. Nagelschmidt, G., Rivers, D., King, E. J., and Trevella, W.: Dust and collagen content of lungs of coal-workers with progressive massive fibrosis. *Br. J. Indust. Med. 20:* 181-191, 1963.
136. Natusch, D. F. S., and Wallace, J. R.: Urban aerosol toxicity: The influence of particle size. *Science 186:* 695–699, 1974.
137. Newhouse, M., Sanchis, J., and Bienenstock, J.: Lung defense mechanisms. *N. Engl. J. Med. 295:* 990–998, 1045–1052, 1976.
138. Niewoehner, D. E., and Cosio, M. G.: See Chapter 9 of this volume.
139. Niewoehner, D. E., Kleinerman, J., and Rice, D. B.: Pathologic changes in the peripheral airways of young cigarette smokers. *N. Engl. J. Med. 291:* 755–758, 1974.
140. Nifong, G. D., Boettner, E. A., and Winchester, J. W.: Particle size distributions of trace elements in pollution aerosols. *Am. Ind. Hyg. Assoc. J. 33:* 569–775, 1972.
141. *Occupational Exposure to Asbestos.* Criteria for a recommended standard. U.S. Dept. of Health, Education, and Welfare, National Institute for Occupational Safety and Health, Rockville, Maryland, 1972.
142. Ortmeyer, C. E., and Abraham, J. L.: Unpublished data.
143. Ortmeyer, C. E., Costello, J., Morgan, W. K. C., Swecker, S., and Peterson, M.: The mortality of Appalachian coal miners, 1963 to 1971. *Arch. Environ. Health 29:* 67–72, 1974.
144. Parkes, W. R.: *Occupational Lung Disorders.* London, Butterworths, 1974.
145. Pintar, K., Funahashi, A., and Siegesmund, K. A.: A diffuse form of pulmonary silicosis in foundry workers. *Arch. Pathol. Lab. Med. 100:* 535–538, 1976.
146. Pratt, P. C.: Role of silica in progressive massive fibrosis in coal workers' pneumoconiosis. *Arch. Environ. Health 16:* 734–737, 1968.
147. Pratt, P.: See Chapter 3 of this volume.
148. Pratt, P. C., and Kilburn, K. H.: Extent of pulmonary pigmentation as an indicator of particulate environmental air pollution. *Inhaled Part. Vap. 2:* 661–670, 1970.
149. Prine, J. R., Brokeshoulder, S. F., McVean, D. E., and Robinson, F. R.: Demonstration of the presence of beryllium in pulmonary granulomas. *Am. J. Clin. Pathol. 45:* 448–454, 1966.
150. Respiratory disease in industry. *J. Occup. Med. 15:* 166–307, 1973.
151. Robinson, F. R., Brokeshoulder, S. F., Thomas, A. A., and Cholak, J.: Microemission spectrochemical analysis of human lungs for beryllium. *Am. J. Clin. Pathol. 49:* 821–825, 1968.
152. Rodnan, G. P., Benedek, T. G., Medsger, T. A., and Cammarata, R. J.: The association of progressive systemic sclerosis (scleroderma) with coal miners' pneumoconiosis and other forms of silicosis. *Ann. Int. Med. 66:* 323–334, 1967.
153. Rosen, S. H., Castleman, B., and Liebow, A. A.: Pulmonary alveolar proteinosis. *N. Engl. J. Med. 258:* 1123–1142, 1958.
154. Rossiter, C. E.: Evidence of dose-response relation in pneumoconiosis. *Trans. Soc. Occup. Med. 22:* 83–87, 1972.
155. Rubin, I. B., and Maggiore, C. J.: Elemental analysis of asbestos fibers by means of electron probe techniques. *Environ. Health Persp. 9:* 81–94, 1974.
156. Rüttner, J. R., Spycher, M. A., and Sticher, H.: The detection of etiologic agents in interstitial pulmonary fibrosis. *Hum. Pathol. 4:* 497–512, 1973.
157. Saccomanno, G., Archer, V. E., Auerbach, O., and Saunders, R. P.: Susceptibility and resistance to environmental carcinogens in the development of carcinoma of the lung. *Hum. Pathol. 4:* 487–495, 1973.
158. Saffiotti, U., and Wagoner, J. K. (eds.): Occupational carcinogenesis. *Ann. N.Y. Acad. Sci. 271:* 1–516, 1976.
159. Samimi, B., Weill, H., and Ziskind, M.: Respirable silica dust exposure of sandblasters and associated workers in steel fabrication yards. *Arch. Environ. Health 29:* 61–66, 1974.
160. Sanchis, J., Dolovich, M., Chalmers, R., and Newhouse, M. T.: Regional distribution and lung clearance mechanisms in smokers and non-smokers. *Inhaled Part. Vap. 3:* 183–191, 1971.
161. Scarano, D., Fadali, A. M., and Lemole, G. M.: Carcinoma of the lung and anthracosilicosis. *Chest 62:* 251–254, 1972.
162. Schrauzer, G. N. (ed.): *Inorganic and Nutritional Aspects of Cancer.* Plenum Press, 1978.

163. Selikoff, I. J.: Widening perspectives of occupational lung disease. *Prev. Med. 2:* 412–437, 1973.
164. Selikoff, I. J., and Churg, J. (eds.): Biological effects of asbestos. *Ann. N.Y. Acad. Sci. 132:* 1–766, 1965.
165. Selikoff, I. J., and Hammond, E. C.: Asbestos bodies in the New York City population in two periods of time. In *Pneumoconiosis. Proceedings of the International Conference, Johannesburg, 1969,* edited by Shapiro, H. A. pp. 99–105. Capetown, Oxford University Press, 1970.
166. Selikoff, I. J., Hammond, E. C., and Churg, J.: Asbestos exposure, smoking, and neoplasia. *JAMA 204:* 106–112, 1968.
167. Selikoff, I. J., Key, M. M., and Lee, D. H. K. (eds.): Coal workers' pneumoconiosis. *Ann. N.Y. Acad. Sci. 200:* 5–861, 1972.
168. Shapiro, H. A. (ed.): Pneumoconiosis: Proceedings of the *International Conference, in* Johannesburg, 1969. Capetown, Oxford University Press, 1970.
169. Siegesmund, K. A., Funahashi, A., and Pintar, K.: Identification of metals in lung from a patient with interstitial pneumonia. *Arch. Environ. Health 28:* 345–349, 1974.
170. Solomon, A., Goldstein, B., Webster, I., and Sluis-Cremer, G. K.: Massive fibrosis in asbestosis. *Environ. Res. 4:* 430–439, 1971.
171. Sorokin, S. P., and Brain, J. D.: Pathways of clearance in mouse lungs exposed to iron oxide aerosols. *Anat. Rec. 181:* 581–626, 1975.
172. Spencer, H.: The pneumoconioses and other occupational lung diseases. In *The Pathology of the Lung.* 3rd ed., pp. 371–462. Oxford, Pergamon Press, 1973.
173. Stokinger, H. E. (ed): *Beryllium—Its Industrial Hygiene Aspects.* New York, Academic Press, 1966.
174. Strain, W. H.: Prevalence hazards and modes of action of trace elements. Prepared for the *NIEHS Task Force on Research Planning in Environmental Health Science.* On deposit at the National Library of Medicine, Bethesda, Maryland, 1969.
175. Suratt, P. M., Winn, W. C., Jr., Brody, A. R., Bolton, W. K., and Giles, R. D.: Acute silicosis in tombstone sandblasters. *Am. Rev. Resp. Dis. 115:* 521–529, 1977.
176. Suzuki, Y., and Churg, J.: Formation of the asbestos body. A comparative study with three types of asbestos. *Environ. Res. 3:* 107–118, 1969.
177. Tabershaw, I. R. (ed.): *The Toxicology of Beryllium.* U.S. Department of Health, Education and Welfare, PHS, Health Services and Mental Health Administration, NIOSH, 1972.
178. Tapp, E., Curry, A., and Anfield, C.: Sand pneumoconiosis in an Egyptian mummy. *Br. Med. J. 2:* 276, 1975.
179. Thurlbeck, W. M.: *Chronic Airflow Obstruction in Lung Disease.* Vol. 5., Major Problems in Pathology. Philadelphia, W. B. Saunders Co., 1976.
180. Timbrell, V.: The inhalation of fibers. In *Pneumoconiosis. Proceedings of the International Conference, Johannesburg, 1969,* edited by Shapiro, H. A. pp. 99–105. Capetown, Oxford University Press, 1970.
181. Timbrell, V., Griffiths, D. M., and Pooley, F. D.: Possible biological importance of fibre diameters of South African amphiboles. *Nature 232:* 55–56, 1971.
182. Timbrell, V., and Skidmore, J. W.: The effect of shape on particle penetration and retention in animal lungs. *Inhaled Part. Vap. 3:* 49–57, 1970.
183. Tomenius, L.: A study on tracheobronchial deposition and 2-hour retention in rabbits. *Environ. Physiol. Biochem. 5:* 1–7, 1975.
184. Tucker, A. D., Wyatt, J. H., and Undery, O.: Clearance of inhaled particles from alveoli by normal interstitial drainage pathways. *J. Appl. Physiol. 35:* 719–732, 1973.
185. Turner-Warwick, M.: A perspective view on widespread pulmonary fibrosis. *Br. Med. J. 2:* 371–376, 1974.
186. UICC/Cincinnati classification of the radiographic appearances of pneumoconioses. A cooperative study by the UICC Committee. *Chest 58:* 57–67, 1970.
187. Wagner, J. C., Wusteman, F. S., Edwards, J. H., and Hill, R. J.: The composition of massive lesions in coal miners. *Thorax 30:* 382–388, 1975.
188. Walton, W. H. (ed.): *Inhaled Particles and Vapours III.* Unwin Brothers, Limited, London, 1970.
189. Walton, W. H. (ed.): *Inhaled Particles IV.* Unwin Brothers, Limited, London, 1977.
190. Watson, A. J., Black, J., Doig, A. T., and Nagelschmidt, G.: Pneumoconiosis in carbon electrode makers. *Br. J. Ind. Med. 16:* 274–285, 1959.

191. Wells, A. B., and Lamerton, L. F.: Regenerative response of the rat tracheal epithelium after acute exposure to tobacco smoke: A quantitative study. *J. Natl. Cancer Inst. 55:* 887–891, 1975.
192. Wells, O. C.: *Scanning Electron Microscopy.* New York, McGraw-Hill, 1974.
193. West, J. B. (ed.): *Regional Differences in the Lung.* New York, Academic Press, 1976.
194. Weston, J. T., Liebow, A. A., Dixon, M. G., and Rich, T. H.: Untoward effects of exogenous inhalants on the lung. *J. Forens. Sci. 17:* 199–279, 1972.
195. Whitwell, F., Newhouse, M. L., and Bennett, D. R.: A study of the histological cell types of lung cancer in workers suffering from asbestosis in the United Kingdom. *Br. J. Ind. Med. 31:* 298–303, 1974.
196. Whitwell, F., and Rawcliffe, R. M.: Diffuse malignant pleural mesothelioma and asbestos exposure. *Thorax 26:* 6–22, 1971.
197. Wilding, L. P., and Drees, L. R.: Biogenic opal in Ohio soils. *Soil Sci. Soc. Am. Proc. 35:* 1004–1010, 1971.
198. Woldseth, R.: *X-ray energy spectrometry.* Berkeley, Kevex Corp., 1973.
199. Wolman, M.: *Pigments in Pathology.* New York, Academic Press, 1969.
200. Wyatt, J. P.: Occupational lung diseases and inferential relationships to general population hazards. *Am. J. Pathol. 64:* 197–216, 1971.
201. Yesner, R.: Personal communication.
202. Yesner, R., Gelfman, N. A., and Feinstein, A. R.: A reappraisal of histopathology in lung cancer and correlation of cell types with antecedent cigarette smoking. *Am. Rev. Resp. Dis. 107:* 790–797, 1973.
203. Zaidi, S. H.: *Experimental Pneumoconiosis.* Baltimore, The Johns Hopkins Press, 1969.
204. Zenker, F. A.: *Staubinhalations Krankheiten der Lungen.* 1866.
205. Ziskind, M., Jones, R. N., and Weill, H.: Silicosis. *Am. Rev. Resp. Dis. 113:* 643–665, 1976.

Chapter 7

The Cell Biology of Mucus Secretion in the Lung

LYNNE REID

Mucus has an important protective role in the lung. Irritation increases its production: arguing teleologically it is presumed that this is to help in dilution, trapping, and removal of noxious vapors and particulate agents. Since excessive production of mucus is found in several diseases and is associated with structural changes in the airways and sometimes also with serious impairment of respiratory function, the events of mucus secretion are important both in health and disease.

NATURE OF MUCUS SECRETION

The special rheologic features of bronchial mucus arise from the epithelial acid glycoproteins.[3] A glycoprotein is a conjugated protein in which a polypeptide core is covalently linked to oligosaccharide side chains, often branched, without a repeating unit and with a relatively low proportion of sugar residues.[7] Three glycoproteins had been described, and were designated sialomucin, sulphomucin, and fucomucin, although each contained sialic acid and the first two contained sulphate also.[6] However, the histochemical results did not fit with this picture since individual cells might make only a sialylated molecule.[15] On the other hand, the variety of molecular pattern found within granule and cell was greater than suggested by biochemical investigation. It seems that the biochemical data were in large part the result of the methods used to solubilize the native mucus. Since sputum is not suitable for biochemical analysis, various methods of pretreatment are commonly used, varying from ultrasonication to chemical degradation. More recently, other techniques have improved our understanding of the molecular structure.[5, 30] By density gradient ultracentrifugation the mucus glycoprotein can be separated from other macromolecules, in particular from the serum protein components, and in an undegraded form. Purification in this way gives a homogeneous, but polydisperse substance of high molecular weight, between 3 and 7 $\times 10^6$ (Table 1). The glycoprotein molecule can be compared to a porcupine or to the brush end of a bottle brush (Fig. 1). It now seems that there are naked peptide regions lacking oligosaccharide side chains or quills and that at these sites disulphide bonds are found.[31] Action by substances such as dithiothreitol (DTT), which reduce these bonds, indicates that perhaps ten or so are present in the macromolecule. The subunit is, therefore, still large.

TABLE 1. ANALYTICAL COMPOSITION* OF BRONCHIAL GLYCOPROTEINS ISOLATED FROM SPUTUM BY DENSITY-GRADIENT METHODS

Sputum number	12	13	14	17	20
Diagnosis	CB	CB	CB	IA + Bhoea	EA
Fucose	8	8	7	14	7
Galactose	21	21	17	26	20
N-Acetyl glucosamine	22	24	23	22	18
N-Acetyl galactosamine	9	8	9	11	14
Glucose	—	0.4	0.7	1.2	0.5
Mannose	0.6	0.7	1.3	1.4	1.5
N-Acetyl neuraminic acid	23	12	16	1	11
Amino acids	19	23	23	22	30
Total	103	97	97	99	102

* Expressed as gm of component/100 gm of glycoprotein. CB, chronic bronchitis, IA + Bhoea, intrinsic asthma associated with bronchorrhoea; EA, extrinsic asthma.

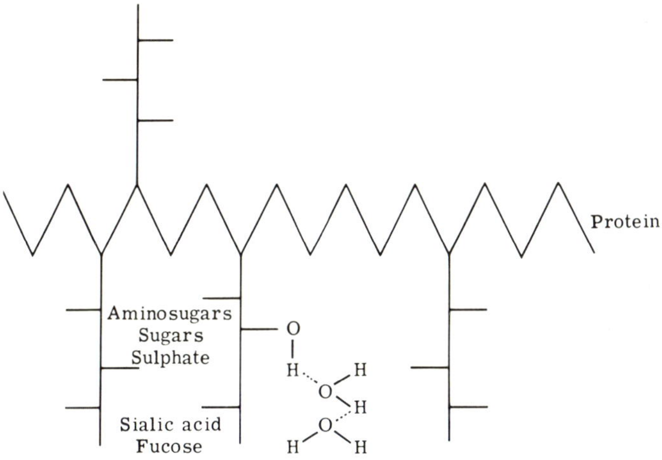

FIG. 1. A diagramatic illustration of a glycoprotein molecule. This is a polypeptide core covalently linked to repeating oligosaccharide side chains. Sialic acid, fucose and sulphate may be attached to the side chain.

A similar pattern has been reported for gastric mucus by Snary et al.[33] and for bovine cervical mucus by Silberberg.[32] The size of the unit and of the macromolecule seems to be smaller for gastrointestinal than for bronchial mucus.

SECRETORY CELLS OF AIRWAY EPITHELIUM

The airway cells that secrete the mucus glycoprotein are found in the submucosal glands and in the surface epithelium. The volume of the submucosal glands is greater than of the secretory cells in the surface epithelium.

In histologic sections a gland consists of the tubules that are seen in cross-section—the acini. Three-dimensional reconstruction of the gland has shown that a collecting duct is an important part of the gland (Fig. 2).[23] It is usually missed in single sections because it passes obliquely from the airway surface. Since most sections of bronchial gland are cut at right angles to the airway, this structure, which is 1 mm long, is seen on cross-section only as another tubule. Furthermore, because of the structure of its lining, it does not stain for mucus and appears uniformly eosinophilic. This is seen ultrastructurally to be due to the many mitochondria that pack the cells. Secreting tubules open from the duct. Reconstruction (Fig. 2B) shows that their proximal part is always lined by mucus-secreting cells; their distal part by serous cells. A serous cell has recently been recognized in the surface epithelium[9] (Fig. 3). In the airways of the rat it is found centrally, while the Clara cell is found distally. Each has discrete electron-dense granules in contrast to the electron-lucent granules of the mucous cell which is rare at all levels. Two secretory cells can be identified in the tracheobronchial glands, the serous and the mucous cell.[22] In the surface epithelium these same two cell types can be identified, as well as the Clara cell.

HISTOCHEMICAL IDENTIFICATION OF GLYCOPROTEIN

Histochemically, differences in the oligosaccharide side chains of the glycoprotein can be identified. The periodic acid Schiff (PAS) reaction stains the sugar part of the glycoprotein, Alcian blue (AB) stains the acid radicals.[11, 15] Epithelial glycoproteins may be either sialylated or sulphated. At pH 1, Alcian blue stains

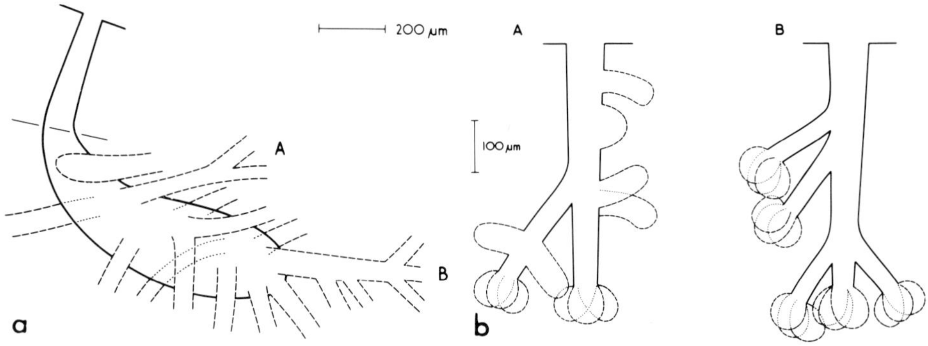

FIG. 2. Reconstruction of (*a*) gland drawn to scale showing collecting duct with tubules arising from it and (*b*) of tubules *A* and *B*. Serous cells, *broken line;* mucous cells, *continuous line.*

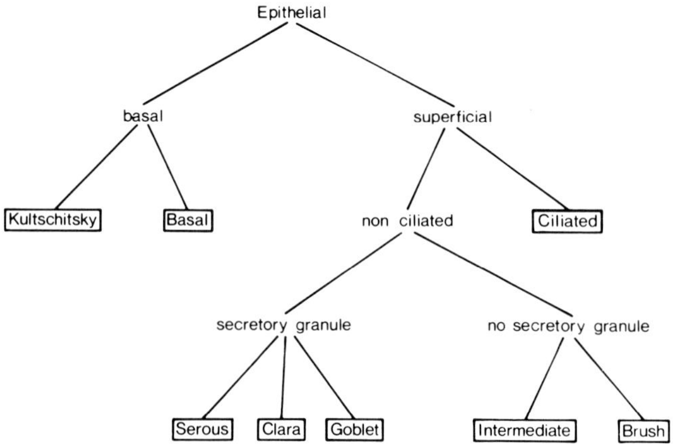

FIG. 3. Classification of eight epithelial cell types identified in airway epithelium. Of the secretory cells the serous cell is normally present in the proximal airways of the rat, the Clara cell in the distal.

TABLE 2. IDENTIFICATION OF EPITHELIAL GLYCOPROTEINS IN CONSECUTIVE TISSUE SECTIONS USING VARIOUS AB-PAS TECHNIQUES

Stain	Group identified
AB(pH 2.6)-PAS	All acid glycoprotein stains blue
Sialidase AB(pH 2.6)-PAS	Sialylated glycoprotein resistant to sialidase and sulphated glycoprotein stain blue
AB(pH 1.0)-PAS	Sulphated glycoprotein stains blue

TABLE 3. COMBINATION OF ACID RADICALS IDENTIFIED WITHIN SINGLE CELLS OF RAT AIRWAY EPITHELIUM

Type of acid glycoprotein	Individual cell type				
	I	II	III	IV	V
Sialylated glycoprotein					
sialidase sensitive	+	+			
sialidiase resistant		+	+	+	
Sulphated glycoprotein				+	+

TABLE 4. SPECIES VARIATION IN GLYCOPROTEIN TYPE WITHIN MUCOUS AND SEROUS CELLS OF SUBMUCOSAL GLAND

Species	Cell type	Neutral glycoprotein	Acid glycoprotein		
			Sialylated		Sulphated
			Sensitive	Resistant	
Rat (Sprague-Dawley)	mucous	±	−	+	+
	serous	+	+	+	+
Mouse	mucous	+	+	−	−
Cat	mucous	±	−	+	+
	serous	+	−	+	+
Dog	mucous	+	−	+	+
	serous	+	−	−	−
Pig	mucous	+	+	+	+
	serous	+	−	+	+

only the sulphate ester; at pH 2.6, it stains all acid radicals. Sialidase digestion removes the sialidase-susceptible sialic acid and leaves behind the resistant form. By staining a series of consecutive sections with these techniques, the various types of glycoprotein molecules with or without an acid radical (Table 2) can be identified.

Quantification makes it possible to assess the proportion of tracheobronchial glands that makes a given type of glycoprotein molecule. In the case of goblet cells the number of secretory cells can be counted and related to the total number of cells present. The various types of secretory cells can be expressed by reference to either total cells or total secretory cells. In the glands, point counting indicates the proportion of the gland occupied by the various types of cells.

By histochemical methods several acid radicals may be identified in the cells of one species. One cell may contain only one type, or more than one may be recognized. Only certain mixtures seem to occur. Table 3 illustrates the range of intracellular mixture found for the cells of the rat airway. A wide species difference is found (Table 4). Within any one species considerable variation may be found between the goblet cells at various airway levels. In man, the distribution of the various histochemical types is similar in the submucosal glands at the various airway levels.[19, 20]

CHANGES IN DISEASE

Chronic bronchitis is still defined as chronic mucous hypersecretion. In man, enlargement of the tracheobronchial mucous glands is the characteristic finding, together with an increase in the number of mucus-secreting cells in the surface epithelium at all levels.[25] Glycoprotein precursors containing acid radicals are increased; in particular, those containing sulphate ester or sialidase-resistant sialic acid.[21]

ORGAN CULTURE

The application of Trowell's method[37] of organ culture to the bronchial tree has contributed to the understanding of the control of bronchial mucous synthesis and its discharge.[28] Explants of tissue 1 cm in length and 1 mm wide and deep are cut from the bronchial mucosa of resected surgical specimens. Radioactive precursors of glycoprotein can be added to the organ culture medium to follow uptake, synthesis, and discharge.[34] If drugs also are added, their effect on this cycle can be followed.[35]

The general pattern of metabolic activity in the airway cells is similar to other secretory cells.[24] The peptide core is synthesized in the rough endoplasmic reticulum; oligosaccharide side chains are synthesized and added in the cisternae of the Golgi apparatus. It may be that the first sugar is added in the endoplasmic reticulum. Within this pattern, differences are found between the serous and mucous cells (Table 5).[28] In both types of cells, the granules show a similar range of staining characteristics, pointing to a similar chemical constitution. The serous cells have a lower specific activity over the granule, pointing to a lower concentration within the granule (Fig. 4). The serous cells discharge steadily but the cell granules stay discrete; the mucus-secreting cells discharge intermittently but more completely.

The cycle of the cell is quickly complete in that the precursor is taken up, incorporated into glycoprotein, and discharged within four hours. Investigation of a wide variety of drugs (Table 6) showed that secretion is increased by parasympathomimetic drugs and is reduced but never prevented by their antagonists. Hypertrophied glands are more sensitive to a given dose of a stimulating drug and less tolerant to an inhibiting one.

More recently, by reflectance microscopy, the concentration of the radioactive precursor within the cell has been taken into account, and by the use of various pharmacologic agents, the control of precursor uptake, synthesis, and discharge have been separately analyzed to determine whether synthesis and discharge are coupled.[4] It seems that over a matter of some hours synthesis and discharge are independent of each other.

ANIMAL MODELS OF DISEASE

The use of laboratory animals has made it possible to investigate intracellular events more closely, particularly under experimental conditions, after exposure to irritants[17, 18] or to drugs.[26, 27, 36] The stigmata described for chronic bronchitis have been produced in a variety of animals by a variety of agents. By studying

TABLE 5. SEROUS AND MUCOUS CELLS OF BRONCHIAL SUBMUCOSAL GLAND

	Differences	
	Serous	Mucous
Granules	(a) Sialo-, sulphomucin, and neutral glycoprotein (b) Electron-dense and discrete	Sialo- and sulphomucin separate or combined, no neutral glycoprotein Electron-lucent and confluent
Discharge	Merocrine into canaliculi and small lumen	Many granules together, like toothpaste, into large lumen
Position	Terminal or lateral end of main secretory tubule	Central in secretory tubule
Transformation	In airway epithelium, irritation changes serous to mucous	Mucous to serous transformation not found
Disease	Present in normal numbers	Hypertrophy of mucous acini in chronic bronchitis
Endoplasmic reticulum	60% endoplasmic reticulum throughout cell	30% endoplasmic reticulum mainly at cell base
Threonine uptake	Faster into Golgi than into mucus	
^{3}H-threonine and ^{3}H-glucose		Higher concentration in mucous than in serous cell
	Similarities	
	Secretory granules contain acid glycoprotein Drain into same tubule Same response to drugs Each cell divides Present both in gland and airway epithelium Granules contain threonine and glucose in 1:1 ratio Synthetic pathways are similar	

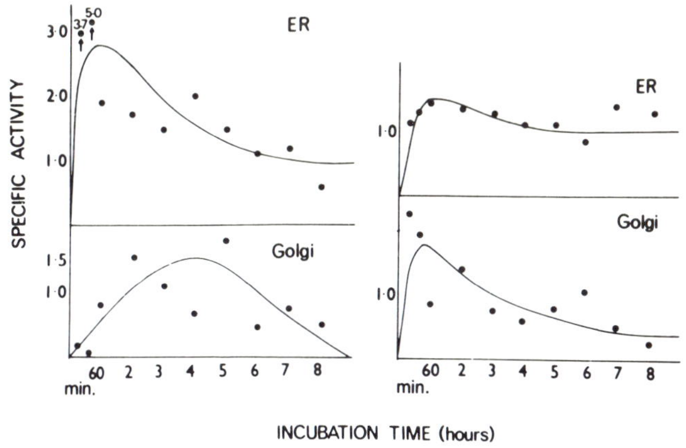

FIG. 4. Specific activity over endoplasmic reticulum and Golgi apparatus of mucous (*left*) and serous cells (*right*) after adding radioactive threonine to the organ culture medium. Slower passage to the Golgi apparatus is seen in the mucous cell.

the early effects of irritation it has been possible to trace the cell transformations that are responsible for shift in cell population.

Cell turnover is another aspect of epithelial function related to the change in cell population (Fig. 5).[2] Mitotic activity has been established for the various

TABLE 6. EFFECT OF PARASYMPATHOMIMETIC AND PARASYMPATHOLYTIC DRUGS ON SECRECTORY INDEX OF MUCOUS CELLS*

Parasympathomimetic drugs	Concentration (μg/ml)		
	1	10	100
Acetylcholine	+18	+38	
	+19	+41	
	+23		
	+25		
	+38		
	+40		
	+41		
	+43		
	+48	+72	
	+50		
	+84	+152	+180
	+92	+133	+156
		+143	
	+140		
Pilocarpine	+46	+54	
		+28	
Carbachol	+36	+48	
Parasympatholytic drugs	**Concentration (μg/ml)**		
	0.5	5	50
Atropine	−18	−29	−35
	−29		
	−58		
	−59		
	−73		
		−20	−31
		−33	
		−43	
		−55	
		−60	
		−71	
Hyoscine	−36	−48	

* The values present % increase (+) or decrease (−) in the secretory index as compared with the corresponding control tissue. Each row of values represents different specimens from the same bronchus.

airway levels in the rat, both male and female (Fig. 5)[2] and in the hamster.[16] The pathway followed by the cells as they differentiate is not established for certain, but it seems likely that the basal cell develops into the intermediate cell which has electron-lucent cytoplasm. This cell then differentiates either into a brush, ciliated, or Clara cell. Increasing density of the cytoplasm occurs as a cell develops into a serous or a mucous cell. Under basal conditions the distribution of the various cell types, and of the types of acid glycoprotein that they contain, differ at the various airway levels but they are relatively stable. Stimulation by irritants or drugs leads to a shift within the total cell population and within the types of secretory cells.

These changes are illustrated by describing the effect of tobacco smoke on the airway epithelium with or without the addition to the tobacco of phenylmethyloxadiazole (PMO).[13, 14] Tobacco produced an increase in the number of goblet cells, but if PMO had been added to the tobacco, this increase did not occur (Fig. 6). On the other hand, PMO had no effect on the glycoprotein shift (Fig. 7). Tobacco alone caused an increase in the cells containing acid glycoprotein and a relative reduction in those free from acid radicals. This same shift occurred after PMO in a cell population with a normal concentration of secreting cells: the "new" type of cell represented a transformation of secretory cells already present. The effect of tobacco also represented in part a change in secretory cells already present and in part a change from intermediate or undifferentiated cells into secretory ones. It is of interest that the concentration of ciliated cells was also increased and that ciliated and secretory cells both increased at the expense of the intermediate cells.[8]

In the proximal airways the new mucous cells represented a transformation of serous cells, at the periphery a transformation of Clara cells. In addition to

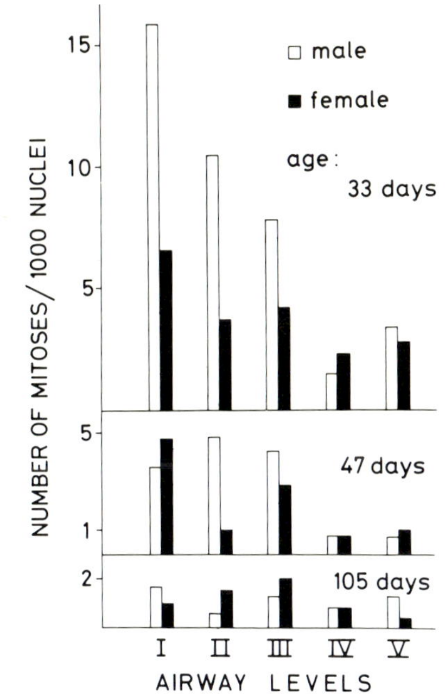

FIG. 5. Mitotic Index (number of mitoses per 1000 nuclei) in male and female colchicine-treated rats of 3 age groups and at 5 airway levels. Levels I to III, trachea; level IV, main bronchus; level V, distal airway.

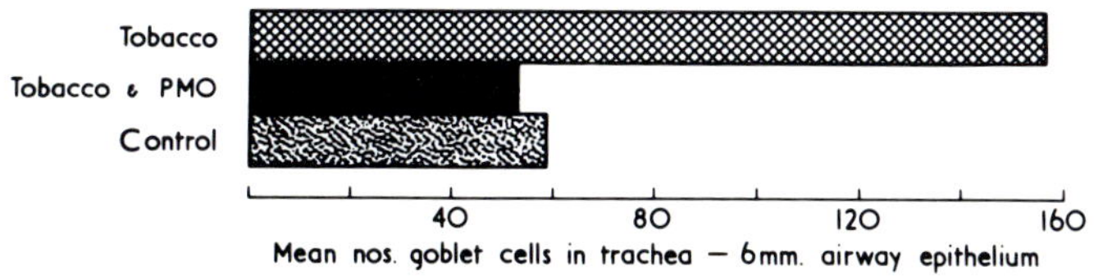

FIG. 6. Goblet cell number in a 6-mm length of trachea taken from animals exposed to: (*i*), smoke from tobacco; (*ii*), smoke from tobacco to which phenylmethyloxadiazole (*PMO*) had been added; and (*iii*), either control or sham exposed.

counting the proportion of the various types of cells, transitional forms could be identified by electron microscopy. The small, discrete, electron-dense granule of the serous cell developed into the large confluent and electron-lucent granule of the mucus-secreting cell.

In these experiments, as after the administration of the drugs described below, when acid glycoprotein appears within a cell it appears first at the apex; when a new type of acid radical appears, it also is first identified at the cell apex[10, 11] after the granules are separated from the Golgi apparatus. It seems that it is at the apex that the membrane is first "turned on" and the activity of new enzymes becomes apparent. Since the membrane is derived from the Golgi apparatus, these are doubtless Golgi membrane enzymes.

Not only is there a shift in the chemical type of glycoprotein contained within the cell, but also in the amount; cells that contained a small amount of secretion soon contained a large amount. Analysis of the shift in the cell population, using an analogue computer, suggests a number of ways in which an individual cell may change (Fig. 8). Other irritants can produce this effect and in other species. The effect of several drugs has been analyzed in a similar way. Isoprenaline sulphate increased the size of the submucosal glands as it did of the salivary glands.[36] More unexpectedly, it increased the number of goblet cells (Fig. 9).[36] To exclude infection as the cause, these experiments were repeated under germ-free conditions; the same increase in mucus-secreting cells occurred in the airway

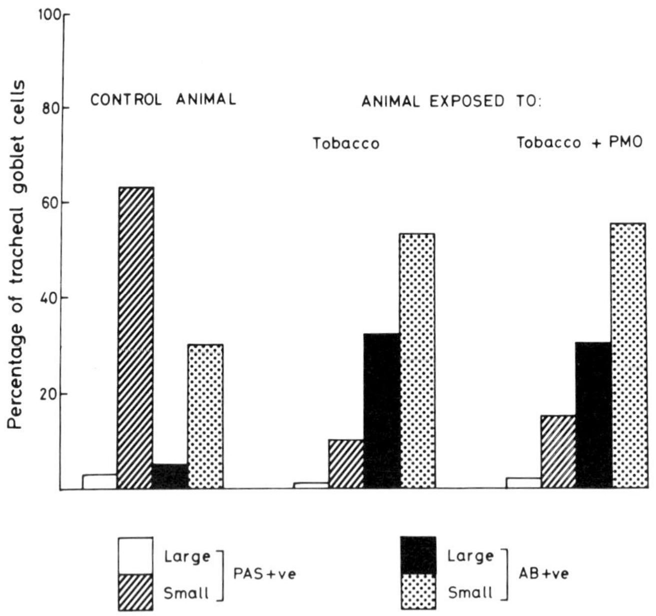

FIG. 7. Distribution of histochemical types of secretory cells in the experimental groups as under Figure 6. AB+ve cells, cells staining with Alcian blue, containing acid glycoprotein. PAS+ve cells, cells staining by periodic acid Schiff reaction indicate that no acid is identified in glycoprotein precursor. *Small* and *large* refer to the amount of secretory product within the cell. The histochemical shift is similar in both populations although it is only in *tobacco alone* that the secretory cell number is increased.

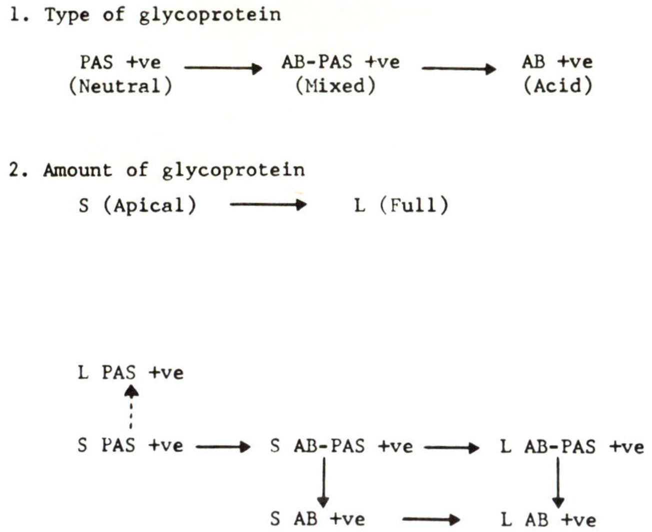

FIG. 8. "Irritation" produces a shift in the epithelial secretory cell population both in type of glycoprotein (*1*) and in amount (*2*). A flow chart shows the way a cell may transform. Abbreviations as in Figure 7; *S*, small, *L*, large.

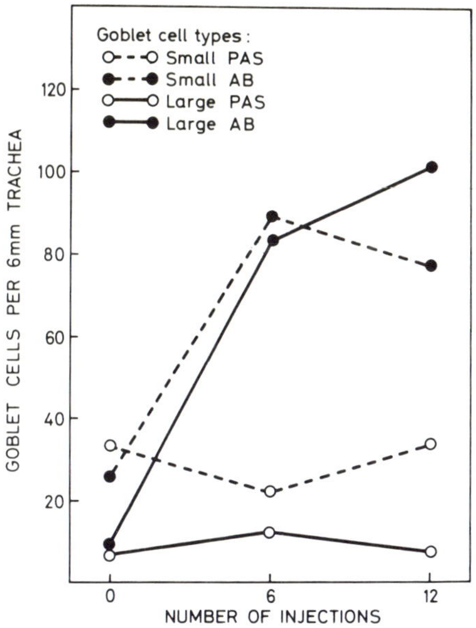

FIG. 9. An increase in total goblet cell number is produced in the trachea by isoprenaline sulphate; it is the cells containing acid glycoprotein (AB+ve) that are increased.

epithelium. Isoprenaline sulphate produced a similar gland hypertrophy in the pig.[1] In the same species, infection with *Mycoplasma hyorrhinis* in one lobe produced a diffuse gland hypertrophy throughout the airways.[12] These experiments show that infection, drugs, and irritants can each produce gland hypertrophy.

REVERSIBILITY

Reversal of the changes produced by isoprenaline sulphate[12] and by exposure to tobacco smoke has been demonstrated.[10] Three months after stopping the drug, gland size and goblet cell number had each returned to normal. It seems that the intracellular acid glycoprotein quickly shifts back toward the normal, following, in reverse, the way the changes had developed (Fig. 10). The increase in number of secretory cells can be related to increased mitotic activity. The speed of recovery has not yet been related to the turnover of the cell population, nor is the relation between the intracellular events and the total secretion entirely formulated.

The origin of the sol and gel phases of secretion is by no means clear. One hypothesis for which there is some evidence would be that the sol consists of the secretion of serous cells, either in gland or surface epithelium, and that mucous cells secrete the discrete viscid gobs that sit on the tips of the cilia. Recently, studies of the sol and gel have shown that the mucus glycoprotein is similar in both but that its concentration in the sol is less.

The variety of the molecular types seen as glycoprotein precursors in the granules and the variety of mixtures within the cells doubtless reflect the variety of oligosaccharide side chains attached to the polypeptide chain. It is particularly in the degree of sialylated and sulphated glycoprotein that they vary.[29]

Increase in the concentration of sialic acid is associated with increased viscosity. If viscid mucus is a protection against noxious agents, then it may be considered desirable that irritation by such substances stimulate the cells to produce more secretion and that of a more viscid form. Shifts in the cell population as a whole and in the intracellular events of a single cell are quickly able to achieve this.

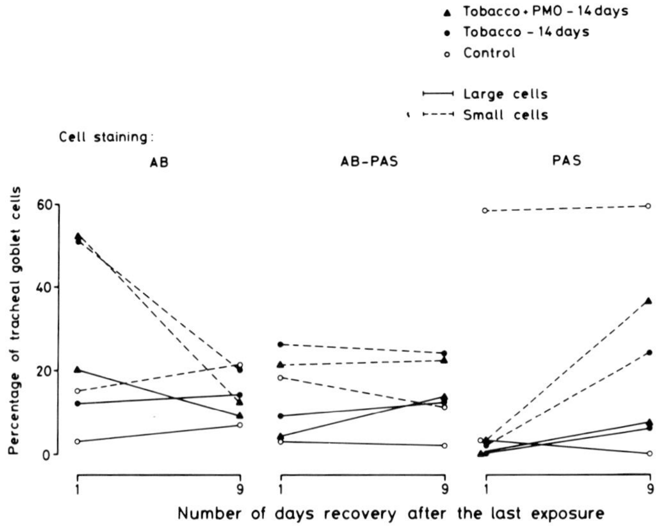

FIG. 10. When exposure to tobacco smoke ceases, cells containing acid glycoprotein decrease in number; those cells containing neutral glycoprotein increase.

REFERENCES

1. Baskerville, A.: The development and persistence of bronchial-gland hypertrophy and goblet-cell hyperplasia in the pig after injection of isoprenaline. *J. Pathol. 119:* 35–47, 1976.
2. Bolduc, P.: Cell turnover of the bronchial and alveolar lining in the rat lung in various types of hypertrophy. Doctoral thesis, University of London, 1976.
3. Charman, J., Lopez-Vidriero, M. T., Keal, E., and Reid, L.: The physical and chemical properties of bronchial secretion. *Br. J. Dis. Chest 68:* 215–227, 1974.
4. Coles, S.: The nature and control of glycoprotein secretion by the human bronchial glands. Doctoral thesis, University of London, 1976.
5. Creeth, J. H., Bhaskar, K. R., Horton, J., Das, I., Lopez-Vidriero, M. T., and Reid, L.: The separation and characterisation of bronchial glycoproteins by density gradient methods. *Biochem. J. 167:* 557–569, 1977.
6. Degand, P., Roussel, P., Lamblin, G., Durand, G., and Havez, R.: Données biochimiques et rheologiques dans l'expectoration. I: Définition biochimique des mucines dans l'expectoration. *Bull. Physiopath. Resp. 9:* 199–217, 1973.
7. Gottschalk, A.: Definition of glycoproteins and their delineation from other carbohydrate-protein complexes. In *Glycoproteins: Their Composition, Structure and Function,* edited by Gottschalk, A., Chapter 2, pp. 24–30. Amsterdam, London, and New York, Elsevier Publishing Co., 1972.
8. Jeffery, P. K.: Goblet cell increase in rat bronchial epithelium arising from irritation or drug administration—An experimental and electron microscopic study. Doctoral thesis, London University, 1973.
9. Jeffery, P. K., and Reid, L.: New observations of rat airway epithelium: A quantitative and electron microscopic study. *J. Anat. 120:* 295–320, 1975.
10. Jones, R.: Modification of mucus in animal models of disease. International Symposium of Mucus in Health and Disease, September 13–16, 1976. Surrey, England, University of Guildford, 1977.
11. Jones, R.: The glycoproteins of secretory cells in airway epithelium. In *Respiratory Tract Mucus, Ciba Foundation Symposium.* Amsterdam, Elsevier/Excerpta Medica/North-Holland, pp. 175–188, 1978.
12. Jones, R., Baskerville, A., and Reid, L.: Histochemical identification of glycoproteins in pig bronchial epithelium: (a) normal and (b) hypertrophied from enzootic pneumonia. *J. Pathol. 116:* 1–11, 1975.
13. Jones, R., Bolduc, P., and Reid, L.: Protection of rat bronchial epithelium against tobacco smoke. *Br. Med. J. 2:* 142–144, 1972.
14. Jones, R., Bolduc, P., and Reid, L.: Goblet cell glycoprotein and tracheal gland hypertrophy in rat airways: The effect of tobacco smoke with or without the anti-inflammatory agent phenylmethyloxadiazole. *Br. J. Exp. Pathol. 54:* 229–239, 1973.
15. Jones, R., and Reid, L.: The effect of pH on Alcian blue staining of the epithelial acid glycoproteins. II: Human bronchial submucosal gland. *Histochem. J. 5:* 19–27, 1973.
16. Kleinerman, J.: Inhalation carcinogenesis. *AEC Symposium Series 18:* 271, 1970.
17. Lamb, D., and Reid, L.: Mitotic rates, goblet cell increase and histochemical changes in mucus in rat bronchial epithelium during exposure to sulphur dioxide. *J. Pathol. Bacteriol. 96:* 97–111, 1968.
18. Lamb, D., and Reid, L.: Goblet cell increase in rat bronchial epithelium after exposure to cigarette and cigar tobacco smoke. *Br. Med. J. 1:* 33–35, 1969.
19. Lamb, D., and Reid, L.: Histochemical types of acidic glycoprotein produced by mucous cells of the trancheobronchial glands in man. *J. Pathol. 98:* 213–229, 1969.
20. Lamb, D. and Reid, L.: Histochemical and autoradiographic investigation of the serous cells of the human bronchial glands. *J. Pathol. 100:* 127–138, 1970.
21. McCarthy, C., and Reid, L.: Intracellular mucopolysaccharides in the normal human bronchial tree. *Quart. J. Exp. Physiol. 49:* 85–94, 1964.
22. Meyrick, B., and Reid, L.: Ultrastructure of cells in the human bronchial submucosal glands. *J. Anat. 107:* 281–299, 1970.
23. Meyrick, B., Sturgess, J. M., and Reid, L.: A reconstruction of the duct system and secretory tubules of the human bronchial submucosal gland. *Thorax 24:* 729–736, 1969.

24. Meyrick, G., and Reid, L.: In vitro incorporation of [^{3}H]threonine and [^{3}H]glucose by the mucous and serous cells of the human bronchial submucosal gland: A quantitative electron microscope study. *J. Cell Biol. 67:* 320–344, 1975.
25. Reid, L.: Bronchial mucus production in health and disease. In *The Lung, International Academy of Pathology Monograph No. 8,* edited by Liebow, A. A., and Smith, D. E. Chapter 8, pp. 87–108. Baltimore, The Williams & Wilkins Co., 1968.
26. Reid , L.: An experimental study of hypersecretion of mucus in the bronchial tree. *Br. J. Exp. Pathol. 44:* 437–445, 1963.
27. Reid, L.: Evaluation of model systems for study of airway epithelium, cilia, and mucus. *Arch. Int. Med. 126:* 428–434, 1970.
28. Reid, L., Meyrick, G., and Coles, S.: Glycoprotein synthetic pathways in, and drug effects on, the human bronchial mucosa in vitro. In *Organ Culture in Biomedical Research, British Society for Cell Biology Symposium,* edited by Balls, M. and Monnickendam, M., p. 463. London, Cambridge University Press, 1976.
29. Reid, L.: Secretory cells. *Fed. Proc., 36:* 2703–2707, 1977.
30. Roberts, G. P.: Isolation and characterisation of glycoproteins from sputum. *Eur. J. Biochem. 50:* 265–280, 1974.
31. Roberts, G. P.: The role of disulfide bonds in maintaining the gel structure of bronchial mucus. *Arch. Biochem. Biophys. 173:* 528–537, 1976.
32. Silberberg, A.: Structure and function of mucus. In *Respiratory Tract Mucus, Ciba Foundation Symposium.* Amsterdam, Elsevier/Excerpta Medica/North-Holland, 1978.
33. Snary, D., Allen, A., and Pain, R. H.: The structure of pig gastric mucus, conformational transitions induced by salt. *Eur. J. Biochem. 24:* 183–189, 1971.
34. Sturgess, J., and Reid, L.: Secretory activity of the human bronchial mucous glands *in vitro. Exp. and Mol. Pathol. 16:* 362–381, 1972.
35. Sturgess, J., and Reid, L.: An organ culture study of the effect of drugs on the secretory activity of the human bronchial submucosal gland. *Clin. Sci. 43:* 533–543, 1972.
36. Sturgess, J., and Reid, L.: The effect of isoprenaline and pilocarpine on (a) bronchial mucus-secreting tissue and (b) pancreas, salivary glands, heart, thymus, liver and spleen. *Br. J. Exp. Pathol. 54:* 388–403, 1973.
37. Trowell, O. A.: The culture of mature organs in a synthetic medium. Problems of maintenance of mature organs in vivo. *Exp. Cell Res. 16:* 118–147, 1959.

Chapter 8

Quantitative Morphology and Structure: Functional Correlations in the Lung

KEITH HORSFIELD

The techniques developed by geologists for estimating proportions of minerals in rocks have been applied with considerable success to the study of both normal and abnormal lung structure. Point counting and linear intercept methods applied to macroscopic and microscopic sections of lung tissue have allowed estimates to be made of numbers of structures and their dimensions, and to quantitate lesions in lungs and airways. Notable advances were made by Weibel[20] and Dunnill[3, 4] in the early 1960's. Weibel studied five human lungs and found that the alveolar surface area was about 70 m^2, the total number of alveoli was 300×10^6, that the capillary surface area approximated alveolar surface area, that the average air-blood distance in the alveolar wall was approximately 1 μm, and that the proportion of lung formed by alveolar duct increased with age while the proportion formed by alveoli decreased. Besides introducing widely accepted methods for quantitating emphysema[3] and bronchial wall components,[5] Dunnill indicated that there were only 20×10^6 alveoli in a newborn infant's lung, that alveolar multiplication was rapid in the first two years of life, had slowed by age 4 years, and had probably stopped by age 8 years.[4] Since then work has mostly been an amplification of their data, with emphasis on variations due to stature and age. In brief, the following have been the major amplifications. Alveolar surface area shows a wide range of 40–100 m^2, and is primarily determined by lung size—tall subjects have large lungs that have a large surface area.[17] Surface area decreases with age, starting perhaps at age 25,[17] and this is a reflection of the alterations in the internal geometry of the lung with age as noted by Weibel[20] and confirmed by others.[15, 18] Stature also determines the number of alveoli and a range of 250–450 $\times 10^6$ has been found in adult humans.[1] The total number of airways, both bronchi and bronchioles, remains the same irrespective of stature and lung volume, and thus these airways are larger in taller subjects.[12]

The observed variation in alveolar number in adults suggests that the conclusions reached from Dunnill's data about the rate and time of cessation of alveolar multiplication may not necessarily be correct. For example, he found 290×10^6 alveoli in an 8-year-old child and, since this was considered to be the adult complement at the time of his observation, it was assumed that alveolar multiplication had ceased by this age. However, it could be that this child was destined to have the number of alveoli at the upper limit of the normal range (450×10^6), so it is possible that only two-thirds of alveoli are formed by age 8. A much wider variation of alveolar number has recently been reported in children as might be anticipated from the wide range in adults.[18] A final amplification of Weibel's original observations is that there is a loss of alveolar wall tissue with increasing age beyond 20 years. The mechanism of this is unknown, but it is likely loss of capillary bed.[18]

A basic assumption in this approach is that the structures to be studied are distributed randomly in three-dimensional space. While this may hold true for the alveoli and alveolar ducts it is certainly not true of the conducting airways, which together make up a highly organized structure. Studies of the conducting airways have therefore utilized other techniques such as injection with radioopaque materials and radiologic demonstration of their morphology, or resin casting of the airways followed by dissolution of the lung tissue. When airway casts are studied, as many of the larger proximal branches are counted and measured as is reasonably possible within the time available, and samples of the more numerous peripheral airways may be broken off for study. The two sets of data thus obtained, proximal and distal, can be joined to give a continuous picture.

The lung is often thought of as consisting of three components—a *conducting zone* in which gas is transported but no gas is exchanged; a *transitional zone* in which there is both gas exchange and transport; and a *respiratory zone* in which gas is exchanged. In my view, the subdivision into a transitional zone and a respiratory zone is artificial since gas transport and gas exchange occur in both areas. It is true, however, that there are three sets of airway structure—one nonalveolated, one partly alveolated, and one completely alveolated. The conducting zone consists of bronchi (airways with cartilage in their walls) and bronchioles whose walls contain neither cartilage nor alveoli. Bronchioles are intimately connected to the elastic tissue and collagen of the alveolar walls. Thus dimensions of bronchioles are greatly influenced by the volume of the lung and the elastic recoil pressures within the lung. We have found it useful to describe the "lobular bronchiole" for quantitative purposes.[9] This bronchiole is the first airway distal from the trachea that is less than or equal to 0.7 mm in internal diameter. It is usually three orders (see below) proximal to the terminal bronchiole. The latter is the last purely conducting airway and the structure distal to it is known as the acinus, which is the gas-exchanging unit of the lung. The proximal few branches within the acinus have both alveolated and nonalveolated epithelium in their walls. They are the respiratory bronchioles. Distal to them are the entirely alveolated structures—alveolar ducts which lead into the terminal structures of the lung, the alveolar sacs.

In order to present airway data, to make calculations from them, and to make comparisons within and between species, some method of classification of airway data is required. The most generally used is that of Weibel,[20] in which generations are counted down from the trachea, itself designated generation zero. Weibel's model of the conducting airways consists of sixteen symmetric dichotomously branching generations: it has been widely used as a basis for physiologic calculation.[6, 13, 14]

The great value of Weibel's model is the ease with which it can be used; for example, the number of structures in any generation n is given by 2^n. Thus there are 2^{16} or 65,536 terminal bronchioles and the same number of acini, since each terminal bronchiole supplies one acinus, and 131,071 conducting airways. If the summed cross-sectional area of the airways at any level and their distance from the carina are represented as a single tube in longitudinal section a trumpet-shaped figure is obtained (Fig. 1, *left*). This model has been used in several attempts to compute the movement of gas by convection and diffusion in the airways.[13]

The overall shape of the airway system can be related to the physical process concerned with the movement of gas molecules within them. Considering for convenience the movement of oxygen from air to blood, there are three distinct physical processes involved: (1) convective flow in the conducting airways brought about by a transpulmonary pressure difference; (2) mixing of fresh inspired gas with residual alveolar gas by molecular diffusion; and (3) crossing the alveolar-capillary membrane by diffusion in the tissue phase.

The acinus is situated, on average, about 25 cm from the larynx and convective flow enables large volumes of gas to be transported rapidly over this distance. From the proximal alveolar ducts to the alveolar walls is a distance of about 2.6 mm, and oxygen diffuses over this distance during inspiration. The total mass transferred by this process is proportional to the cross-sectional area available, which is 10^4 cm^2 in the alveolar sacs, and to the diffusion coefficient of oxygen in nitrogen, which is 0.25 cm^2/sec. Finally, oxygen transverses the alveolar-capillary membrane by diffusion through the tissue, a distance of about 1 μm, with an

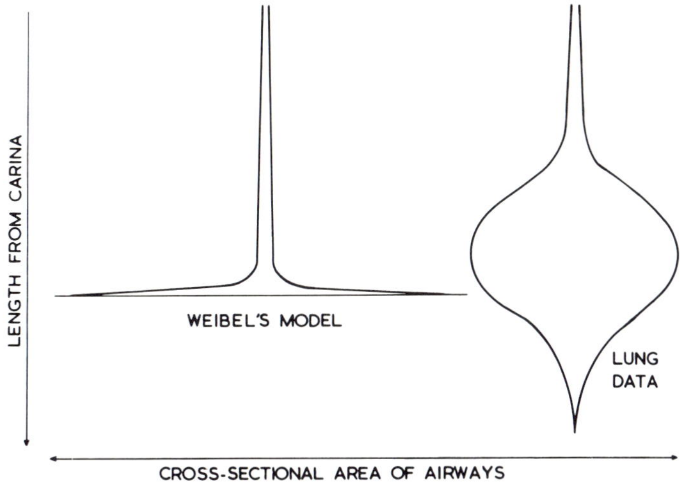

FIG. 1. The airways represented as a single structure shown in longitudinal section: (*left*), Weibel's symmetrical model;[20] (*right*), the data of Horsfield and Cumming.[10] The figures represent plots of the summed cross-sectional area of all the airways at any given distance from the carina (abscissa) versus distance from the carina (ordinate). No scales are given—the objective is simply to show how the two shapes differ.

available area of about 70 m^2. Here diffusion is much slower, possibly approximating the rate in water, in which the diffusion coefficient for oxygen is 0.00193 cm^2/sec. It is interesting to note that the surface area offered by the erythrocytes in the pulmonary capillaries is approximately equal to that of the alveolar-capillary membrane.

These three processes, from above downwards, are progressively less efficient; *i.e.,* less oxygen is transported across unit area in unit time. This increasing inefficiency is compensated by the successively shorter distances over which each process operates and the increasing cross-sectional area available. Figures 2 and 3 summarize these features.

That the symmetric models which are almost universally used do not accurately represent the real structure is self-evident on inspection of a bronchial tree cast, for there is a considerable degree of asymmetry. If generations are counted down from the trachea airways of different size and function are assigned to the same generation, and this therefore results in an inappropriate classification. Branches of asymmetric trees can be better grouped by counting orders, which is done by starting at the periphery and counting upwards towards the trachea. In the method described by Horsfield and Cumming[9] the order increases by one at each junction (Fig. 4A), whilst in that described by Strahler[10] the order only increases when two branches of the same order meet (Fig. 4, B and C).

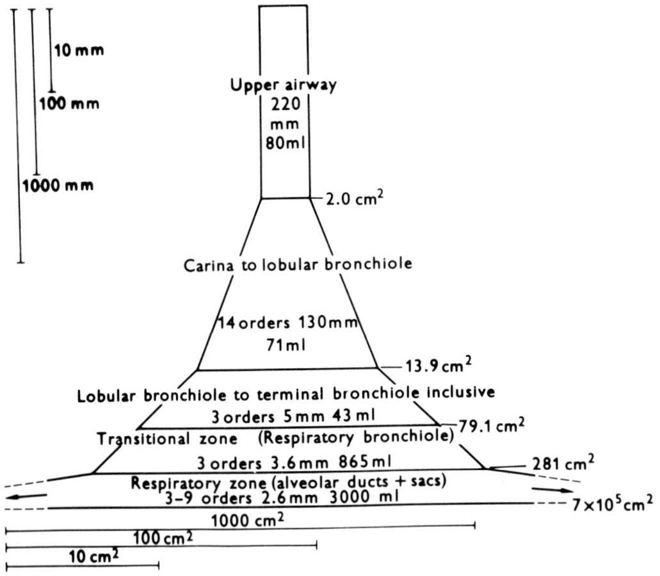

FIG. 2. The functional anatomy of the airways. The airways are divided into five groups, for each of which are indicated the number of orders, their summed length in millimeters, volume in milliliters, and summed cross-sectional area in square centimeters at the distal end of the group. The lengths and cross-sectional areas are drawn on a separate, but identical, logarithmic scale for each group. Mass flow is dominant down to the end of the transitional zone and diffusion in the gas phase is dominant within the respiratory zone. Diffusion in the tissue phase occurs across the alveolar-capillary membrane, indicated by the lower horizontal line (after Thurlbeck and Wang[19]). (Reproduced from Horsfield, K.: The relation between structure and function in the airways of the lung. *Brit. J. Dis. Chest 68:* 159, 1974.)

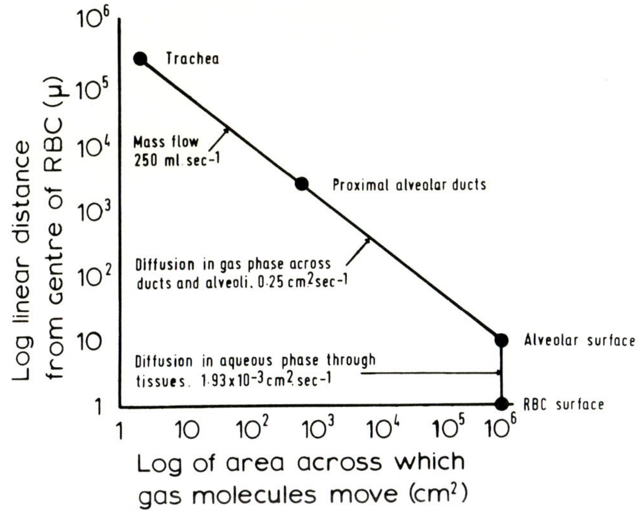

FIG. 3. An illustration of the relation between anatomic dimensions and the physical processes by which gas molecules are transported in different regions of the airways, from the trachea down to the erythrocyte. Progressing from the trachea downwards the following points may be noted: (1) the physical process by which gas molecules are transported becomes less efficient; (2) the linear distance over which each successive physical process operates becomes shorter; (3) the available cross-sectional area increases.

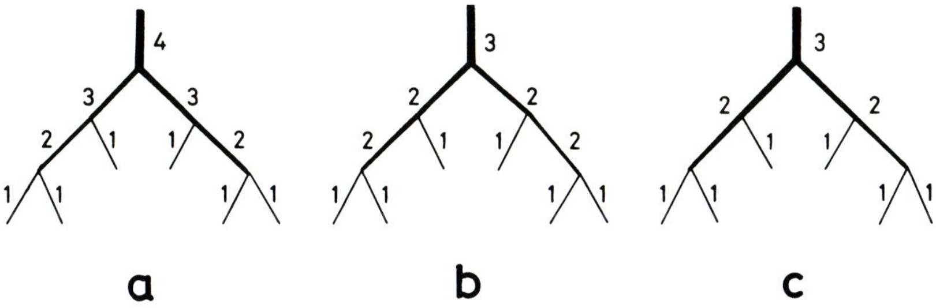

FIG. 4. Orders in a branching tree. (*a*) Horsfield's method. The orders increase by one at each junction. (*b*) Strahler's method, stage 1. Orders increase by one when two identically ordered branches meet. (*c*) Strahler's method, stage 2. Contiguous branches of the same order are combined to make only one branch. (Reproduced by permission, from Horsfield, K.: Some mathematical properties of branching trees with application to the respiratory system. *Bull. Math. Biol. 38:* 307, 1976.)

A study of a cast of the human bronchial tree analyzed in terms of Horsfield orders gave an estimate of about 28,000 terminal bronchioles.[9] The total number of branches down to and including a given order in a dichotomously branching tree is $2u-1$, where u is the number of branches in that order. This gives an estimated 55,999 (say 56,000) conducting airways. These figures are less than half those suggested by the symmetric model, a discrepancy which casts doubt on some of the calculations based on symmetric models. Thus calculations of airways resistance or viscous pressure drop[14] will be too low, since there are fewer than half as many branches in parallel in the real structure than in the model.

One way of expressing the asymmetry is by measuring the pathlength from the carina to each lobular branch (2 or 3 orders proximal to a terminal bronchiole).

The distribution of pathlengths is shown in Figure 5. It ranges from 7–22 cm, with a mode at about 12 cm. This three-fold range is a good indication of the degree of asymmetry.

When considering diffusion problems in the airways it may be important to take asymmetry into account. Figure 6 shows a diagrammatic representation of the diffusion of nitrogen back up the airways following the inspiration of a breath of oxygen. It may be seen that nitrogen can enter airways, larger than would be anticipated from the study of a symmetric model, by diffusion along short asymmetric branches. This may be part of the explanation for the rapid fall in Fowler dead space on breath-holding.

The asymmetric bronchial tree has a different length versus cross-sectional area relation than the model, resembling a turnip more than a trumpet (Fig. 1, *right*). Those who use the symmetric model must take into account the ways in which it diverges from reality and assess whether they could affect the relevance of their results.

The number of branches in each order of an airway cast can be counted, and the diameter and length of each branch measured. Using a semilogarithmic scale,

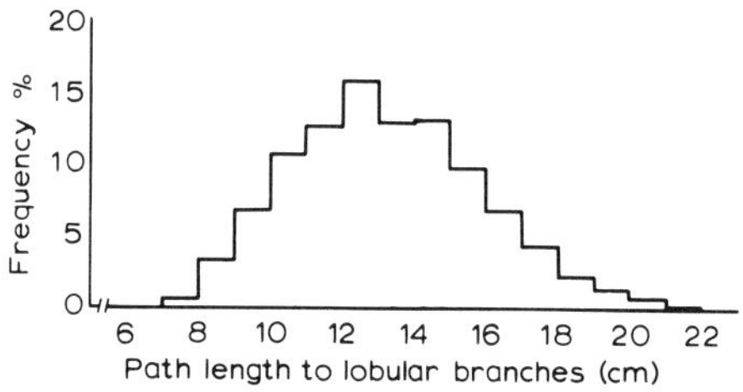

FIG. 5. Frequency distribution (percent) of pathlengths from carina to lobular branches in the human bronchial tree. Lobular branches are 2 to 3 orders proximal to the terminal bronchioles. (Reproduced by permission, from Horsfield, K., and Cumming, G.: Morphology of the bronchial tree in man. *J. Appl. Physiol. 24:* 378, 1968.)

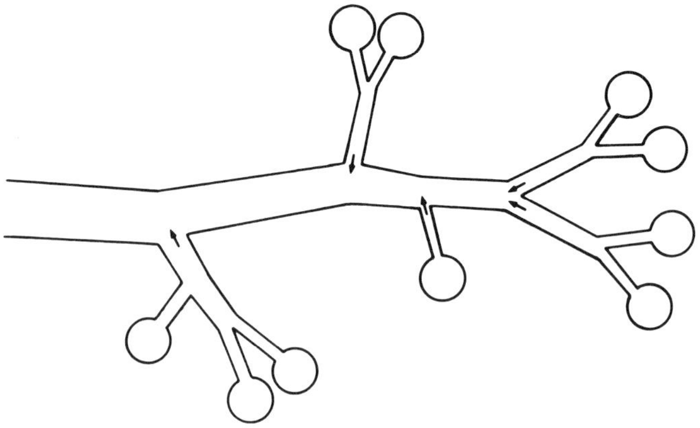

FIG. 6. A representation of asymmetric airways. After the inspiration of a breath of pure oxygen, nitrogen in the residual gas diffuses back up the airways, as indicated by the *arrows*. Because of the asymmetry nitrogen can reach the larger airways more rapidly than expected.

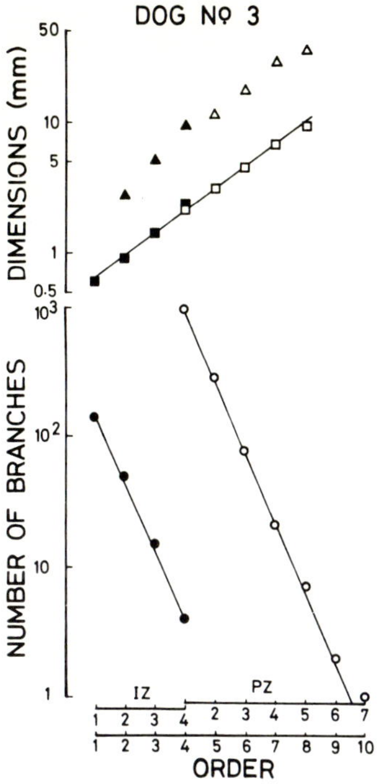

FIG. 7. Morphologic data from a cast of a dog's lung, by Strahler orders. *IZ,* intermediate zone, with bronchi of 0.5 to 2.0 mm diameter; *PZ,* proximal zone with bronchi of 2.0 mm diameter and greater; *open symbols,* PZ data; *closed symbols,* IZ data; circles, numbers; squares, mean diameters; triangles, mean lengths. (Reproduced by permission, from Horsfield, K., and Cumming, G.: Morphology of the bronchial tree in the dog. *Resp. Physiol. 26:* 177, 1976.)

number, mean diameter, and mean length of branches in each Strahler order are plotted against order in Figure 7; the data are from a dog lung. Each of these variables gives a linear plot, and thus successive orders show a geometric increase in mean dimensions and a geometric decrease in numbers. The factor by which the number decreases with order is the branching ration R_b, and the factors by which mean diameter and mean length increase with order are the diameter ratio R_d, and the length ratio R_l, respectively. In this particular lung R_d is nearly equal to R_l, *i.e.,* the two plots are nearly parallel, and furthermore $R_b = R_d^3$. Thus $R_b = R_d^3 = R_l^3$. In the human lung these equations are closely approximated, as shown by the following values:

R_b	$R_b^{1/3}$	R_d	R_l
2.805	1.410	1.427	1.402

These values may be utilized to investigate viscous pressure dissipation in the airways, using Poisseuille's equation. While this approach is admittedly too simplistic (see also the work of Pedley, Schroter, and Sudlow[14]), the results are nevertheless of interest.

For any branch the difference in pressure $\Delta P = R\mathring{V}$ where R is the resistance and $\mathring{V}$ the flow. From Poisseuille's equation R is proportional to L/D^4, where L is the length of the branch and D its diameter. Thus in arbitrary units:

$$\Delta P = \frac{L\mathring{V}}{D^4}$$

For a branch one order higher:

$$\Delta P_1 = \frac{L_1\mathring{V}_1}{D_1^{\,4}}$$

But

$$L_1 = LR_l$$
$$D_1 = DR_d$$
$$\mathring{V}_1 = \mathring{V}R_b$$

The first two of these follow by definition; the third follows because if there are $1/R_b$ as many branches in the higher order, each has to carry R_b times more flow. By substitution:

$$\Delta P_1 = \frac{LR_l \times \mathring{V}R_b}{D^4 \times R_d^{\,4}}$$

R_b and R_l cancel with $R_d^{\,4}$ to give:

$$\Delta P_1 = \frac{L\mathring{V}}{D^4}$$

This is the same as ΔP, and hence the viscous pressure dissipation is equal in each order. The particular interest in this result lies in the concept developed by geomorphologists[11, 16] that entropy production is minimal when energy losses in each order are equal. This raises the possibility that the design of the bronchial tree is such as to minimize work of breathing, given the other constraints such as volume and tissue mass available for that organ.

The factors which determine the value of the ratios are probably different for each one. R_d may be modeled during growth of the airways in response to airflow and the pressure developed in the airways. R_l may be determined partly by growth and it is also affected by the shape of the chest. Geometrically it would be expected to have a cube root relation to the volumes of lung units, which are in turn related directly to R_b. R_b itself is decided before birth because all the branches of the bronchial tree are present at about 5 months' gestation.[2] There are differences in the value of R_b between species, the reasons for which are not understood.

REFERENCES

1. Angus, G. E., and Thurbeck, W. M.: Number of alveoli in the human lung. *J. Appl. Physiol. 32:* 483–485, 1972.
2. Bucher, U., and Reid, L.: Development of the intrasegmental bronchial tree: The pattern of branching and development of cartilage at various stages of intra-uterine life. *Thorax 16:* 207–218, 1961.
3. Dunnill, M. S.: Quantitative methods in the study of pulmonary pathology. *Thorax 17:* 320–328, 1962.

4. Dunnill, M. S.: Postnatal growth of the lung. *Thorax 17:* 329–333, 1962.
5. Dunnill, M. S., Massarella, G. R., and Anderson, J. A.: A comparison of the quantitative anatomy of the bronchi in normal subjects, in status asthmaticus, in chronic bronchitis, and in emphysema. *Thorax 24:* 176–179, 1969.
6. Green, M.: How big are the bronchioles? *St. Thomas's Hospital Gazette 63:* 136–139, 1965.
7. Horsfield, K.: The relation between structure and function in the airways of the lung. *Br. J. Dis. Chest 68:* 145–160, 1974.
8. Horsfield, K.: Some mathematical properties of branching trees with application to the respiratory system. *Bull. Math. Biol. 38:* 305–315, 1976.
9. Horsfield, K., and Cumming, G.: Morphology of the bronchial tree in man. *J. Appl. Physiol. 24:* 373–383, 1968.
10. Horsfield, K., and Cumming, G.: Morphology of the bronchial tree in the dog. *Respir. Physiol. 26:* 173–182, 1976.
11. Leopold, L. B., and Langbein, W. B.: The concept of entrophy in landscape evolution. *Geological Survey Professional Paper 500-A:* pp. A1–A20, 1962.
12. Matsuba, K., and Thurlbeck, W. M.: The number and dimensions of small airways in nonemphysematous lungs. *Am. Rev. Resp. Dis. 104:* 516–524, 1971.
13. Paiva, M., Lacquet, L. M., and van der Linden, L. P.: Gas transport in a model derived from Hansen-Ampaya anatomical data of the human lung. *J. Appl. Physiol. 41:* 115–119, 1976.
14. Pedley, T. J., Schroter, R. C., and Sudlow, M. F.: The prediction of pressure drop and variation of resistance within the human bronchial airways. *Resp. Physiol. 9:* 387–405, 1970.
15. Ryan, S. F., Vincent, T. N., Mitchell, R. S., Filley, G. F., and Dart, G.: Ductectasia: An asymptomatic pulmonary change related to age. *Med. Thorac. 22:* 181–187, 1965.
16. Stall, J. B., and Yang, C. T.: *Hydraulic geometry of 12 selected stream systems of the United States.* University of Illinois, Water Resources Center, Research Report No. 32, 1970.
17. Thurlbeck, W. M.: The internal surface area of nonemphysematous lungs. *Am. Rev. Resp. Dis. 95:* 765–773, 1967.
18. Thurlbeck, W. M., and Angus, G. E.: Growth and aging of the normal human lung. *Chest 67:* 3S–7S, 1975.
19. Thurlbeck, W. M., and Wang, N. S.: The structure of the lung. In *MTP International Review of Science: Respiratory Physiology,* series 1, Vol. 2. London, Butterworths, 1974.
20. Weibel, E. R.: *Morphometry of the Human Lung.* Berlin, Springer-Verlag, 1963.

Chapter 9

Chronic Obstructive Lung Disease: The Role of Airway Disease, with Special Emphasis on the Pathology of Small Airways*

DENNIS E. NIEWOEHNER AND MANUEL G. COSIO

It is standard teaching that the pathology of chronic obstructive pulmonary disease (COPD) can be separated into two major components: (1) disease affecting lung parenchyma (emphysema), and (2) disease directly involving the conducting airways.‡ It is generally thought that either type of disease, if sufficiently severe, may alone cause significant airflow obstruction. These entities coexist in most cases of COPD and they may share common etiologies. Therefore, it is not easy to distinguish the relative functional importance of emphysema and chronic airway disease in most patients with COPD.

The importance of emphysema as a cause of expiratory airflow obstruction is well established. Emphysema is easily recognized at routine autopsy examination and its extent can be accurately quantitated by one of several methods. Several large clinical and pathologic correlative studies have shown a consistent though far from perfect relationship between the extent of emphysema observed at

* Financial assistance for research by D.E.N. was provided by Grant No. HL 16542 from the National Heart and Lung Institute, and Research Career Development Award No. 1 KO4 HL 00102.

‡ The use of the same terms to describe clinical, physiologic, and pathologic entities is a problem which hampers the understanding of obstructive lung disease. In this discussion the term COPD is used to indicate a clinical syndrome with characteristic physiologic abnormalities, particularly a reduction in expiratory flow rates. Excluded from this definition are patients with bronchiectasis, chronic asthma, and cystic fibrosis. Emphysema refers to an anatomic lesion "characterized by abnormal, permanent enlargement of the air spaces distal to the terminal bronchiole, accompanied by destruction of their walls" which is the definition agreed upon by an expert committee.[1] We depart from the recommendations of this same committee with regard to the use of "chronic bronchitis." Chronic bronchitis has come to be defined as a clinical entity characterized by cough and excess sputum production, even though it is properly a pathologic term meaning bronchial inflammation. The pathologist has no inclusive term to describe the various lesions of the conducting airways associated with COPD. In this discussion the term chronic airway disease is used for the entire complex of pathologic changes in the airways, including the bronchioles, which are commonly associated with COPD. The term chronic mucus hypersecretion will be used to indicate chronic sputum production. It is realized that this deviates from standard usage, but as shown in the ensuing discussion, we feel that the standard clinical definition of chronic bronchitis may not be very useful. As far as possible, the use of the term chronic bronchitis will be avoided.

autopsy and the severity of clinical and physiologic impairment in the patients.[5, 31, 37, 45, 47] Animal models in which proteolytic enzymes are used to induce alveolar destruction have also been helpful in understanding the physiologic consequences of emphysema. Depending upon the method by which these enzymes are administered, an emphysema-like lesion may be produced in which there is little or no morphologic evidence of airways injury.[8, 32, 36] The functional changes produced by these experimental lesions qualitatively resemble those observed with COPD in humans. At the present time no one seriously questions that emphysema is an important and possibly an essential lesion in causing severe COPD. It may seem strange that we will not be reviewing the morphology of emphysema in detail. In our view this is unnecessary. There have been no major advances in the morphology of emphysema since the subject was reviewed at the last long course.[§] A recent detailed review of the morphology of emphysema is available.[46] The main facts seem clear cut. Where there is controversy about the morphology of emphysema, this stems from subjective description and assertion and thus resolution is difficult.

The situation with regard to chronic airway disease is far less clear. As reviewed below, a variety of lesions is observed throughout the bronchial tree of patients with COPD. However, until recently it has not been possible for even the expert pathologist to relate any specific lesion or combination of lesions to airflow obstruction in a consistent manner. Animal models have not been helpful because no one has succeeded in producing an experimental airways lesion which causes significant irreversible obstruction to airflow. The lesions of the airways presumed to cause airflow obstruction have been difficult to identify and characterize.

Though much remains to be done in this area, significant progress has been made in recent years through the efforts of many different groups of investigators. The purpose of this discussion is to review some of the relevant studies which have helped to identify the lesions in the conducting airways which cause airflow obstruction in COPD.

LESIONS OF AIRWAYS IN PATIENTS WITH COPD

A variety of pathologic changes is observed in the bronchial tree of patients with COPD. These lesions include acute and chronic inflammatory infiltrates in the walls of large and small airways, enlargement of the bronchial mucus glands, fibrosis, goblet cell metaplasia in the epithelium, increased amounts of luminal mucus, distortions in the shape of airways, pigment within and surrounding the walls of airways, and desquamation of the lining epithelium. Previous investigators provided excellent descriptions of these lesions and little can be added in a qualitative way to this earlier work.

In 1954 Reid[39] published her comprehensive description of airway pathology observed in lungs from patients with productive cough and airflow obstruction. She distinguished those abnormalities found in early cases from those in advanced disease. Hypertrophy of the mucus secreting elements, both bronchial mucus glands and epithelial goblet cells seen in early disease was considered to be the primary event. In advanced cases additional pathologic lesions were observed,

§ *IAP Monographs in Pathology, No. 8, The Lung,* Averill A. Liebow and David E. Smith, editors, The Williams & Wilkins Co., Baltimore.

particularly in the membranous bronchioles. These included purulent bronchiolitis, microabscess formation, and deformity of airway lumens with alternating regions of stenosis and dilatation. Enlargement of mucus glands in the walls of proximal bronchi was thought to be more important than increases in the number of epithelial goblet cells as a cause of sputum production. Enlargement of the bronchial mucus glands was considered to be the major pathologic criterion for the diagnosis of chronic bronchitis (Chronic mucus hypersecretion). Because excess mucus production was thought to be such an essential feature of chronic bronchitis, the clinical disease was defined by an expert committee in terms of cough and sputum production.[1]

In a subsequent paper in 1960 Reid described a method for quantitating the extent of mucus gland enlargement (the Reid Index).[40] Many studies investigating various aspects of the morphology, epidemiology, and the pathogenesis of bronchial mucus gland enlargement followed.

While pathologic changes in the large airways were emphasized, other pathologists described abnormalities in the peripheral airways of patients with COPD. Laennec,[18] in his original observations on the emphysematous lung, commented upon pathologic alterations in the distal airways, and he considered that air trapping and obstruction could be attributed principally to these lesions. In 1953 Spain and Kaufman[43] provided detailed descriptions of peripheral airway pathology in severely emphysematous lungs. They observed that many noncartilaginous bronchioles had thickened walls and were inflammed. Smooth muscle was hypertrophied and focal areas of mucosa were ulcerated. They also commented upon the deformity of the bronchiolar lumen resulting from alternating regions of stenosis and dilatation.

Similar pathologic lesions were observed by McLean[30] who emphasized the role of mucus plugging in peripheral airways as a possible cause of airflow obstruction. He observed acute and chronic inflammation in many bronchioles and speculated that extension of this inflammatory process into surrounding lung parenchyma was a factor in the pathogenesis of emphysema. Inflammation in the bronchioles was postulated to arise from exposure to a variety of infectious and chemical agents. Healing was thought to result in fibrosis, which in McLean's view accounted for the distortion in the shape of the airway, and which in some instances caused complete obliteration of the lumen.

Unquestionably, the best general description of peripheral airway pathology in COPD was provided by Leopold and Gough[19] in a paper published in 1957. They studied 140 lungs with generalized emphysema, of which 75 were considered to have predominantly the centrilobular type. In virtually all cases of centrilobular emphysema they observed widespread inflammation and fibrosis in the conducting airways. The inflammatory changes consisted largely of lymphocyte and plasma cell infiltrations. An increased density of reticulin fibers and occasionally a loss of elastic fibers were observed in the smaller airways. Metaplasia of the lining epithelium was frequently observed. Extensive mural fibrosis was not a common finding and when present usually involved the "supplying" bronchiole to the centrilobular lesion. ("Supplying" bronchioles by their definition are either the proximal respiratory bronchiole or the terminal bronchiole.)

Leopold and Gough[19] examined many supplying bronchioles by serial sections. Though it is not clear what they considered normal, and values are not given, the authors state that a modest reduction in luminal area was observed in 60% of the airways examined. Severe reduction (to less than two-thirds of normal) was unusual, being present in only 11 of the 60 airways examined in serial sections. In the remaining airways, luminal dimensions were considered normal despite the presence of inflammation in the walls of the airway. It was also their impression that the size of the emphysematous space bore little relationship to the degree of pathologic narrowing in the supplying bronchiole. These studies indicate that chronic imflammation is common in distal airways of lungs with centrilobular emphysema, but luminal stenosis is an inconstant finding and when present is usually modest in extent.

In contrast to the findings in centrilobular emphysema, Leopold and Gough[19] observed that inflammation in the membranous and respiratory bronchioles of the 65 lungs with pure generalized (panlobular) emphysema was uncommon. In these lungs chronic inflammatory reactions were observed more frequently in the large and medium-sized bronchi.

Anderson and Foraker in 1962[2] used quantitative methods to study the pathology of the peripheral airways. In histologic sections from both normal and emphysematous lungs, they selected the single smallest bronchiole in each lung. The luminal area of this single airway was determined by planimetry. Bronchiolar lumens were consistently smaller in the emphysematous lungs compared to bronchioles from normal lungs. However, since only a single airway in each lung was studied, it is not possible from their studies to determine the extent of these stenotic lesions. These investigators also comment upon the frequency with which patchy inflammatory reactions are observed in the peripheral airways.

Subsequently, Linhartová, in collaboration with Anderson and Foraker,[21] quantitated irregularities in the luminal shape of membranous bronchioles from severely emphysematous lungs. From reconstructions of serial histologic sections, they determined that the lumens of normal bronchioles are nearly cylindrical and have smooth internal surfaces. In contrast, peripheral airways in emphysematous lungs have irregular surfaces and the lumens are distorted. Regions of stenosis alternate with areas of dilatation along the longitudinal axis of the airway.

Bronchographic methods have also been used to demonstrate airway abnormalities in patients with COPD. The bronchographic appearance of "peripheral pooling" was commented upon in early studies. It was originally thought that these "pools" represented bronchiolar ectasia, but subsequent studies by Leopold and Seal[20] conclusively demonstrated that these radiologic features represent centrilobular emphysematous lesions. Other bronchographic abnormalities described in the peripheral airways of patients with COPD include abrupt cutoffs which suggest mucus plugs, multiple areas of stenosis, mucosal irregularities, and a failure of the distal airways to taper in a normal manner.[41]

PHYSIOLOGIC AND PATHOLOGIC CORRELATION FROM AUTOPSY STUDIES

The pathologic studies described above have been important in identifying and describing the different lesions in patients with COPD. An equally important consideration is the functional significance of each specific lesion. Numerous efforts have been made to correlate physiologic and clinical abnormalities with abnormal airway morphology.

Before describing the results of these correlative studies, it is important to comment briefly upon methods. The results of correlative studies may be influenced greatly by the exactness with which morphologic features are measured. Even if the reproducibility of the method has been adequately evaluated, it is frequently not possible to determine independently whether the measurement in question is an appropriate one. In the case of emphysema there appears to be little problem. This lesion is easily identified, there is general agreement that it is a functionally relevant abnormality, and quantitative estimates of its severity by experienced people are reasonably reproducible,[44] Thus, methodology is probably not a significant limiting factor in correlating emphysema with functional variables.

The methodologic problems in evaluating airway lesions are much greater, and it is not certain that all of the functionally relevant lesions have even been identified. Except for mucus gland enlargement, other lesions of chronic bronchitis, such as inflammation, fibrosis, and luminal mucus, are not easy to quantitate. Subjective and nonquantitative scoring methods are prone to error and the reproducibility of these scoring methods must be carefully examined. There is a formidable sampling problem in the bronchial tree, because of the enormous number of airways, which are non-randomly distributed. The number of airways evaluated, particularly the peripheral airways, may be critical to the accuracy of the method employed. The use of necropsy material also presents a problem in interpretation. Inflammation and mucus plugging may occur during the terminal illness and not reflect the preterminal state of the airways. Negative results obtained from comparing airflow obstruction and the morphologic lesions of chronic bronchitis must be viewed with these considerations in mind.

The physiologic consequences of bronchial mucus gland enlargment have been most thoroughly investigated. The interest in this morphologic feature was a natural outgrowth of the importance attached to it by previous pathologic studies. Correlative studies are facilitated by the ease and accuracy with which the volume of gland mass can be quantitated by histologic methods.

Thurlbeck[46] recently reviewed and summarized the studies which have evaluated bronchial gland enlargement with respect to physiologic airflow obstruction. Except for one study involving coal miners done by McKenzie and co-workers[29] which may be a special case, relationships between the extent of bronchial mucus gland enlargement and various physiologic abnormalities have been nonexistent or present only at a very low level of significance. Similar conclusions have been reached in studies of structure-functional correlations in postmortem lungs.[33, 35, 46] While these studies do not exclude the possibility that mucus gland enlargement has a role in the pathogenesis of COPD, the idea that bronchial gland hyperplasia *per se* causes significant airflow obstruction either by encroachment on bronchial lumen or by excess mucus production remains an unproven hypothesis.

There are relatively few studies in which lesions other than bronchial gland enlargement are correlated with physiologic studies obtained before death. Martin and associates[23] measured the Reid Index of mucous gland enlargement, and evaluated the extent of inflammation and fibrosis in the large airways which they termed the bronchitis index. In the small airways they measured the lumen-to-bronchiole diameter ratio as an index of peripheral airways disease, though they do not mention how many airways were evaluated in each lung. The intercorrelations among the Reid Index, the bronchitis index, and the lumen-to-bronchiole diameter were very poor. No significant relationship between any of these morphologic features and pulmonary function tests could be demonstrated except for a weak correlation between the Reid Index and the airflow velocity index ($r = -0.37$) and between the lumen-to-bronchiole ratio and the residual volume to total lung capacity ratio ($r = -0.46$).

Karpick and associates[17] compared morphologic findings in patients who died from respiratory failure mostly secondary to COPD, to the findings in patients dying of nonrespiratory causes. In 79% of patients dying of respiratory failure (but only 34% of controls), goblet cell metaplasia was observed in more than 20% of the bronchioles examined. They postulated that luminal mucus secondary to the increased number of goblet cells might be a major cause of airflow obstruction in acute respiratory failure. They also compared pulmonary function tests obtained before the terminal illness with pathologic findings at autopsy. Neither the Reid Index nor the extent of goblet cell metaplasia in bronchioles correlated with either maximal midexpiratory flow rates (MMF) or the ratio of the forced expiratory volume at one second to the forced expiratory volume ($FEV_{1.0}/FEV$). The extent of goblet cell metaplasia also did not correlate with the Reid Index.

Recently Mitchell and his co-workers[31] reported the results of their extensive correlative studies in COPD. Instead of physiologic data, the clinical severity of COPD was based upon a complex clinical and laboratory evaluation. The extent of emphysema was determined from inflated and fixed lung sections. Pathologic studies also included an evaluation of inflammation, fibrosis, and goblet cell metaplasia in both large and small airways, bronchial mucus gland enlargement, and the number and diameter of membranous bronchioles. A close relationship was observed between the severity of COPD as judged clinically and the extent of anatomic emphysema. The clinical severity of COPD and the various indices of airway disease in general correlated only at low levels of significance or not at all. These authors concluded that the pathologic changes in the airways were relatively unimportant as a determinant of clinical COPD in comparison with emphysema.

Thus, correlative studies using autopsy specimens have not shown a consistent relationship between chronic bronchitis and the extent of clinical and physiologic impairment in COPD. Whether these largely negative results indicate that chronic airway disease is unimportant as a cause of airflow obstruction or whether they merely reflect methodologic problems in its morphologic evaluation is impossible to determine.

LOCALIZATION OF SITE OF AIRFLOW RESISTANCE IN NORMAL AND DISEASED LUNGS

An increase in total pulmonary resistance (R_L) measured during tidal breathing is characteristically observed in patients with COPD. The increase in R_L in turn is related both to the clinical severity of the disease and to the degree of airflow obstruction as determined by spirometry.[37, 38] The increase in R_L must be caused by narrowing of airway lumens. Important questions relate to the site and mechanism of this abnormal narrowing.

Bronchioles are elastic structures whose dimensions partly depend upon the tethering effect of surrounding lung parenchyma. With emphysema there is a loss of lung elastic recoil and presumably a secondary loss of radial traction about each intrapulmonary airway. At the same lung volume, airway length and diameter presumably would be less in an emphysematous lung than in a normal lung. The increase in R_L usually observed in severely emphysematous lungs might be attributed entirely to the loss of this tethering effect. If so, we would anticipate a close correlation between the extent of emphysema and the increase in R_L. This has not been found. Physiologic-morphologic correlative studies in patients with COPD by Park and associates[37] and by Boushy and his colleagues[5] show that although R_L was increased in emphysematous lungs there was no correlation between the increase in R_L and the amount of emphysema within the group studied. Similarly emphysema lesions produced in laboratory animals without evidence of airway injury cause little or no change in R_L.[32, 36] These observations strongly suggest that factors in addition to emphysema are responsible for the increased R_L in patients with COPD. It is reasonable to suspect that one of these factors is intrinsic pathology of the airways.

A major advance in understanding the pathophysiology of chronic airways obstruction resulted from the work of Hogg, Macklem, and Thurlbeck[14] in Montreal. They attempted to localize the site of increased R_L in lungs at necropsy, using physiologic methods. Catheters were passed retrograde into the bronchial tree and out through the pleura. The proximal end of the catheter was wedged in the lateral wall of intermediate sized airways. The lungs were oscillated at high frequencies with a loudspeaker attached to the airway opening and resistive pressure drops were partitioned between the central airways and the peripheral airways of less than 2 mm internal diameter.

By this method, mean resistance of the central airways in five normal lungs was 0.51 cm H_2O/liter/sec and of the peripheral airways in the same lungs was only 0.18 cm H_2O/liter/sec. Peripheral resistance in seven lungs with varying grades of emphysema was variably increased but on the average was 20 times greater than in normal lungs. The increased peripheral resistance in the diseased lungs was not closely related to the extent of emphysema and the resistance of the central airways in the same lungs was increased only slightly.

This study has had an enormous influence on investigative work in COPD. It provided the first direct evidence that disease in the peripheral airways, not the central bronchi, is mainly responsible for the increased R_L observed in COPD. Because the lesions responsible for this increased peripheral resistance were thought to comprise a variety of lesions, not all inflammatory, these investigators coined and popularized the term "small airways disease." These same investigators also introduced novel and interesting ideas concerning the pathophysiology and natural history of COPD.

If their concept that peripheral resistance is negligible in normal lungs is correct, then considerable disease might be present in the membranous bronchioles without having any appreciable effect on routine ventilatory function tests. It is possible that pathologic changes might be present for many years in the peripheral airways in a subclinical form with overt clinical disability representing the terminal stages of the disease. Clinical studies have shown that once disability is evident, COPD worsens at a fairly predictable rate which is not affected by available therapy,[7, 13] The concept that disease might be present for a long period in a subclinical form was exciting because it offered the hope that if diagnosed earlier, the disease might be more amenable to therapy.[22]

In recent years much effort has been devoted to developing and evaluating tests of small airways function which are thought capable of detecting early disease. These tests include the single breath oxygen test (from which is calculated the slope of phase III and the volume at which phase IV commences, the "closing volume"), the frequency dependence of dynamic compliance, the flow-volume curve, and the use of gas mixtures other than air. There has also been renewed interest in expiratory flow rates at mid and low lung volumes as measured by conventional spirometry. Numerous clinical studies have suggested that these tests may be more sensitive in detecting minimal disease than conventional tests such as the vital capacity or the ratio of the forced expiratory volume (FEV) at one second to the FEV. Whether these newer tests are more specific for small airways function than older tests is open to conjecture.

The concept that peripheral airways resistance is negligible in normal lungs but predominates in COPD has another corollary. If this concept is correct, it is necessary to postulate extensive dimensional changes in the lumens of peripheral airways with advanced disease. Studies by the Montreal group indicate that peripheral airways resistance in single normal lungs is approximately 0.20 cm H_2O/liter/sec (or 0.10 cm H_2O/liter/sec for both lungs). It is common to observe values for R_L in the range of 5–10 cm H_2O/liter/sec or greater in patients with COPD. If this increase in R_L reflects largely small airways disease, the resistance of these airways must be increased by a factor of 50–100. For laminar flow in cylindrical tubes, resistance varies as the fourth power of diameter. For a 50- to 100-fold increase in resistance of the peripheral airways it is necessary to postulate approximately a 3-fold decrease in average luminal diameter. Such large changes in diameter should be easy to detect morphologically.

Bignon and his associates[3, 4, 11] performed the first detailed morphometric studies on peripheral airways in lungs from patients with COPD. Most patients did not have extensive physiologic studies but most had chronic respiratory failure and many died of the disease. Bignon *et al.* measured the internal diameter of 75–100 membranous bronchioles on histologic sections from each lung. They expressed their results as the percentage of airways with internal diameters less than 350 μm. In five normal lungs this value did not exceed 20%. Values in the diseased lungs were highly variable but the percentage of airways less than 350 μm was between 20 and 50% in the majority of cases. The average change in small airway diameter in the diseased lungs compared to the normal lungs was very modest. These investigators also observed a poor correlation between the extent of emphysema in any particular lung and the degree of bronchiolar narrowing.

Using similar methods, Matsuba and Thurlbeck[25, 26] came to similar conclusions. They studied 20 emphysematous lungs from patients known to have symptomatic COPD and compared results from these lungs to 20 nonemphysematous lungs. They observed significant though subtle differences between the two groups. In the emphysematous lungs the proportion of airways less than 400 μm internal diameter was slightly increased compared to the nonemphysematous group. The range of values in both groups was relatively large and the average difference was very small. They also measured the proportion of the total area on the histologic sections occupied by small airways lumen and found it to be decreased from 0.0142–0.0087 in the emphysematous lungs, a more significant but still modest difference.

In a subsequent report these same investigators studied small airways in nonemphysematous lungs from patients with a long history of productive cough.[27] The extent of physiologic disturbance in these individuals is not fully described, but none had severe COPD. The average small airway diameter in the subjects with productive cough was significantly reduced in comparison with those subjects without cough. However, the relative difference (0.81 mm *vs.* 0.66 mm) is again small.

These quantitative morphologic studies indicate that the extent of bronchiolar narrowing in patients with COPD is, on the whole, relatively slight, a conclusion in accord with the earlier observation of Leopold and Gough.[19] These observations raise a troublesome question. If resistance in the peripheral airways is very small in normal lungs but very large in COPD, it is difficult to understand how such minor changes in diameter can account for such large functional differences.

One explanation for this seeming paradox is that the measurements of average bronchiolar diameter made at total lung capacity (the volume at which available measurements were made) are not particularly relevant. It has been shown that these measurements are meaningful in normal lungs (see below) but there is no assurance that the same is true in abnormal lungs. For example, alternating regions of stenosis and dilatation have been demonstrated in severely diseased lungs by serial histologic sections and by bronchographic methods. Despite gross distortions in shape, the average luminal diameter along the longitudinal axis of such an airway might not be changed. Similarly, it may not be possible to infer accurately the functional properties of diseased airways from static observations. Membranous bronchioles normally decrease in diameter with lung deflation. It is possible that disease causes these airways to narrow and close at abnormally high lung volumes even though dimensions are unchanged at full inflation. Even with these considerations in mind, it seems surprising that greater changes in average bronchiolar diameter are not found in severely diseased lungs.

Functional and morphologic correlative studies performed by Niewoehner and co-workers[33, 35] on postmortem human lungs may also provide an explanation for this paradox. Lungs were obtained from victims of sudden death and care was taken to exclude lungs with edema, infection, or excessive bronchial secretions. Tests of mechanical function were performed within a few hours after death. These tests included pressure-volume curves, total pulmonary resistance, maximal expiratory flow rates, the frequency dependence of dynamic compliance, and the single breath nitrogen test. The values obtained from postmortem lungs agree closely with comparable measurements in age-matched live subjects. Quantitative morphologic studies used in these studies included the measurement of large (lobar and segmental) airway and intermediate-sized (2.5–4.0 mm) airway diameter and measurements of bronchial gland mass, mean bronchiolar diameter, and severity of emphysema as assessed by the average distance between alveolar walls.

The most significant result from these studies is that in a group of normal and nearly normal lungs all tests of ventilatory function correlate closely with mean

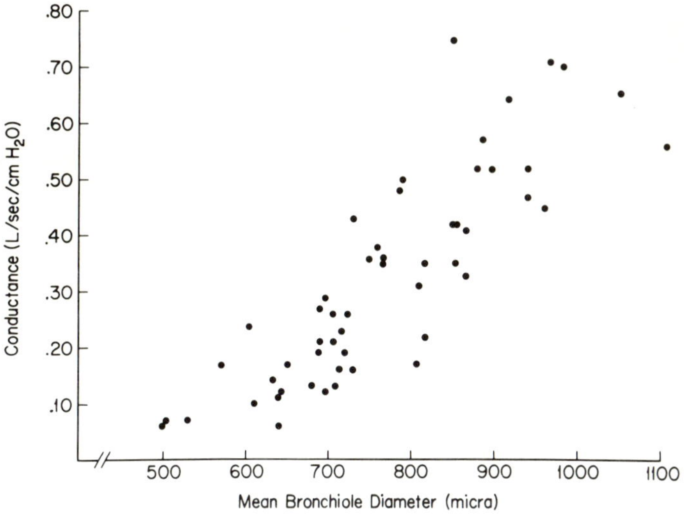

FIG. 1. As the mean bronchiole diameter increases, so does the airway conductance of the lung. Conductance is the reciprocal of airway resistance.

bronchiolar diameter and not with the diameter of either large or intermediate sized airways or with the extent of bronchial gland enlargement. An example of this relationship is shown in Figure 1 on which total pulmonary conductance (the reciprocal of resistance) is plotted against mean bronchiolar diameter. The closeness of the relationship is evident from inspection and confirmed by the correlation coefficient (+0.85). Similar relationships are observed in comparing bronchiolar diameter with maximal expiratory flow rates, with the frequency dependence of dynamic compliance, and with both the slope of phase III and the "closing volume" calculated from the single breath nitrogen test.

The results of these studies strongly suggest that even in the normal lung the peripheral airways are important determinants of ventilatory function. While varying slightly in their relative sensitivity, all ventilatory tests evaluated are quite sensitive to minor differences in luminal diameter of the peripheral airways. This does not exclude the possibility that peripheral resistance in some normal lungs may be relatively low. It may be seen in Figure 1 that considerable variability in average bronchiolar diameter was observed in normal lungs that were studied. The correlative methods employed in this study do not permit airflow resistance to be directly partitioned between central and peripheral components in individual lungs. It is possible that those lungs with the largest peripheral airways do in fact have a relatively low peripheral resistance. However, this is clearly not true for the group as a whole and the evidence suggests that in many, if not most, normal lungs the peripheral component of airflow resistance is considerably larger than previously thought.

If the interpretation of these findings is correct, it has subtle though important implications concerning the pathophysiology of COPD. It lends further support to the idea that small airways disease is the functionally important lesion in COPD. If the contribution of the bronchioles to total airflow resistance is significant in the normal lung, it follows that ventilatory function would be even more vulnerable to pathologic changes in those airways. This concept differs from that of Hogg and associates,[14] chiefly in terms of the extent of bronchiolar disease required to produce significant functional abnormalities for the whole lung.

That minor degrees of pathologic narrowing might cause considerable functional change can be appreciated graphically in Figure 1. Close inspection shows that a 2-fold decrease in average bronchiolar diameter results in an approximate 10- to 15-fold decrease in total conductance. Very small changes in airway caliber cause large changes in airflow conductance. In view of this relationship the seemingly insignificant changes in small airway diameter observed by Leopold and Gough, by Matsuba and Thurlbeck, and by Bignon and his associates take on added functional importance and may largely explain the increased R_L usually observed in COPD.

SMALL AIRWAYS DISEASE IN CIGARETTE SMOKERS

The concept that disease might occur in the peripheral airways long before COPD becomes clinically evident has been confirmed from both physiologic and pathologic studies. It is well established that cigarette smoking is causally related to COPD. Because clinically obvious COPD does not occur until after many years of exposure to cigarette smoke, young smokers might be a logical group in which to identify and characterize early disease.

Several clinical studies have documented the presence of subtle functional abnormalities in young smokers by a variety of physiologic tests. Seely and her co-workers[42] found that maximal expiratory flow rates, particularly at low lung

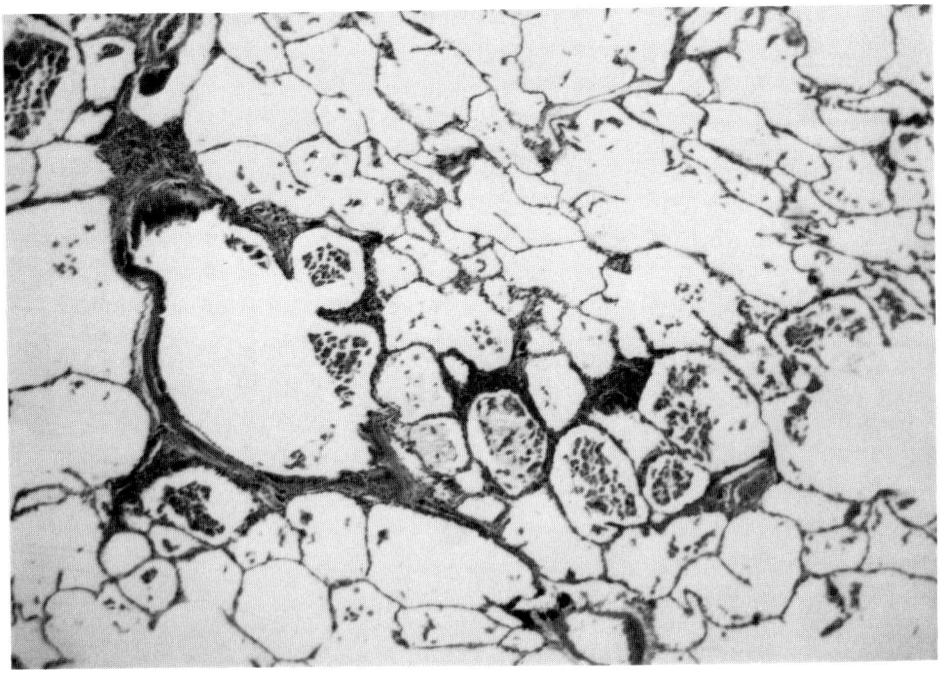

FIG. 2. Section through the junction of a terminal bronchiole and a respiratory bronchiole illustrates a typical early lesion caused by cigarette smoking in a 34-year-old man. Aggregates of pigmented macrophages can be seen in the respiratory bronchiole and in adjacent alveoli. There is mild inflammation of the bronchiolar walls. × 40.

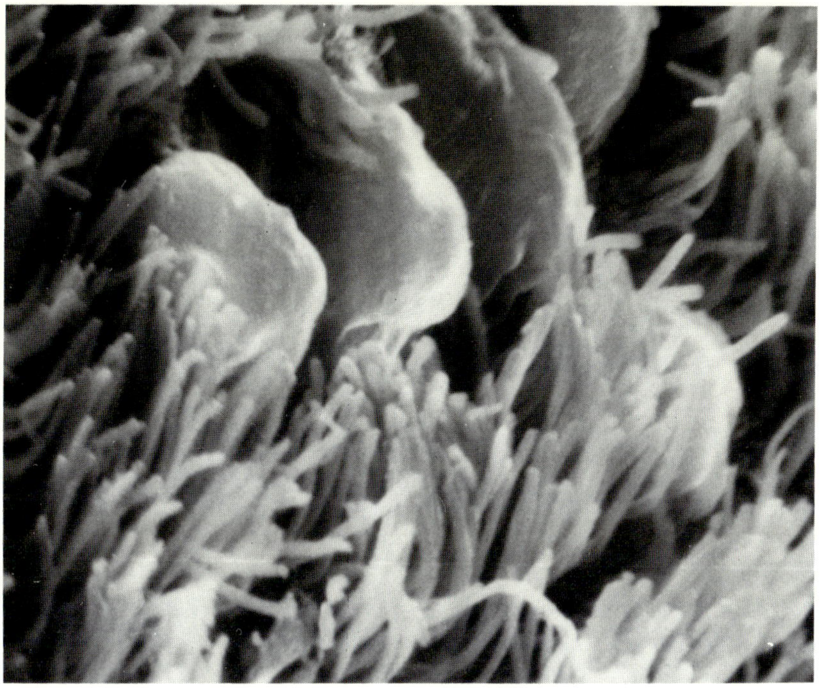

FIG. 3. Scanning electron micrograph of epithelial surface in a bronchiole of a 25-year-old nonsmoker. The Clara cells are nonciliated and are best seen towards the top of the picture where their smooth surfaced projections are obvious. × 5000. (Courtesy of Dr. Richard V. Ebert)

volumes, are reduced in teenage smokers. Frequency dependence of dynamic compliance was observed in young adult smokers by Ingram and O'Cain.[15] McCarthy and his colleagues[28] first demonstrated an increase in the closing volume of asymptomatic smokers. Buist and her colleagues[6] have evaluated the closing volume as a screening test for large populations and found a large percentage of abnormal values in cigarette smokers.

The pathologic changes which may be responsible for these minimal functional abnormalities in young smokers have been investigated recently. One of us (D.N.) in collaboration with Jerome Kleinerman and Donald Rice,[34] studied 39 lungs from youthful victims of sudden death. A characteristic lesion was observed in the respiratory bronchioles of all 19 smokers, but was seen in only 5 of 20 nonsmokers. This lesion, which we termed "respiratory bronchiolitis," consists of clusters of brown pigmented alveolar macrophages with edema, fibrosis, and epithelial hyperplasia in adjacent bronchiolar and alveolar walls (Fig. 2). In addition, an increased number of mural inflammatory cells and desquamated epithelial cells was observed in the bronchioles of smokers.

The inflammatory lesion in the respiratory bronchiole is of interest also because centrilobular emphysema occurs at the same anatomic site. As has been previously suggested, inflammation may be important in the pathogenesis of emphysema. Alveolar wall destruction is thought to be caused by enzymatic digestion of connective tissue elements. Lung macrophages contain a variety of proteases which when introduced into the tracheobronchial tree of laboratory animals produce an emphysema-like lesion.[16, 24] It is interesting to speculate that the release of proteases by macrophages over a long period may destroy adjacent alveolar walls and cause emphysema.

Other pathologic lesions in the bronchial tree caused by cigarette smoking were identified by Ebert and Terracio.[12] They studied bronchi from older smokers who underwent surgery. By use of light and scanning electron microscopy, they demonstrated an increase in the number of goblet cells and a decrease in the number of Clara cells from smokers (Figs. 3 and 4). The significance of the decreased number of Clara cells is not clear. These cells are thought to have a secretory function and the secretion may be the "hypophase" on which the surface active layer of the lung lies. Ebert and Terracio[12] and others[17] have advanced the hypothesis that the disappearance of Clara cells and their replacement by goblet cells may result in the bronchioles becoming lined by a film of mucus. Normally, bronchioles behave as though they are lined by surface active material and osmiophilic material, consistent in appearance with surfactant, has been observed lining the bronchioles. Replacement of the surfactant layer by a film of mucus would render the bronchioles unstable since, under these conditions, the surface activity of the lining layer would not diminish markedly as the airways narrowed on expiration. They would thus close unduly easily and open with great difficulty leading to functional obstruction that would not be recognized by morphologic examination of the lungs. Since Clara cell secretion may also be important in ciliary clearance, their loss may partly explain impaired clearance of

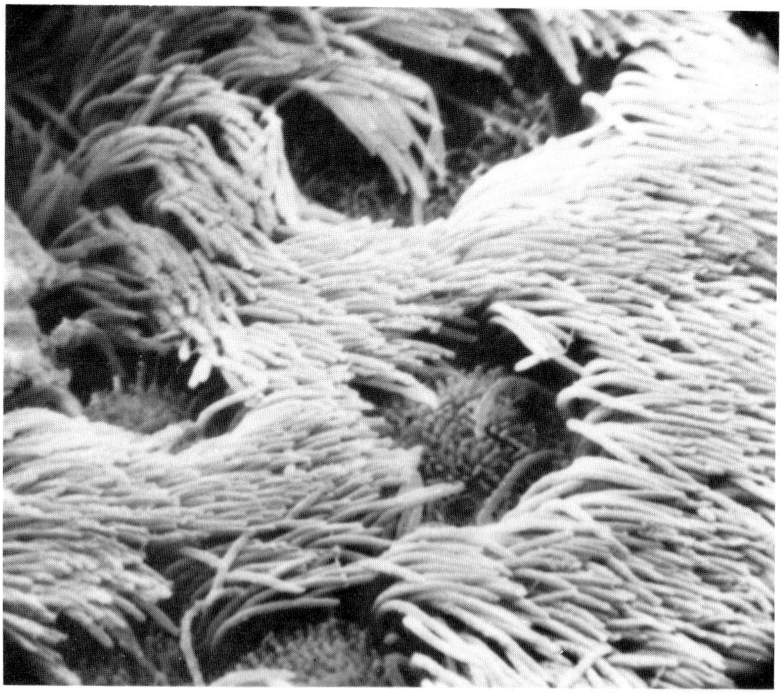

FIG. 4. Scanning electron micrograph of epithelial surface in a bronchiole of a 53-year-old cigarette smoker. Clara cells are absent and many goblet cells were seen by light microscopy. × 5000. (Courtesy of Dr. Richard V. Ebert)

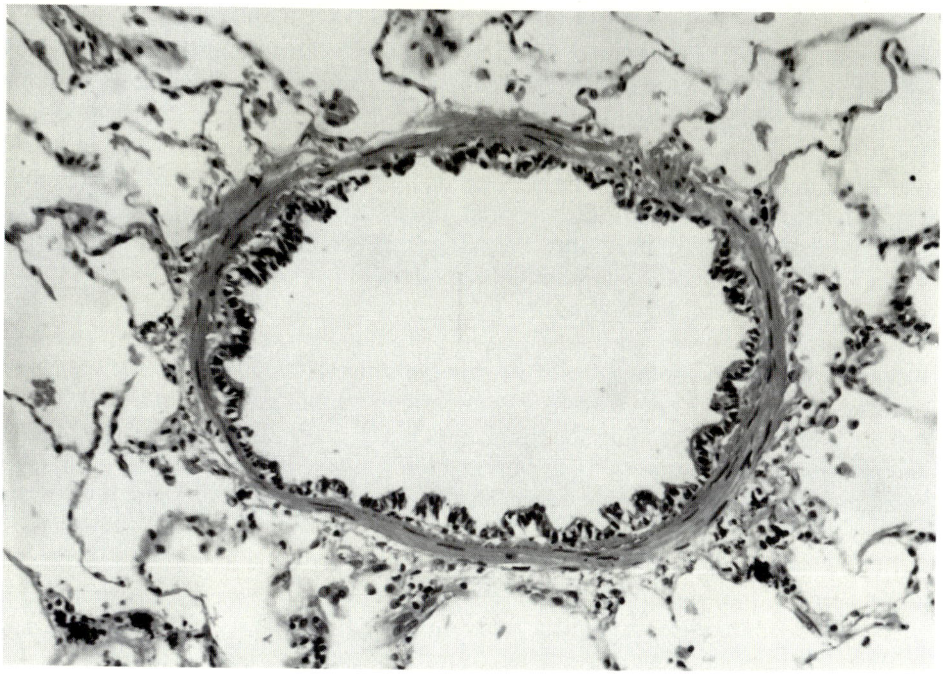

FIG. 5. Normal bronchiole in an inflation fixed human lung. × 100.

radioactive particles which Camner and Philipson[9] demonstrated in some cigarette smokers.

PHYSIOLOGIC AND PATHOLOGIC STUDIES IN PATIENTS UNDERGOING THORACOTOMY

Recent studies by Cosio and his collaborators,[10] using lung tissue obtained at surgery, have provided the first convincing evidence that pathologic changes in bronchioles do cause significant obstruction to airflow. The use of surgical specimens for pathologic studies avoids the uncertainties concerning possible changes caused by the terminal illness. It also permits physiologic and pathologic studies to be done closer together in time. A variety of pulmonary function tests were performed on 36 patients between 24 and 73 years of age shortly before surgery. A few subjects had normal pulmonary function tests but most had minimal to moderately severe COPD. Since surgery was a condition for selection into the study, none had severe clinical disease.

The amount of emphysema, if any, was quantitated from thick lung slices from the surgical specimens. Multiple histologic sections were studied by observers who had no knowledge of the physiologic data. They evaluated the following morphologic features in bronchioles: (1) luminal mucus; (2) squamous and goblet cell metaplasia in the epithelium; and (3) inflammation, fibrosis, pigment deposition, and smooth muscle hypertrophy in the airway wall. A numerical value was assigned for each specific abnormality in each case. The intraobserver and interobserver reproducibility of the composite score for each lung by this method was found to be excellent ($R = 0.91$ and 0.87, respectively).

There is a remarkably close relationship (R = 0.87) between composite scores for the physiologic disturbances and the pathologic changes in the small airways for the patients in this study. When considering individual morphologic lesions, mural inflammation and fibrosis had the greatest functional significance and epithelial metaplasia was somewhat less important. The amount of luminal mucus was totally unrelated to the extent of physiologic dysfunction. Mild to moderate emphysema was observed in 12 cases and, not unexpectedly, its severity paralleled the severity of the peripheral airways disease. However, functional abnormalities in this group of patients with mild to moderately severe COPD related much more closely to small airway pathology than to the extent of emphysema.

This study also provided interesting information concerning the progression of disease in the bronchioles (Figs. 5–8). The characteristic lesions associated with minimal functional change were a mononuclear inflammatory infiltrate in the airway wall with mild squamous and goblet cell metaplasia in the epithelium. Large numbers of pigmented macrophages, similar to those seen in young cigarette smokers, were commonly observed in respiratory bronchioles and in adjacent alveoli.

Inflammation in the peripheral airways was prominent with all stages of physiologic impairment, but this feature tended to be more severe with minimal dysfunction and less prominent in more advanced disease.

With increasing airflow obstruction mural fibrosis and pigment deposition were more conspicuous. More advanced disease was also characterized by increasing epithelial metaplasia. As demonstrated by morphometry, there was a progressive

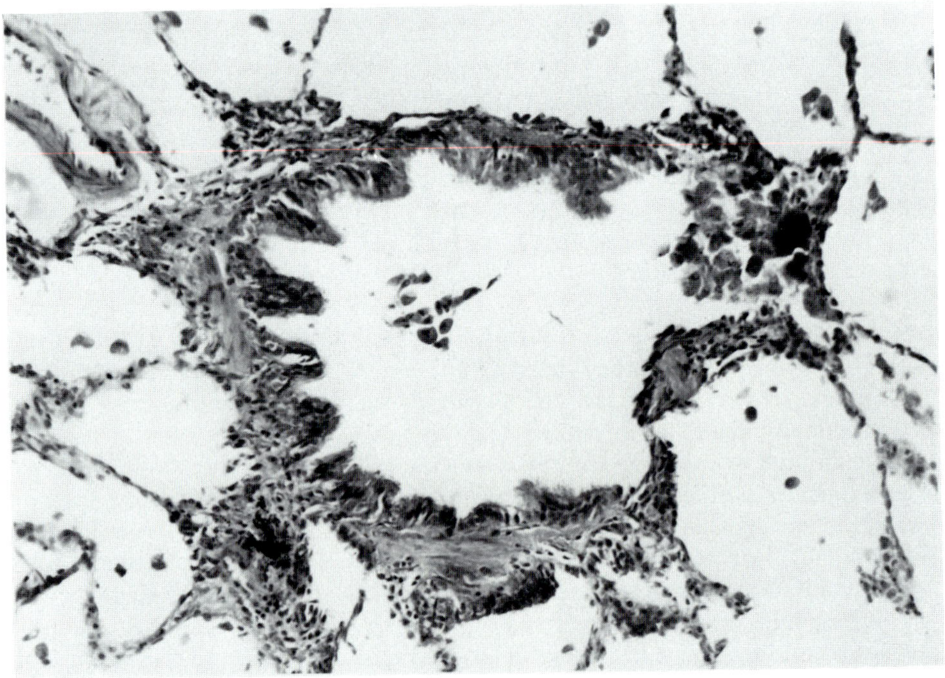

FIG. 6. Minimal inflammation in the wall of a bronchiole from a patient with mild airflow obstruction. A few macrophages are also present. × 100.

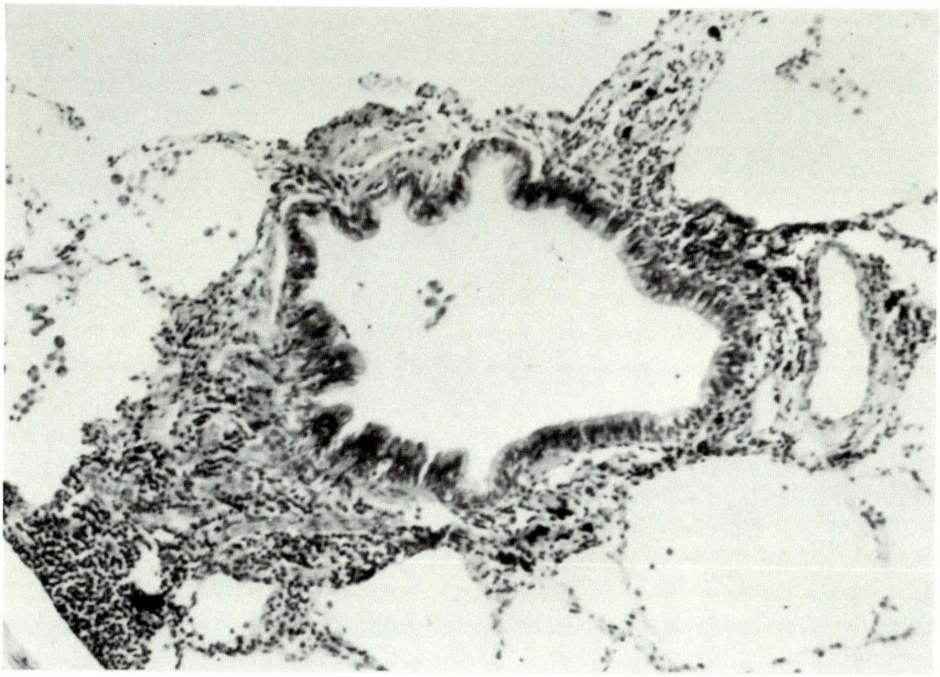

FIG. 7. Severe bronchiolar inflammation and early fibrosis in a patient with more advanced physiologic abnormalities. × 100.

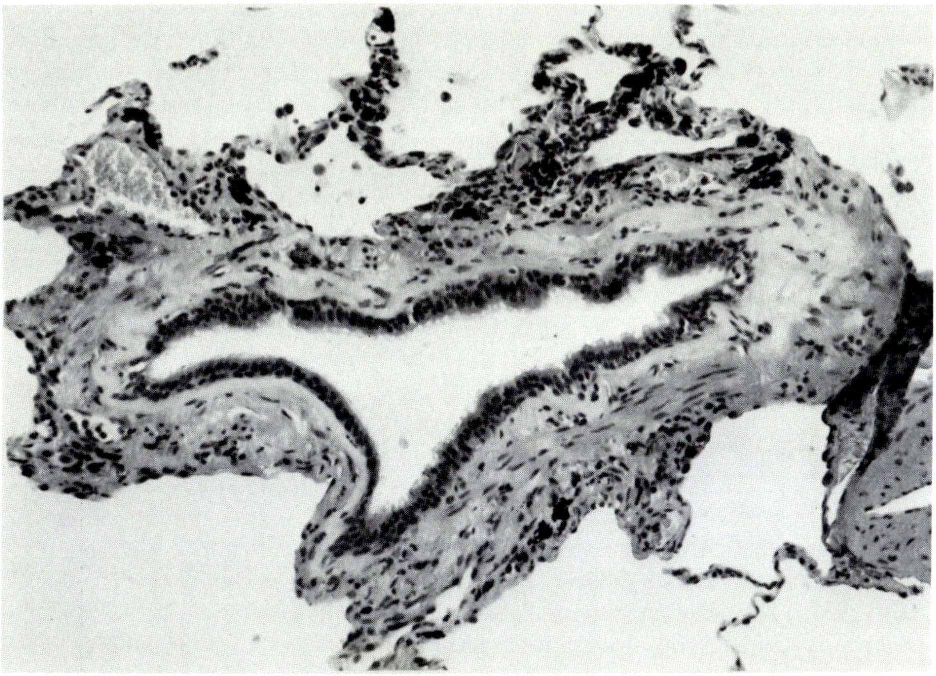

FIG. 8. Fibrosis and deformation of a bronchiole from a patient with severe airflow obstruction. × 100.

increase in average wall thickness, but an objective assessment of luminal diameters of the membranous bronchioles did not show narrowing except in the most severely diseased lungs. Deformities in airway shape were commonly observed in more advanced disease. Minimal amounts of luminal mucus were observed in nearly every case but there was no increase with progression of the disease.

CONCLUSIONS AND PERSPECTIVE

A variety of lesions occurs at all levels of the bronchial tree in patients with COPD. Bronchial mucus gland enlargement has been considered the most important of these lesions and has been the conventional pathologic criterion for the diagnosis of chronic mucus hypersection. Efforts to correlate bronchial mucus gland enlargement with other airway lesions or with physiologic abnormalities have been largely unsuccessful.

Physiologic studies in which airflow resistance was partitioned between central and peripheral airways provided an important clue concerning the site of the functionally relevant lesions in chronic bronchitis. Other studies indicate that the resistance in the peripheral airways of normal lungs may be much greater than previously thought, so that relatively minor morphologic changes observed in bronchioles may have profound functional consequences. Early descriptive studies and more recent quantitative studies indicate that alterations in the dimensions of the small airways are modest even in severe COPD.

There is now both functional and morphologic evidence that disease in the peripheral airways is the earliest manifestation of COPD. Recent studies also indicate that inflammation and fibrosis in the small airways may be the most important anatomic causes of mild to moderately severe airflow obstruction.

Fatal COPD in the absence of significant emphysema is unusual though it does occur. However, severe anatomic emphysema may be present without significant disability on the part of the patient. It seems reasonable to believe that the causes of early COPD are due mainly to lesions in the small airways. In severe disease the cause of airflow obstruction is multifactorial and two very important causes are peripheral airways disease and emphysema. The relative importance of each in severe COPD still is not clear.

An hypothesis concerning the natural history of COPD, particularly in those cases associated with cigarette smoking, is shown graphically in Figure 9. The earliest lesion identified is inflammation in the respiratory bronchiole. With further injury inflammatory lesions in the bronchioles become more evident and there are associated epithelial abnormalities. At this stage there is little change in the static dimensions of the small airways. Minimal functional abnormalities may occur from small changes in the elastic properties of the bronchiolar walls, from pathologic changes in smooth muscle tone, or from subtle alterations in the functional properties of the epithelial lining material. With cumulative injury over a long period, chronic inflammation leads to fibrosis and perhaps an increase in the amount of smooth muscle. These lesions are very likely irreversible. At this stage deformities in airway shape and decreases in average luminal diameter first become evident. Emphysematous lesions in the respiratory bronchiole and in adjacent parenchyma appear at about the same time, possibly in response to the same inflammatory lesions. The progression of these irreversible lesions,

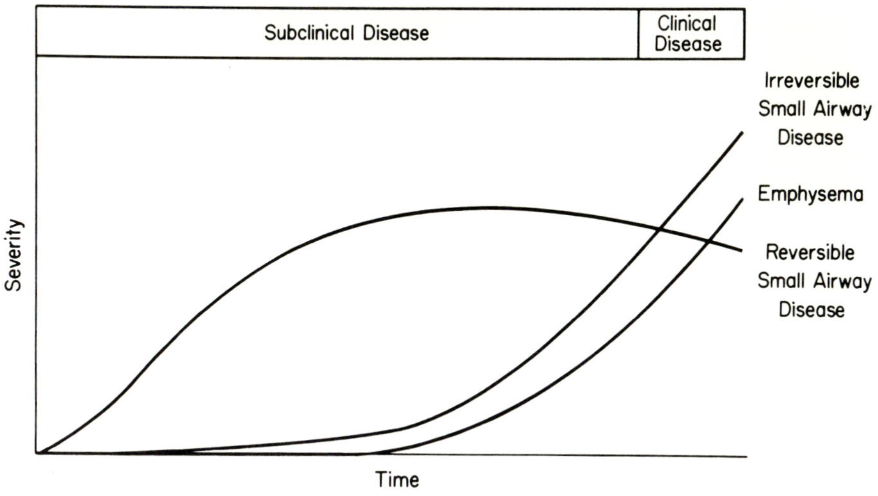

FIG. 9. A proposed natural history for COPD.

perhaps in combination with aging and with other unidentified factors, eventually give rise to severe airflow obstruction.

REFERENCES

1. American Thoracic Society: Chronic bronchitis, asthma, and pulmonary emphysema. A statement by the Committee on Diagnostic Standards for Nontuberculous Respiratory Diseases. *Am. Rev. Resp. Dis. 85:* 762–768, 1962.
2. Anderson, A. E., Jr., and Foraker, A. G.: Relative dimensions of bronchioles and parenchymal spaces in lungs from normal subjects and emphysematous patients. *Am. J. Med. 32:* 218–226, 1962.
3. Bignon, J., Khoury, F., Even, P., Andre, J., and Brouet, G.: Morphometric study in chronic obstructive bronchopulmonary disease. Pathologic, clinical and physiologic correlations. *Am. Rev. Resp. Dis. 99:* 669–695, 1969.
4. Bignon, J., Andre-Bougaran, J., and Brouet, G.: Parenchymal, bronchiolar, and bronchial measurements in centrilobular emphysema. Relation to weight of right ventricle. *Thorax 25:* 556–567, 1970.
5. Boushy, S. F., Aboumrad, M. H., North, L. B., and Helgason, A. H.: Lung recoil pressure, airway resistance, and forced flows related to morphologic emphysema. *Am. Rev. Resp. Dis. 104:* 551–561, 1971.
6. Buist, A. S., van Fleet, D. L., and Ross, B. B.: A comparison of conventional spirometric tests and the test of closing volume in an emphysema screening center. *Am. Rev. Resp. Dis. 107:* 735–743, 1973.
7. Burrows, B., and Earle, R. H.: Course and prognosis of chronic obstructive lung disease. A prospective study of 200 patients. *N. Engl. J. Med. 280:* 397–404, 1969.
8. Caldwell, E. J.: Physiologic and anatomic effects of papain on the rabbit lung. *J. Appl. Physiol. 31:* 458–465, 1971.
9. Camner, P. and Philipson, K.: Tracheobronchial clearance in smoking—Discordant twins. *Arch. Environ. Health 25:* 60–63, 1972.
10. Cosio, M., Corbin, R., Ghezzo, H., Loveland, M., Martin, R., Dosman, J., Macklem, P., and Hogg, J.: Structure-function relationships in small airway obstruction. *Am. Rev. Resp. Dis. 113(Part 2):* 225, 1976 (Abstr.).
11. Depierre, A., Bignon, J., Lebeau, A., and Brouet, G.: Quantitative study of parenchyma and small conductive airways in chronic nonspecific lung disease: Use of histologic stereology and bronchial casts. *Chest 62:* 699–708, 1972.

12. Ebert, R. V., and Terracio, M. J.: The bronchiolar epithelium in cigarette smokers. Observations with the scanning electron microscope. *Am. Rev. Resp. Dis. 111:* 4–11, 1975.
13. Emirgil, C., Sobol, B. J., Varble, A., Waldie, J., and Weinheimer, B.: Long-term course of chronic obstructive pulmonary disease. A new view of the mode of functional deterioration. *Am. J. Med. 51:* 504-512, 1971.
14. Hogg, J. C., Macklem, P. T., and Thurlbeck, W. M.: Site and nature of airway obstruction in chronic obstructive lung disease. *N. Engl. J. Med. 278:* 1355–1360, 1968.
15. Ingram, R. H., Jr., and O'Cain, C. F.: Frequency dependence of compliance in apparently healthy smokers versus non-smokers. *Bull. Physio-path. Resp. 7:* 195–210, 1971.
16. Janoff, A., Rosenberg, R., and Galdston, M.: Elastase-like esteroprotease activity in human and rabbit alveolar macrophage granules (35426). *Proc. Soc. Exp. Biol. Med. 136:* 1054–1058, 1971.
17. Karpick, R. J., Pratt, P. C., Asmundsson, T., and Kilburn, K. H.: Pathological findings in respiratory failure: Goblet cell metaplasia, alveolar damage, and myocardial infarction. *Ann. Int. Med. 72:* 189–197, 1970.
18. Laennec, R. T. H.: A treatise on the diseases of the chest and on mediate auscultation. Translated by Sir John Forbes. 4th ed. London, Longmans, 1834.
19. Leopold, J. G., and Gough, J.: The centrilobular form of hypertrophic emphysema and its relation to chronic bronchitis. *Thorax 12:* 219–235, 1957.
20. Leopold, J. G., and Seal, R. M.: The bronchographic appearance of "peripheral pooling" attributed to the filling of centrilobular emphysematous spaces. *Thorax 16:* 70–77, 1961.
21. Linhartová, A., Anderson, A. E., Jr., and Foraker, A. G.: Topology of nonrespiratory bronchioles of normal and emphysematous lungs. *Human Pathol. 5:* 729–735, 1974.
22. Macklem, P. T.: Obstruction in small airways—A challenge to medicine (editorial). *Am. J. Med. 52:* 721–724, 1972.
23. Martin, C. J., Katsura, S., and Cochran, T. H.: The relationship of chronic bronchitis to the diffuse obstructive pulmonary syndrome. *Am. Rev. Resp. Dis. 102:* 362–369, 1970.
24. Mass, B., Ikeda, T., Meranze, D. R., Weinbaum, G., and Kimbel, P.: Induction of experimental emphysema: Cellular and species specificity. *Am. Rev. Resp. Dis. 106:* 384–391, 1972.
25. Matsuba, K., and Thurlbeck, W. M.: The number and dimensions of small airways in nonemphysematous lungs. *Am. Rev. Resp. Dis. 104:* 516–524, 1971.
26. Matsuba, K., and Thurlbeck, W. M.: The number and dimensions of small airways in emphysematous lungs. *Am. J. Pathol. 67:* 265–284, 1972.
27. Matsuba, K., and Thurlbeck, W. M.: Disease of the small airways in chronic bronchitis. *Am. Rev. Resp. Dis. 107:* 552–558, 1973.
28. McCarthy, D. S., Spencer, R., Greene, R., and Milic-Emili, J.: Measurement of closing volume as a simple and sensitive test for early detection of small airway disease. *Am. J. Med. 52:* 747–753, 1972.
29. McKenzie, H. I., Glick, M., and Outhred, K. G.: Chronic bronchitis in coal miners: Ante-mortem-post-mortem comparisons. *Thorax 24:* 527–535, 1969.
30. McLean, K. H.: The pathogenesis of pulmonary emphysema. *Am. J. Med. 25:* 62–74, 1958.
31. Mitchell, R. S., Stanford, R. E., Johnson, J. M., Silvers, G. W., Dart, G., and George, M. S.: The morphologic features of the bronchi, bronchioles, and alveoli in chronic airway obstruction: A clinicopathologic study. *Am. Rev. Resp. Dis. 114:* 137–145, 1976.
32. Niewoehner, D. E., and Kleinerman, J.: Effects of experimental emphysema and bronchiolitis on lung mechanics and morphometry. *J. Appl. Physiol. 35:* 25–31, 1973.
33. Niewoehner, D. E., and Kleinerman, J.: Morphologic basis of pulmonary resistance in the human lung and effects of aging. *J. Appl. Physiol. 36:* 412–418, 1974.
34. Niewoehner, D. E., Kleinerman, J., and Rice, D. B.: Pathologic changes in the peripheral airways of young cigarette smokers. *N. Engl. J. Med. 291:* 755–758, 1974.
35. Niewoehner, D. E., Knoke, J., and Kleinerman, J.: Peripheral airways as a determinant of ventilatory function in the human lung. *J. Clin. Invest. 60:* 139–151, 1977.
36. Park, S. S., Goldring, I. P., Shim, C. S., and Williams, M. H., Jr.: Mechanical properties of the lung in experimental pulmonary emphysema. *J. Appl. Physiol. 26:* 738–744, 1969.
37. Park, S. S., Janis, M., Shim, C. S., and Williams, M. H., Jr.: Relationship of bronchitis and emphysema to altered pulmonary functions. *Am. Rev. Resp. Dis. 102:* 927–936, 1970.
38. Penman, R. W. B., O'Neill, R. P., and Begley, L.: Lung elastic recoil and airway resistance as factors limiting forced expiratory flow. *Am. Rev. Resp. Dis. 101:* 528–535, 1970.

39. Reid, L. McA.: Pathology of chronic bronchitis. *Lancet 1:* 275–278, 1954.
40. Reid, L.: Measurement of the bronchial mucous gland layer: A diagnostic yardstick in chronic bronchitis. *Thorax 15:* 132–141, 1960.
41. Scott, K. W. M., and Steiner, G. M.: Postmortem assessment of chronic airways obstruction by tantalum bronchography. *Thorax 30:* 405–414, 1975.
42. Seely, J. E., Zuskin, E., and Bouhuys, A.: Cigarette smoking: Objective evidence for lung damage in teen-agers. *Science 172:* 741–743, 1971.
43. Spain, D. M., and Kaufman, G.: The basic lesion in chronic pulmonary emphysema. *Am. Rev. Tuberc. 68:* 24–30, 1953.
44. Thurlbeck, W. M., Dunnill, M. S., Hartung, W., Heard, B. E., Heppleston, A. G., and Ryder, R. C.: A comparison of three methods of measuring emphysema. *Human Pathol. 1:* 215–226, 1970.
45. Thurlbeck, W. M., Henderson, J. A., Fraser, R. G., and Bates, D. V.: Chronic obstructive lung disease. A comparison between clinical, roentgenologic, functional and morphologic criteria in chronic bronchitis, emphysema, asthma and bronchiectasis. *Medicine* (Baltimore) *49:* 81–145, 1970.
46. Thurlbeck, W. M.: *Chronic Airflow Obstruction in Lung Disease.* Vol. 5, *Major Problems in Pathology,* J. L. Bennington, consulting ed. Philadelphia, W. B. Saunders Co., 1976.
47. Watanabe, S., Mitchell, M., and Renzetti, A. D., Jr.: Correlation of structure and function in chronic pulmonary emphysema. *Am. Rev. Resp. Dis. 92:* 221–227, 1965.

Chapter 10

Bronchial Asthma*

J. C. HOGG

Bronchial asthma is a condition which has defied precise definition.[44] Most physicians would agree, however, that it is typically characterized by dyspnea associated with wheezing that is caused by mechanical obstruction in the airways. The main difficulty in defining asthma is that physicians of different disciplines observe different aspects of the disease. The pathologist has usually studied the lungs of patients who died in status asthmaticus, an unusually severe manifestation of asthma that can result in death. Fortunately, the vast majority of the patients who have asthma never suffer from status asthmaticus so that most clinicians who treat asthma are much more familiar with the acute attacks, which are much easier to manage. With regard to pathogenesis, there is substantial evidence that favors a decisive role of the immunologic system in some forms of asthma, and indeed, most attacks occur in atopic patients. However, a significant number of asthmatic patients have attacks which occur either spontaneously or are precipitated by factors which irritate the airways and do not appear to have any immunologic basis. This fact raises important questions concerning the neurologic control of bronchial smooth muscle and whether or not asthma occurs primarily in patients that have hyperreactive airways because the control of their bronchial smooth muscle is abnormal.[27]

CLASSIFICATION

The complexities of the disease make it difficult to classify. The classification presented in Table 1 is modified from one proposed by Rose, Hogg, and Macklem[41] and will unquestionably be revised as knowledge increases. A reasonable classification must take into account both the patients in whom the etiology is clearly immunologic in nature and also those in whom immunologic mechanisms cannot be involved. Although these two categories were once labeled extrinsic and intrinsic asthma, this oversimplification is no longer justified. The largest group consists of individuals whose attacks are mediated by reagin. These patients usually have an atopic background and their asthma is frequently preceded either by atopic dermatitis or by allergic rhinitis. They often have a family history of allergy and exhibit immediate wheal and flare response to skin tests. Their spasmodic attacks of asthma are related to food, drugs, or allergens suspended in

* Supported by Grant No. MA-4219 from the Medical Research Council of Canada.

TABLE 1*

Type of asthma	Precipitating factor	Skin test	Bronchial provocation
Reagin mediated	Specific antigen challenge	Type I	Immediate
Non-reaginic	Respiratory tract infection	Usually negative	Nonspecific Hyperreactive airways
Aspirin sensitive	Interference with prostaglandin synthesis by aspirin	Negative	Nonspecific Hyperreactive airways
Exercise induced	Exercise: may occur alone or with other forms of asthma	Negative	
Cold air sensitive	Cold air or other irritants: may occur with other forms of asthma	Negative	
Allergic bronchopulmonary aspergillosis	Antigen challenge	Type I and III	Immediate and delayed
Industrial asthma	Chemical challenge	Type I and III	Immediate and delayed

* Modified from Rose, Hogg, and Macklem (Ref. 41).

the air. Between attacks these patients may be largely symptom-free and their symptoms may become perennial and occur whenever the allergen to which they are sensitive appears in the environment.

The second large group is the so-called non-atopic variety of asthma. The asthmatic attacks often coincide with respiratory tract infection. In some patients the precipitating infection appears to be localized in the paranasal sinuses, but in others it may occur as a complication of chronic bronchitis. The terms "chronic bronchitis with wheezing" or "chronic infective asthma" have been used to describe this latter condition. Skin tests are usually negative, but eosinophilia is common.

A third important group of patients with asthma is that of those who present with chronic hyperplastic rhinitis, with or without polyp formation, and who have a marked sensitivity to aspirin.[43] The symptoms often precede the development of intolerance to aspirin by months, or even years. It has been suggested that agents such as aspirin and a variety of other nonsteroidal, anti-inflammatory compounds induce asthma by inhibiting the biosynthesis of prostaglandins,[16] but this hypothesis remains to be proven.

Asthma that can be induced by exercise has been investigated extensively in recent years and is of great interest. Its precise mechanism is unknown, and it does not appear to be precipitated by either the breathing pattern of exercise or the fall in P_{CO_2}.[26] However, water loss from the respiratory mucosa may be an important factor in precipitating the attacks.[8] It is likely incorrect to think of exercise-induced asthma as an homogeneous entity as it may occur as a complication of several forms of asthma. The precipitation of asthmatic attacks by breathing cold air is well documented, but again it seems likely that this represents a nonspecific factor which can produce bronchospasm in airways that have been rendered hyperirritable by allergy or infection.

An important group of patients with asthma has been described by Pepys.[34] These patients appear to develop both type I and type III reactivity to aspergillus, and they appear to have similar reactions in their airways. When they receive a bronchial challenge with antigen they may develop both an immediate and a delayed response which occurs 4–6 hours after inhalation of the antigen. Both skin and aerosol challenge tests are therefore characterized by this so-called dual response.

Finally, a variety of industrial agents are also known to be chronic inducers of asthma.[36, 35] These include chemical dusts such as the complex salts of platinum, gases such as Toluene 2–4 diisocyanate, and the fumes of epoxy resins and plastics, wood dust, chemical powder, and the henna dye of hairdressers. A major difficulty in studying all of these compounds has been to differentiate the immunologic aspects from the contribution to the attacks of the irritant effect of the material. The data which favor an immunologic mechanism are that attacks seem to occur only after repeated exposure; sensitivity to the material seems to increase with the passage of time; and that in the majority of cases very minute quantities of the material are required to induce an attack. Unfortunately, not one of these observations provides conclusive proof that the disease is immunologically mediated and all of the observations might be expected in a patient who had hyperreactive airways before exposure.

PATHOPHYSIOLOGY OF ASTHMA

Deposition of Material in Tracheobronchial Tree

The respiratory system is well designed to purify and control temperature and humidity of the air inhaled. The deposition of antigenic or irritating material within the lung is a complex and poorly understood subject,[11] but the understanding of several important features of the airway may help to clarify the mechanisms. The narrowest air passages in the respiratory system are located in the nose and upper airways. When breathing through the nose, the airways resistance is much greater than when breathing through the mouth. The larynx offers about 50% of the total lower airways resistance and the large bronchi account for 30%, so that very little of the resistance is located in the smaller airways. Because of this, the bulk of the lower airway resistance is encountered in the first 10–12 orders of branching, and when air is breathed in, gas velocity is greater in the central portions of the tracheobronchial tree than in the peripheral portions. Large particles, because of their greater mass, will be deposited in the large airways where their momentum due to their velocity and mass is great. Smaller particles that remain in the airstream will be deposited in the more peripheral areas where there is little flow of air. Very small particles with long settling times will not be deposited at all and will be breathed out of the lung on expiration. From this oversimplified discussion, it is obvious that factors such as the rate and depth of breathing can greatly influence antigen deposition by varying the velocities of the antigen particles. Similarly, warming and humidification of the air will induce deposition of antigen as water is absorbed by the particles. As the particles grow in size they develop greater inertial forces which favour impaction, shorter settling times and thus their deposition in the more central airways. Once particles are deposited in the airway, they may be cleared by several mechanisms including the sneeze, cough, mucociliary clearance, and phagocytosis by alveolar macrophages. Although each of these mechanisms is complex and incompletely understood, their collective function can greatly influence how much of the material entering the airways remains in the lungs. Because of the complexities of both deposition and clearance, it is obvious that it is almost impossible to determine the exact dose of antigen that a patient will receive when exposed to a particular antigen, even under the most controlled laboratory conditions.

Sites of Interaction Between Antigen and Mast Cells

The location of mast cells in the tracheobronchial tree are of obvious interest because of their theoretic importance in type I-mediated disease. Although mast cells abound in the airways,[9] most investigators have found them to be concentrated in the submucosal connective tissue, frequently adjacent to blood vessels and nerves, and closely associated with collagen fibrils.[50] Studies of bronchial biopsies by Salvato[42] suggest that the numbers of mast cells were reduced in the lungs of asthmatics in areas where he found a prevalence of degranulated and disrupted cells. The barrier between the airway lumen where antigen first appears and the mast cells in the submucosa is formidable. The antigen must traverse the mucociliary blanket and the epithelium which are joined together by tight junctions. These junctions represent membrane fusion between cells,[51] and in the case of the tracheobronchial epithelium, they are continuous around the cell periphery and are extremely tight.[20, 21] The nature of the mucosal barrier could either prevent or delay entry of antigen into the submucosa after it has been deposited on the surface of the airways. This means that when antigen is breathed in there should be a delay in the response if the antigen molecule has to penetrate the mucosa to the mast cells in the submucosa. The fact that antigen challenge of ascaris sensitive Rhesus monkeys[29] produces rapid shallow breathing within seconds of the onset of challenge strongly suggests that the first reaction to inhaled antigen occurs in the lumen (Fig. 1). The fact that the quantitative study of the numbers of mast cells[18] has shown that there is a small, but significant population of mast cells in the bronchial mucosa and epithelium of macaca fasicularis monkeys suggests that antigen and mast cells meet at the airway surface. Patterson and his colleagues[33] have also shown that it is possible to obtain "basophiloid cells" (? mast cells) from the bronchial washings of both allergic monkeys and man, but the large number of epithelial cells that are also obtained by this procedure makes it difficult to be certain of the exact location of these cells when they were in the lung. In any event, it seems highly likely that these superficial mast cells are the first to react with antigen.

In their study of antigen challenge of sensitive monkeys Pare, Michoud, and Hogg[29] showed that the rapid shallow breathing preceded the increase in airways resistance by an interval of about 40 seconds (Fig. 1). This suggests that rapid shallow breathing and bronchoconstriction may be mediated by separate mechanisms. The importance of bronchial reflexes in asthma has been stressed, and recent data suggest that these reflexes are more important with respect to control of the rapid shallow breathing than bronchoconstriction.[10] Indeed, it seems likely that a few mast cells in the surface of airways could react with antigen and release enough histamine to stimulate the irritant receptors which stimulate the rapid shallow breathing at the start of the attack. There is also recent evidence, both in monkeys[19] and in guinea pigs,[3] that antigen and histamine challenge can

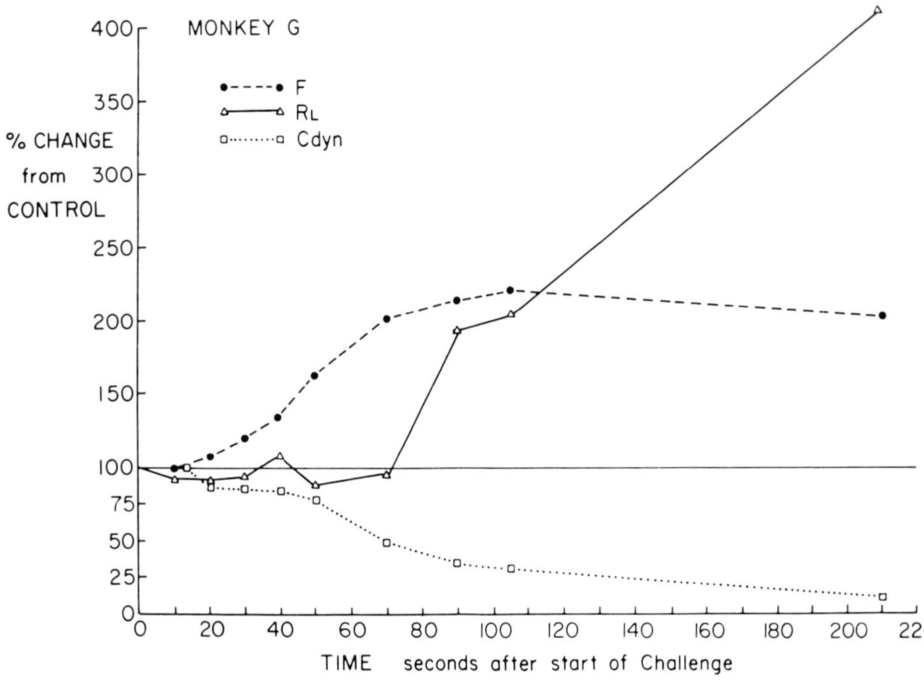

FIG. 1. Data from Pare *et al.*[29] showing physiologic response in an allergic monkey following bronchial challenge. The increase in breathing frequency occurring 20 seconds after onset of challenge suggests that the initial reaction between antigen and antibody occurs in the bronchial lumen. *F*, respiratory frequency; R_L, resistance to airflow in lung; *Cdyn*, dynamic compliance.

increase bronchial epithelial permeability. This has suggested the hypothesis that an initial reaction at the luminal surface can change the mucosal barrier so that more antigen can penetrate to greater numbers of mast cells in the submucosa. The small number of mast cells in the lumen would then be very important, both for the initiation and amplification of the asthmatic attack.

IMMUNOGLOBULINS IN ASTHMA

There are at least three types of immunoglobulin involved in antigen antibody mechanisms related to asthma in man. In atopic asthma it is postulated that antigen combines with IgE antibody which is attached to receptor sites on the surface of mast cells by its FC fragment. A series of events takes place culminating in the release of chemical mediators such as histamine, slow-reacting substance of anaphylaxis (SRS-A), and eosinophilic chemotactic factor (ECF-A).[2, 22, 23, 28] Histamine and SRS-A are thought to produce smooth muscle constriction, either by direct or reflex action or both, and ECF-A is thought to be responsible for the eosinophilia which occurs in the bronchial wall. A second group of mediators[37] is also released and these consist of prostaglandins E and F and the kinins. Just why some individuals form IgE antibody to a variety of antigens and others do not is unknown but genetic factors seem likely to play a role.

It has been suggested that in non-atopic children, IgA antibody is formed to allergens by preference and that these IgA molecules remove antigen determinants which are no longer available to IgE-producing plasma cells. Thus, a deficiency in IgA antibody would permit the production of high IgE levels with reaginic activity.[49] This concept is partially supported by evidence that a low or even absent serum IgA level has been found in atopic populations, and by the fact that the incidence of atopy was much greater in IgA-deficient patients as compared to normal subjects.[45]

It is also possible that a heat-stable, short-lived variety of IgG, or so-called short-term anaphylactic IgG antibody, also plays a role in asthma. Recent studies by Bryant, Burns, and Lazarus[4] have identified an IgG heat-stable immunoglobulin of a short-lived, homocytotropic variety that may be responsible for asthma in a group of dust-sensitive, asthmatic patients.

A third antibody system which seems capable of inducing airways obstruction in man is the conventional IgG, in addition to IgE. The best example of this is allergic bronchopulmonary aspergillosis.[34] This dual system accounts for the presence of both type I and type III reactions. In this situation it is presumably the interaction of IgE and aspergillus antigen, in addition to the activation of complement by IgG and aspergillus antigen complexes which is responsible for the release of mediators; but a great deal remains to be clarified.

Immunopharmacology

In recent years Austen[2, 22, 23, 28] and Lichtenstein[24, 25] and their co-workers have investigated the mechanism and control of the antigen-mediated release of mediators from human lung fragments and from circulating human leukocytes. Their data suggested the possibility that the release of mediators was monitored via the cyclic nucleotides and they showed that stimuli which raised the intracellular levels of cyclic AMP decreased the amount of mediator release, while stimuli that lowered the intracellular levels of cyclic AMP increased the amount of mediator release. They also showed that there was a possible push-pull mechanism between the raising of cyclic AMP and the lowering of cyclic GMP. They postulated that various agents controlled the release of mediators from target cells by their action on the cyclic nucleotides. This concept has been summarized in a recent monograph,[2] and the information concerning the control of mediator release has provided insights into the pharmacology and pathophysiology of asthma. However, it does not provide a complete explanation for the pathophysiology of asthma, as the action of mediators cannot explain all aspects of this complex disease.

Morphology

Although the study of the morphology of the airways in asthma has been dominated by autopsy studies, some biopsy studies have been carried out. The results of the immunofluorescent studies designed to localize the antibodies thought to be responsible for precipitating attacks have been somewhat disappointing, and there is a large discrepancy between data and theory. For example, Callerame *et al.*[6, 7] found staining for IgE in 5 of 11 biopsies and in 6 of 7 autopsy specimens. IgM predominated, but IgA and IgG as well as C_3 were found. In further studies, there was no difference in the number of IgE-containing plasma cells between atopic and non-atopic specimens, although curiously, the average number of these cells in lung specimens from asthmatic persons was lower than that found in normal controls. The report of heavy staining of IgE found in lung basement membrane by Gerber, Paronetto, and Kochwa[17] and the fact that IgE was located on other cells is interesting, but needs to be confirmed. The presence of IgG, M, or A may be explained on the basis of chronic, intercurrent infection or could be present due to an increased capillary permeability caused by mediators released by the activation of mast cells by IgE.

Unfortunately, there are practically no studies that have carefully examined the sequence of events following deposition of antigen in the tracheobronchial tree. Indeed, the most-often quoted studies on the pathology of asthma have dealt almost entirely with patients who died in status asthmaticus. The major gross features of the pathology of status asthmaticus are the presence of mucous plugs, the absence of any significant emphysema, and occasional areas of bronchiectasis.[12, 13] Bronchiectasis is a particularly common feature of bronchopulmonary aspergillosis where it is usually central in location, more common in the upper airways, and unlike classical bronchiectasis in that the peripheral airways seem to be preserved. The airway plugging in the asthmatic lung is due to the dense exudate in the bronchial lumen.[12, 13] This exudate is heterogeneous and has mucous, serous, and cellular components. The mucous component arises from both excess production by the hypertrophied mucous glands[13] and the increase in the number of goblet cells. Decreased clearance of mucus caused by sloughing of the mucosa due to submucosal edema must also contribute to the mucus found in the tracheobronchial tree. The serous component of the exudate arises from the intense inflammatory reaction in the submucosa, and the cellular component is made up of eosinophils and tracheobronchial epithelial cells that are sloughed into the airway lumen. The changes in the bronchial wall at postmortem are striking and consist primarily of hyperplasia of the mucous glands and an increase in the amount of bronchial smooth muscle.[14] The fact that some of these morbid anatomic changes are present during life can be established by examination of the sputum. This shows the Curschmann spirals which represent casts of the small airways that are made up of the nonmucoid elements of the exudate and the Charcot-Leyden crystals which are derived from the eosinophils in the exudate. The so-called creola bodies which are found in the sputum result from the sloughing of epithelium into the lumen.

Hyperreactivity of Airways

An important nonimmunologic feature of patients with asthma is that their airways hyperreact to bronchoconstrictor agents and to nonspecific irritants.[11, 30, 47] When these materials are administered in bronchial provocation tests, the increase in pulmonary resistance or decrease in maximum expiratory flow rates are much greater than those expected for normal subjects, and they occur with much smaller doses of the inhaled material. As some of these stimuli are inert, *e.g.,* cold air and citric acid, the immune mechanism is clearly not responsible for this response. Several theories have been put forward to account for this hyperreactivity, all of which are interesting and none of which are conclusively proven. The first is an abnormality of the bronchial epithelium which could result in a greater absorption of bronchoconstricting materials into the submucosa. For example, cigarette smoking[46] has been shown to change epithelial permeability in the guinea pigs, and it has subsequently been shown that irritants such as ether anesthesia[40] and mediators of bronchoconstriction such as histamine and methacholine[3] can do the same thing. The recent study of Empey and others[15] is of interest in this regard because they showed that bronchial hyperreactivity to histamine and citric acid aerosols increased markedly during upper respiratory tract infection, and this hyperreactivity decreased when the infection disappeared. Since atropine aerosol blocked the increase in resistance to both of these substances, it was suggested that the rapidly-adapting airway receptors were stimulated more readily during the infection. These data are consistent with the hypothesis originally put forward by Nadel[27] that the airways hyperreactivity seen in asthmatics is mediated by the cholinergic nervous system and results from a "sensitization" of the irritant receptors in the airway epithelium. Whether or not the "sensitization" of the irritant receptors is due to epithelial damage changing bronchial permeability and allowing higher concentrations of irritants to reach the submucosa is an interesting hypothesis that remains to be tested.

Another possibility is that hyperreactivity may be explained by an abnormality in the control of the bronchial smooth muscle. This abnormality could arise from a defect in autonomic control or from a defect in the nonadrenergic inhibitor system. This latter system is part of the "purinergic" nervous system[5] which in the gastrointestinal tract is responsible for the wave of inhibition which precedes the peristaltic wave. This system is controlled by ganglia, and absence of the ganglia results in spastic states of the colon and rectum as in Hirschprung's disease. This system has been demonstrated *in vitro* in the airway smooth muscle of both guinea pig[39] and man,[38] and it is conceivable that a defect in the nonadrenergic inhibitory system may play an important role in the pathophysiology of asthma. Such a defect would interfere with the normal bronchodilating mechanism and could result in hyperreactivity. An older hypothesis for hyperreactivity is that the control of the bronchial smooth muscle is normally balanced by the activities of the sympathetic and parasympathetic nervous system and that bronchial hyperreactivity occurs when there is abnormal parasympathetic activity.

Finally, it is impossible to leave the discussion of asthma without mentioning the concept that increased α-adrenergic activity in the presence of partial β-adrenergic blockade might be the cause of some forms of asthma. This is the basis of the so-called β-adrenergic blockade theory of asthma which was originally put forward by Szentivanyi.[48] In support of this theory Patel and Kerr[32] found that administered phenylephrine with and without the prior administration of propranol produced a significant reduction in FEV_1 and specific airways conductance in asthmatic but not in control patients. The β-adrenergic blockade theory received further support from the observations of Parker and Smith[31] on the level of cyclic AMP in peripheral leukocytes. They found, as compared with normal patients, that all patients with asthma had lower levels of cyclic AMP in their leukocytes and the more severe the asthma, the lower the level. In addition, they found that the cells from asthmatic patients responded to catecholamines and theophylline to a much lesser degree. These findings have been confirmed for circulating lymphocytes, both in reagin-mediated and non-reagin-mediated asthma. The importance of this mechanism to clinical asthma is somewhat hypothetical and awaits further clarification.

SUMMARY

In summary, Figure 2 shows a working hypothesis concerning asthma that tries to take into account the events that occur in the airway lumen, in the bronchial mucosa, and in the nerves and smooth muscle of the airway wall. The speed of onset of attacks following antigen challenge[29] and the fact that the mucosal barrier is formidable[20, 21] make it reasonable to assume that the very small percentage of the total number of airways mast cells that are present in the lumen[18, 19] are the first to interact with antigens. The fact that mediators thought to be released from mast cells by antigen challenge have been shown to change mucosal permeability[3] makes it possible that the initial reaction between antigen and mast cell at the surface will allow more antigen to penetrate the mucosal barrier and gain access to the much larger number of mast cells in the submucosa. This amplification step may well explain why bronchial smooth muscle spasm

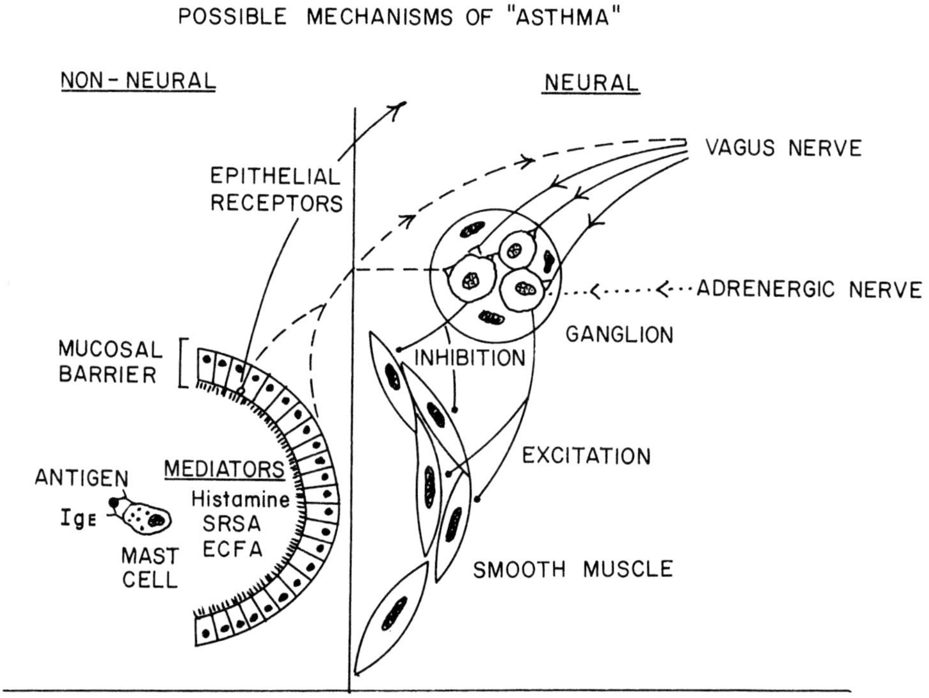

FIG. 2. A working hypothesis for asthma stressing the importance of events in the airway lumen, mucosa, and wall of the bronchus. Reagin-mediated attacks are probably triggered in the bronchial lumen where inhaled antigen reacts with IgE on the small number of mast cells in the bronchial lumen. The mediators released cause rapid shallow breathing by stimulating the irritant receptors present in the bronchial mucosa. Bronchial smooth muscle constriction may be produced by direct action of the mediators on the smooth muscle, by reflex bronchoconstriction, or both. The reactivity of the smooth muscle is determined by neuromuscular factors and hyperreactivity of the airways smooth muscle may be explained by an imbalance in adrenergic and cholinergic innervation, by a defect in the nonadrenergic inhibitor system, or by an abnormality of the smooth muscle itself. Mediator release at the surface also causes a change in mucosal permeability that amplifies the reaction by allowing more antigen to penetrate to the larger number of mast cells in the submucosa. This change in permeability might also increase airway sensitivity as it would allow more mediator to penetrate to the nerve endings.

caused by antigen lasts much longer than that induced by histamine. Once the mucosal barrier is breached it also seems possible that the subsequent challenge with mediators may provoke a greater response after challenge than before. Indeed, this may be part of the mechanism for the "sensitization" of the irritant receptor which Empey and his colleagues[15] have shown to be associated with mucosal damage. Finally, the third important area is the neurologic and pharmacologic control of bronchial smooth muscle. It seems that bronchial hyperreactivity could be explained by an abnormality of the purinergic nervous system as Richardson[38, 39] has suggested, or that airways hyperreactivity may be due to an imbalance between adrenergic and cholinergic control of the smooth muscle. It is also possible that the smooth muscle of asthmatic subjects is abnormal, but little information exists concerning this possibility. Finally, it remains to be determined if asthma can be explained by links between the factors controlling mediator release and those involved in the neurologic control of the bronchial smooth muscle. It may be that such a linkage is the key to understanding asthma, but it is also possible that these two factors function completely independently.

Acknowledgements: The help of Dr. John Richardson in preparing this manuscript, and in particular, his permission to use the diagram relating to the control of smooth muscle, which forms part of Figure 2, is acknowledged.

REFERENCES

1. Altshuler, B.: Behaviour of airborne particles in the respiratory tract, In *Circulatory and Respiratory Mass Transport.* A CIBA Foundation Symposium, edited by Wolstenholme, G.E.W., and Knight, J., pp. 215–235, Little, Brown & Co., Boston, 1969.
2. Austen, K. F., Lewis, R. A., Wasserman, S. I., and Goetzl, E. J.: Generation and release of chemical mediators of immediate hypersensitivity in human cells. American College of Chest Physicians, Park Ridge, Illinois, 1975.
3. Boucher, R., Ranga, V., Pare, P. D., Inoue, S., Moroz, L. A., and Hogg, J. C.: The effect of histamine and methacholine on respiratory mucosal permeability. Abstract. American Thoracic Society, May, 1976.
4. Bryant, D. H., Burns, M. W., and Lazarus, L.: Identification of IgG antibody as a carrier of reaginic activity in asthmatic patients. *J. Allergy Clin. Immunol. 56:* 417–428, 1975.
5. Burnstock, G.: Purinergic nerves. *Pharmacol. Rev. 24:* 509–581, 1972.
6. Callerame, M. L., Condemi, J. J., Bohrod, M. G., and Vaughan, J. H.: Immunologic reactions of bronchial tissues in asthma. *N. Engl. J. Med. 284:* 459–464, 1971.
7. Callerame, M. L., Condemi, J. J., Ishizaka, K., Johansson, S. G. O., and Vaughan, J. H.: Immunoglobulins in bronchial tissues from patients with asthma, with special reference to immunoglobulin E. *J. Allergy 47:* 187–197, 1971.
8. Chen, W. Y., Horton, D. J. and Souhrada, J. F.: Respiratory heat and water loss in exercise-induced asthma. *Physiologist 19:* 152, 1976 (abstr.).
9. Connell, J. T.: Asthmatic deaths. Role of the mast cell. *JAMA 215:* 769–776, 1971.
10. Cotton, D. J., Bleecker, E. R., Fischer, S. P., Graf, P. D.,, Gold, W. M., and Nadel, J. A.: Rapid, shallow breathing after *Ascaris suum* antigen inhalation: Role of vagus nerves. *J. Appl. Physiol. 42:* 101–106, 1977.
11. Curry, J. J.: The action of histamine on the respiratory tract in normal and asthmatic subjects. *J. Clin. Invest. 25:* 785–791, 1946.
12. Dunnill, M. S.: The pathology of asthma, with special reference to changes in the bronchial mucosa. *J. Clin. Pathol. 13:* 27–33, 1960.
13. Dunnill, M. S.: The pathology of asthma in the identification of asthma. In *Identification of Asthma.* A CIBA Foundation Symposia, edited by Ruth Porter and Joan Birch, pp. 35–46, Churchill Livingstone, London, 1971.

14. Dunnill, M. S., Massarella, G. R., and Anderson, J. A.: A comparison of the quantitative anatomy of the bronchi in normal subjects, in status asthmaticus, in chronic bronchitis, and in emphysema. *Thorax 24:* 176–179, 1969.
15. Empey, D. W., Laitinen, L. A., Jacobs, L., Gold, W. M., and Nadel, J. A.: Mechanisms of bronchial hyperreactivity in normal subjects after upper respiratory tract infection. *Am. Rev. Resp. Dis. 113:* 131–139, 1976.
16. Flower, R. J.: Drugs which inhibit prostaglandin biosynthesis. *Pharmacol. Rev. 26:* 33–67, 1974.
17. Gerber, M. A., Paronetto, F., and Kochwa, S.: Immunohistochemical localization of IgE in asthmatic lungs. *Am. J. Pathol. 62:* 339–352, 1971.
18. Guerzon, G., Pare, P. D., and Hogg, J. C.: The distribution of mast cells and eosinophils in Rhesus monkey lungs. *Clin. Res. 24:* 691A, 1976 (abstr.).
19. Hogg, J. C., Pare, P. D., Boucher, R., Michoud, M-C., Guerzon, G., and Moroz, L.: Pathologic abnormalities in asthma, In *Asthma II: Pathology, Pathophysiology and Treatment,* edited by Austen, K. F., and Lichtenstein, L. M., New York, Academic Press, 1977.
20. Inoue, S., and Hogg, J. C.: Intercellular junctions of the tracheal epithelium in guinea pigs. *Lab. Invest. 31:* 68–74, 1974.
21. Inoue, S., and Hogg, J. C.: A freeze-etch study of the tracheal epithelium of normal guinea pigs with particular reference to intercellular junctions. *J. Ultrastruct. Res. 61:* 89–99, 1977.
22. Kaliner, M., and Austen, K. F.: A sequence of biochemical events in the antigen-induced release of chemical mediators from sensitized human lung tissue. *J. Exp. Med. 138:* 1077–1094, 1973.
23. Kaliner, M., Orange, R. P., and Austen, K. F.: Immunological release of histamine and slow reacting substance of anaphylaxis from human lung. IV. Enhancement by cholinergic and alpha adrenergic stimulation. *J. Exp. Med. 136:* 556–567, 1972.
24. Lichtenstein, L. M., and De Bernardo, R.: The immediate allergic response. In vitro action of cyclic AMP-active and other drugs on the two stages of histamine release. *J. Immunol. 107:* 1131–1136, 1971.
25. Lichtenstein, L. M., and Osler, A. G.: Studies on the mechanisms of hypersensitivity phenomena. IX. Histamine release from human leukocytes by ragweed pollen antigen. *J. Exp. Med. 120:* 507–530, 1964.
26. McFadden, E. R., Stearns, D. R., Ingram, R. H., Jr., and Leith, D. E.: Relative contributions of hypocarbia and hyperpnea as mechanisms in postexercise asthma. *J. Appl. Physiol. 42:* 22–27, 1977.
27. Nadel, J. A.: Neurophysiological aspects of asthma. In, *Asthma:Physiology, Immunopharmacology and Treatment,* edited by Austen, K. F., and Lichtenstein, L. M., Chapter 3. New York, Academic Press, 1973.
28. Orange, R. P., Austen, W. G., and Austen, K. F.: Immunological release of histamine and slow-reacting substance of anaphylaxis from human lung. I. Modulation by agents influencing cellular levels of cyclic 3′,5′-adenosine monophosphate. *J. Exp. Med. 134:* 136s–148s, 1971.
29. Pare, P. D., Michoud, M-C., and Hogg, J. C.: Lung mechanics following antigen challenge in *Ascaris suum* sensitive Rhesus monkeys. *J. Appl. Physiol. 41:* 668–676, 1976.
30. Parker, C. D., Bilbo, R. E., and Reed, C. E.: Methacholine aerosol as test for bronchial asthma. *Arch. Intern. Med. 115:* 452–458, 1965.
31. Parker, C. W., and Smith, J. W.: Alterations in cyclic adenosine monophosphate metabolism in human bronchial asthma. I: Leukocyte responsiveness to β-adrenergic agents. *J. Clin. Invest. 52:* 48–59, 1973.
32. Patel, K. R., and Kerr, J. W.: The airways response to phenylephrine after blockade of alpha and beta receptors in extrinsic bronchial asthma. *Clin. Allergy 3:* 439–448, 1973.
33. Patterson, R., McKenna, J. M., Suszko, I. M., Solliday, N. H., Pruzansky, J. J., Roberts, M., and Kehoe, T. J.: Living histamine-containing cells from the bronchial lumens of humans. Description and comparison of histamine content with cells of Rhesus monkeys. *J. Clin. Invest. 59:* 217–225, 1977.
34. Pepys, J.: Immunologic approaches in pulmonary disease caused by inhaled materials. *Ann. N.Y. Acad. Sci. 221:* 27–37, 1974.
35. Pepys, J., Hutchcroft, B. J., and Breslin, A. B.: Asthma due to inhaled chemical agents-persulphate salts and henna in hairdressers. *Clin. Allergy 6:* 339–404, 1976.
36. Pepys, J., Pickering, C. A. C., and Hughes, E. G.: Asthma due to inhaled chemical agents—Complex salts of platinum. *Clin. Allergy 2:* 391–396, 1972.

37. Piper, P. J., and Vane, J. R.: Release of additional factors in anaphylaxis and its antagonism by anti-inflammatory drugs. *Nature 223:* 29–35, 1969.
38. Richardson, J., and Beland, J.: Nonadrenergic inhibitory nervous system in human airways. *J. Appl. Physiol. 41:* 764–771, 1976.
39. Richardson, J. B., and Bouchard, T.: Demonstration of the non adrenergic inhibitor system in the trachea of the guinea pig. *J. Allergy Clin. Immunol. 56:* 473–480, 1975.
40. Richardson, J., Bouchard, T., and Ferguson, C. C.: Uptake and transport of exogenous proteins by respiratory epithelium. *Lab. Invest. 35:* 307–314, 1976.
41. Rose, B., Hogg, J. C., and Macklem, P. T.: The pathogenesis of bronchial asthma. In, *Immunological Diseases,* 3rd ed, edited by Samter, M., Talmage, D. W., Rose, B., Austen, F., and Vaughan, J. H. Little, Brown and Co., Boston 1977.
42. Salvato, G.: Mast cells in bronchial connective tissue of man: Their modifications in asthma and after treatment with the histamine liberator 48/80. *Int. Arch. Allergy Appl. Immunol. 18:* 348–358, 1961.
43. Samter, M., and Beers, R. F., Jr.: Intolerance to aspirin. Clinical studies and consideration of its pathogenesis. *Ann. Int. Med. 68:* 975–983, 1968.
44. Scadding, J. G.: The definition of asthma: General introduction. In, *Identification of Asthma,* A CIBA Foundation Symposium, edited by Ruth Porter and Joan Birch, pp. 13–34, Churchill Livingstone, 1971.
45. Schwartz, D. P., and Buckley, R. H.: Serum IgE concentrations and skin reactivity to anti-IgE antibody in IgA-deficient patients. *N. Engl. J. Med. 284:* 513–517, 1971.
46. Simani, A. S., Inoue, S., and Hogg, J. C.: Penetration of the respiratory epithelium of guinea pigs following exposure to cigarette smoke. *Lab. Invest. 31:* 75–81, 1974.
47. Simonsson, B. G., Jacobs, F. M., and Nadel, J. A.: Role of autonomic nervous system and the cough reflex in the increased responsiveness of airways in patients with obstructive airway disease. *J. Clin. Invest. 46:* 1812–1818, 1967.
48. Szentivanyi, A.: The beta adrenergic theory of the atopic abnormality in bronchial asthma. *J. Allergy 42:* 203–232, 1968.
49. Taylor, B., Norman, A. P., Orgel, H. A,., Stokes, C. R., Turner, M. W., and Soothill, J. F.: Transient IgA deficiency and pathogenesis of infantile atopy. *Lancet 2:* 111–113, 1973.
50. Trotter, C. M., and Orr, T. S. C.: A fine structure study of some cellular components in allergic reactions. I: Degranulation of human mast cells in allergic asthma and perennial rhinitis. *Clin. Allergy 3:* 411–425, 1973.
51. Weinstein, R. S., and McNutt, N. S.: Cell junctions. *N. Engl. J. Med. 286:* 521–524, 1972.

Chapter 11

Present Trends in Lung Cancer

HARRY L. IOACHIM

In the first decade of this century, Lung Carcinoma was an uncommon tumor, in sharp contrast with its present position as the leading cause of death by neoplasia in men. With 93,000 new cases of pulmonary cancer in the male population in 1976,[78] primary carcinoma of the lung now comprises almost 10% of all malignant neoplasms in the USA (Fig. 1). Most industrialized countries have recorded similar increases of over 100% incidence in neoplasms of the lung between 1950 and 1964.[52] While both incidence and mortality of other neoplasms have leveled off or decreased in the last decade, the death rate of lung cancer in men has increased exponentially and is today 18 times higher than 40 years ago (Fig. 2).[78]

ETIOLOGY

As a result of intensive epidemiologic research carried out during the last 20 years in this field, it is now generally accepted that cancer of the lung is a disease of modern civilization and in large part preventable. The incidence of lung neoplasms correlates directly with population density, urbanization, industrialization, tobacco-smoking, and even with the registration of automobiles.[39]

The etiologic factors in lung cancer are divided into personal air pollutants; that is, smoking, and nonpersonal air pollutants which include atmospheric contaminants and industrial exposure.[5] In the first Surgeon General's Report issued in 1964[83] it was stated that "in comparison with non-smokers, average male smokers have a 9- to 10-fold risk and heavy smokers a 20-fold risk to develop lung cancer." At that time, Kreyberg[49] of Oslo had divided carcinomas of the lung into two major groups: type 1, which included squamous and oat cell carcinomas related to smoking, and type 2, including adenocarcinomas and large cell carcinomas with no apparent increase of incidence in smokers. The group largely responsible for the great increase in lung carcinoma was that of white male smokers who generally had Kreyberg type 1 tumors and there was a strong suggestion that cigarette tar acts as a carcinogen with a dose-response relationship.[90]

In the 13 years since the Surgeon General made his report, these conclusions were generally confirmed although it is also accepted that smoking might represent a very common but not very potent carcinogen (74).

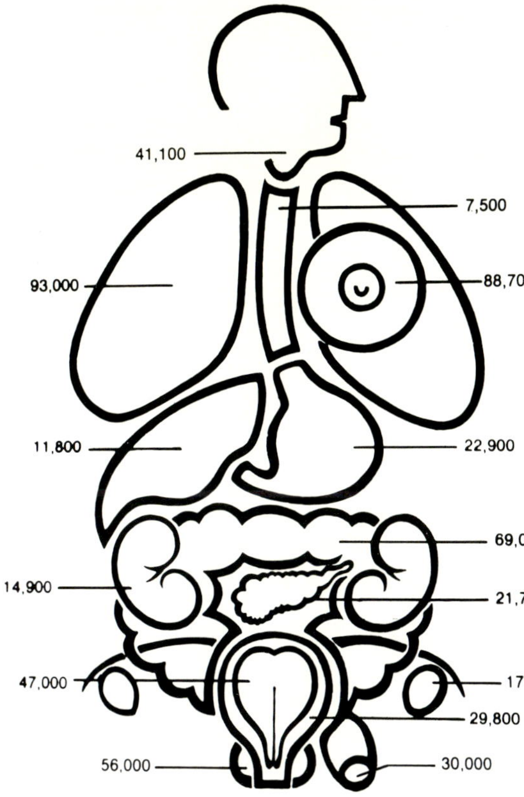

FIG. 1. Cancer incidence 1976 in the U.S.A. expressed as number of new cases per year. (Reproduced by permission, from the American Cancer Society and *Ca-A Can. J. Clin. 27:* 30–31, 1976.)

Today, new trends in the incidence of lung cancer have become evident, partially changing the old patterns[77].

The rates of lung cancer for white males have started to level off, possibly due to the decrease of smoking in certain social groups, notably physicians (Table 1),[18] and perhaps due to the introduction of filter and low tar cigarettes. However, along with this encouraging news comes the startling rise in the incidence of lung cancer in women and in the nonwhite population.[77] In recent years, the increase of pulmonary neoplasms in women is taking place to such an extent that for the first time the rate of increase exceeds that in men.[47] Table 2[35] shows how the male/female ratio for cancer of the lung progressively increased until 1960 and is now decreasing. This is not because males have fewer pulmonary tumors but because lung cancer in women is increasing exponentially (Fig. 3),[78] at a time when it is tending to level off in the male population. It is believed by some,[5] that the mortality by lung cancer follows commencement of smoking by 15 to 20 years. The marked increase in male smokers occurred around World War 1 and by 1920, 46% of American men were smokers with the death rate of lung cancer increasing dramatically in the 40's. Women began smoking substantially around World War

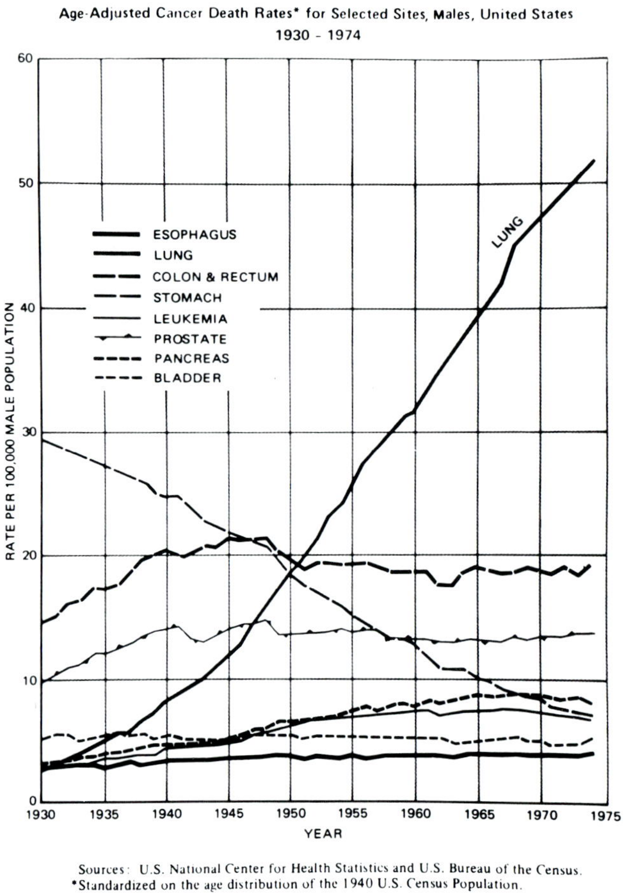

FIG. 2. Cancer death rates for males in the U.S.A. 1930–1974. (Reproduced by permission, from the American Cancer Society and *Ca-A Can. J. Clin. 27:* 30–31, 1976.)

TABLE 1. TREND IN LUNG CANCER MORTALITY OF BRITISH DOCTORS, 1953–1965*

Lung cancer death in doctors	25% decrease
Lung cancer death in general population	26% increase
Ex-smokers in doctors	12% increase
Filter cigarettes in England	1%→61%

* After Doll, R., and Pike, M. C. (Ref. 18).

II and in the 60's 40% of women smoked, leading to the present increase in the female lung cancer mortality figures.

Smoking is probably not the only contributing factor, in the increased frequency of lung cancer. In the post-war years, women have increasingly entered the work force thus being exposed to industrial pollutants while the black population has progressively moved from the country to the inner cities and the hazards of urban life. Table 3 shows a list, certainly incomplete, of industrial pollutants implicated in the etiology of lung cancer.[5] They range from the very potent radioactive emitters[15] to some with no activity. The effect of these carcinogenic agents is cumulative as shown by Selikoff, Churg, and Hammond[79] in the combination of exposure to asbestos and smoking, which increases the risk of lung cancer 90 times as compared with men who neither work with asbestos nor smoke. A similarly potent, carcinogenic activity of smoking in uranium miners was reported by Saccomanno and his co-workers.[74] The decisive importance of air pollutants, personal or nonpersonal, in the etiology of lung cancer is convincingly suggested by a recent Japanese study[95] in which bronchial carcinomas occurring in patients

TABLE 2. LUNG CANCER DEATHS, SEX RATIOS*

Year	M/F
1900	1
1923	1.03
1930	1.7
1940	2.9
1950	4.5
1960	6.6
1965	6.0
1969	5.1

* From Harley, H. R. S.: Cancer of the lung in women. (Ref. 35).

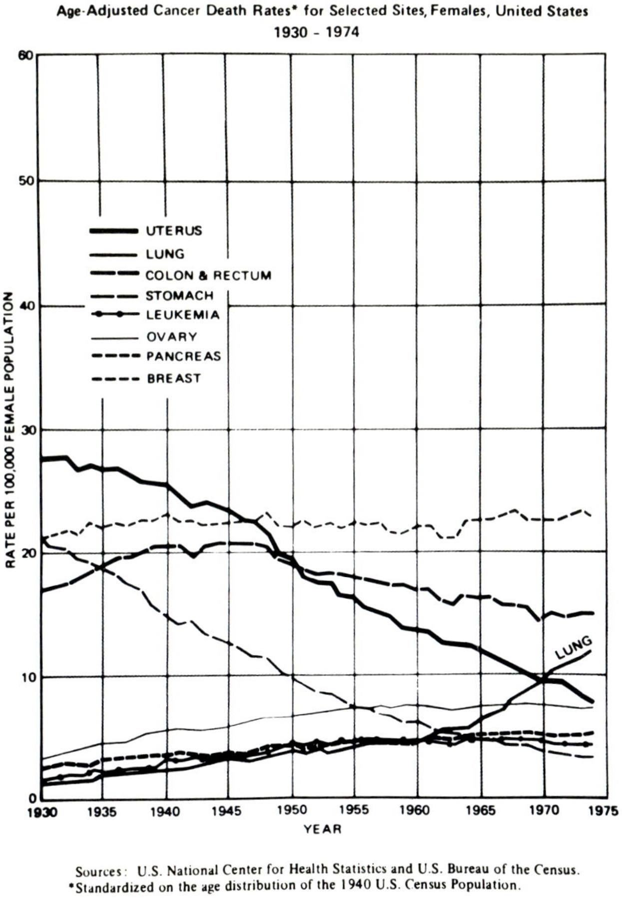

FIG. 3. Cancer death rates for females in the U.S.A. 1930–1974. (Reproduced by permission, from the American Cancer Society and *Ca-A Can. J. Clin. 27:* 30–31, 1976.)

TABLE 3. CARCINOGENS ASSOCIATED WITH LUNG CANCER

X-irradiation	Benzopyrene
Uranium	Iron Oxide
Cobalt	Tar
Chromium	Coal distillates
Nickel	Petroleum distillates
Asbestos	Beryllium
Molybdenum	Arsenic
Vanadium	Bis(chloromethyl)Ether

with pre-existing unilateral lung disease, were observed. Table 4[95] shows that of a total of 46 lung tumors, 37 developed in the healthy lung, the lung able to ventilate and therefore to inhale carcinogens, while only 9 occurred in the diseased lungs. Moreover, 19 of 20 squamous cell carcinomas and all 5 small cell carcinomas, tumors classified by Kreyberg as type 1[49] and supposedly related to exogenous carcinogens, developed in the healthy lung whereas 8 of the 9 tumors that arose in the lung with impaired ventilation were of type 2, tumors believed to be unrelated to environment.

While the role of environmental agents in the etiology of lung neoplasia appears well documented it would be simplistic to conclude that there is a direct cause-effect relationship. In fact, out of a large population exposed to the same carcinogens, only a minority develop lung cancer and the greatest variable in this process is certainly the individual. The decisive importance of genetic factors in carcinogenesis has been repeatedly demonstrated and convincing arguments were furnished by Saccomanno and co-workers,[75] who found that lung cancer did not always develop in miners who had the highest exposure to uranium and tobacco smoke. Some susceptible individuals developed early and sometimes multiple lesions while others showed a remarkable natural resistance with no signs of cellular atypia in their sputum after very long exposure (15 years) to heavy radiation and smoking. Unfortunately, the factors determining individual susceptibility and resistance to lung or other cancers are still largely unknown, representing a research area of much mystery and promise. One day, perhaps, we will be able to screen individuals for the abnormal genotypes that predispose them to certain neoplasms and eliminate potential employees who are at high risk from occupations that are hazardous to them while harmless to others.[62]

DETECTION

If one were to assess the single most important progress made in the management of lung cancer this would probably be in the field of cytopathology of the respiratory tract. While cells from the sputum were examined as early as 1845,[19] exfoliative cytology was only rediscovered in the late 40's under the stimulus of Papanicolaou.[69] Improved technology[45] using cough-induced sputum specimens, bronchial washings, or smears prepared from bronchoscope and brush specimens, has increased the accuracy of screening to almost 100%[17] and made possible, for the first time, the diagnosis of occult lung cancer; that is, cancer still undetectable by X-rays. Symptomatic lung cancer is generally late cancer with a poor 5-year survival.[94] The figures reported by various authors show a survival rate at 24 months that varies between 7 and 55% according to histologic type.[37] Due to the pioneering work of Woolner and McDonald,[88] Saccomanno *et al.*[73] Melamed and co-workers[58] and others, in the field of exfoliative respiratory cytology occult lung cancer is now emerging as a diagnostic entity.[55, 56] Twenty six such cases were detected by 1974 at the Memorial Sloan-Kettering Cancer Center in New York, two-thirds of which had potentially curable tumors and were surgically removed. Of these, two-thirds of the patients were apparently cured.[56]

The Early Lung Cancer Project at the Mayo Clinic reported 41 occult lung cancers detected between 1972–1976 (Table 5), 17 of which were still at the stage of carcinoma *in situ* at the time of surgical removal.[89]

In addition to its important role as a tool in the detection of pulmonary tumors, the examination of exfoliative cytology has changed our concepts about the evolution of lung cancer and provided us with a better understanding of its natural history. Since 1957 Saccomanno and co-workers[76] have followed uranium miners, a group of individuals with a high risk of bronchogenic cancer, with periodic sputum and X-ray examinations. Using a method that they devised, Saccomanno and his associates examined over 50,000 sputum samples collected from 6,000 men. They had thus the unique opportunity to observe the development of bronchogenic carcinoma in man in a series of sputum slides. The changes occurred slowly, over long intervals, and progressed stepwise from squamous metaplasia, to cellular dysplasia, to carcinoma *in situ,* to invasive carcinoma. There was an average period of 4–5 years during which the individuals' exfoliated cells were markedly atypical and represented carcinoma *in situ.* Due to its fast progression and short survival time after diagnosis, it was believed that lung cancer was a rapidly developing tumor with little chance of early diagnosis and treatment. However the studies by Saccomanno *et al.*[74, 76] on the uranium miners showed that an average of 15.9 years elapsed from the beginning of mining to the development of cancer and that 5.7 years was the mean time from the start of moderate atypia to invasive carcinoma. These intervals are much longer than previously suspected and certainly sufficient to permit early detection and application of treatment. These studies also showed that the frequency of squamous

TABLE 4. LUNG CANCER AND PRE-EXISTING UNILATERAL LUNG DISEASE*

Histologic Type	Cases	Healthy	Diseased
Squamous cell carcinoma	20	19	1
Adenocarcinoma	16	9	7
Large cell undifferentiated	5	4	1
Small cell undifferentiated	5	5	0
Total	46	37	9

* After Yoneyama *et al.,* (Ref. 95).

TABLE 5. MAYO LUNG PROJECT, EARLY BRONCHOGENIC CARCINOMA (SPUTUM-POSITIVE, ROENTGEN-NEGATIVE)*

In situ	17
In situ plus microinvasion	16
Invasive	8
Total	41

* After Woolner, L. B. (Ref. 89).

cell carcinomas was greater in older miners and that there was a higher than expected incidence of small cell undifferentiated carcinomas. The latter type of lung cancer has lately emerged as the one most commonly associated with heavy exposures to potent carcinogens.

CLASSIFICATION

The classification of lung tumors according to generally accepted criteria has been strongly advocated by the World Health Organization (WHO) in the interest of international communication and advancement of scientific knowledge.[81] In 1967 under the auspices of WHO, an international panel of experts issued a Histological Classification of Lung Tumors[87] which is presently widely used. However, a search of the literature made by Sobin[81] in 1972 on the subject of histologic classifications of lung tumors revealed that in the 57 papers which he reviewed, 13 different systems of classifications were used.

The WHO classification is a reasonable one, which in the hands of most specialists has repeatedly produced reproducible results.[37, 92–94] To assess the applicability of the WHO classification, a panel of three pathologists, well known experts in this field, reviewed 3,600 biopsies of lung cancer[92] and concluded that the highly differentiated tumors were easily recognizable, the diagnosis being unanimous in 95.7% of the cases.[93] Almost as easily recognized were moderately differentiated tumors with unanimity achieved in 91.4%. However, the poorly differentiated carcinomas were similarly diagnosed by the three panel members in only 46.6% of the cases, making it a highly unreliable category.[93] In another study[23] 5 experienced pathologists read 50 different specimens on two occasions and showed similar rates of disagreement (2–5%) for well differentiated squamous carcinomas and for adenocarcinomas, 23–25% disagreement for undifferentiated small and large cell carcinomas, and 40–42% disagreement for poorly differentiated squamous carcinomas and adenocarcinomas. Between the first and second readings of the same slide by the same pathologist, differences of 2% for the most consistent and 20% for the least consistent reader occurred.[23] A British study[37] on sections of 740 cases of lung cancer concluded that the WHO classification is applicable to primary tumors, bronchial biopsies, and metastatic lymph nodes, and that it is a valuable indicator of cell type. The occasional coexistence of different histologic patterns within the same tumor, certainly raises problems of classification. However, Yesner,[94] based on his personal experience with 10,000 lung cancers, has found that most tumors show a remarkable degree of uniformity in cell type, varying chiefly in the amount of maturation from field to field, as one would expect to find in a growing tissue.

A uniform method of tumor classification is necessary to communicate and to interpret each other's results. The pathologist is in the key position of determining what classification and nomenclature is to be used.[81] His terms of diagnosis become part of the patient's record, find their way into tumor registries and influence the work and results of radiologists, surgeons, and statisticians. As a preliminary phase, WHO panels recommend at least the use of the major categories of lung cancer with less emphasis at the present time on tumor subtyping.

Without entering into morphologic details, the following are some aspects of the major histologic types of lung tumors.

Squamous Cell Carcinoma is the typical bronchogenic carcinoma. It arises in middle and large size bronchi and progresses slowly through the stages of dysplasia and carcinoma *in situ.* Due to its central location, squamous cell carcinoma represents 43% of all positive bronchial biopsies but only 28% of all positive lung biopsies.[94] Fifty-nine percent of squamous cell carcinomas of lung can be diagnosed by bronchial biopsy and its cells are easily recognized in the sputum. It is the most frequent type of lung cancer in males (35.2%[2] to 43.4%[11]), but not in women (12.4%)[11] and the average age of the patients is older than for other carcinomas. It shows the least propensity to metastasis and has the longest survival time. However, squamous cell carcinoma is the lung tumor most likely to develop multiple primary lesions. Their incidence varies between 1 and 20% according to various authors[1, 2, 14, 57] with about 20 to 40% synchronous and 60 to 80% metachronous with the primary tumor. The well-differentiated type presents no problems in microscopic diagnosis which is based on the presence of keratin and intercellular bridges.[51] Less differentiated types can be recognized under the electron microscope by the identification of desmososmes and tonofibrils (Fig. 4). Squamous cell carcinomas elicit the strongest stromal reaction represented by very large infiltrates of lymphocytes and plasma cells.[43, 94] We have found that more differentiated types include more plasma cells[43] which appears to be related to the expression by these tumors of specific tumor-associated antigens.[42–43, 68]

Adenocarcinomas represent only 9% of lung carcinomas in man but 49% of all lung cancers in women.[9] Due to their more peripheral location, only 12% of adenocarcinomas can be diagnosed by bronchial biopsy and they represent about 5% of all positive bronchial biopsies.[94] Conversely, 58% of all peripheral lung tumors are adenocarcinomas.[82] Because of their lack of symptoms and inaccessibility to bronchial biopsy, adenocarcinomas are diagnosed later in their evolution. Although most of them are resectable (up to 98% of adenocarcinomas versus 65% of all other carcinomas), their prognosis is not better and the survival rate at 5 years is 9%, lower than squamous cell carcinomas, which show a 5 year survival of 22% even though this tumor is less frequently resectable. Adenocarcinoma is the most common lung cancer in nonsmokers and has been said to be associated in 45[9] to 67%[13] of cases with pre-existing scars of old infarcts, tuberculosis, or other granulomas. They are more often located in the apical segments of upper lobes and almost never involve segmental or lobar bronchi. In scars, sometimes, the sequence of epithelial cell change from hyperplasia through atypia and neoplasia, can be followed, while the scars can be differentiated from simple fibrosis by the increased amount of elastic fibers and the presence of abundant anthracotic pigment in the dense areas of hyalinized collagen. Microscopically, their diagnosis is based on the presence of glands, papillary formations and mucus secretion. Grading may be difficult, and the secretion of mucus must be ascertained by special stains and not decided on the observation of a rare drop in an otherwise undifferentiated tumor. Multiple patterns, including well formed glandular, cribriform, solid, mucinous, and papillary structures sometimes coexist within the same tumor.[51] Ultrastructurally they are characterized by the presence of microvilli on the cell surface, abundant cytoplasm with many mitochondria, paucity of endoplasmic reticulum and the presence of secretory vacuoles[8] (Fig. 5). Adenocarcinomas are highly aggressive and invade lymph nodes in 50%, blood vessels in 40%, pleura in 77% and perineural spaces in 35% of cases.

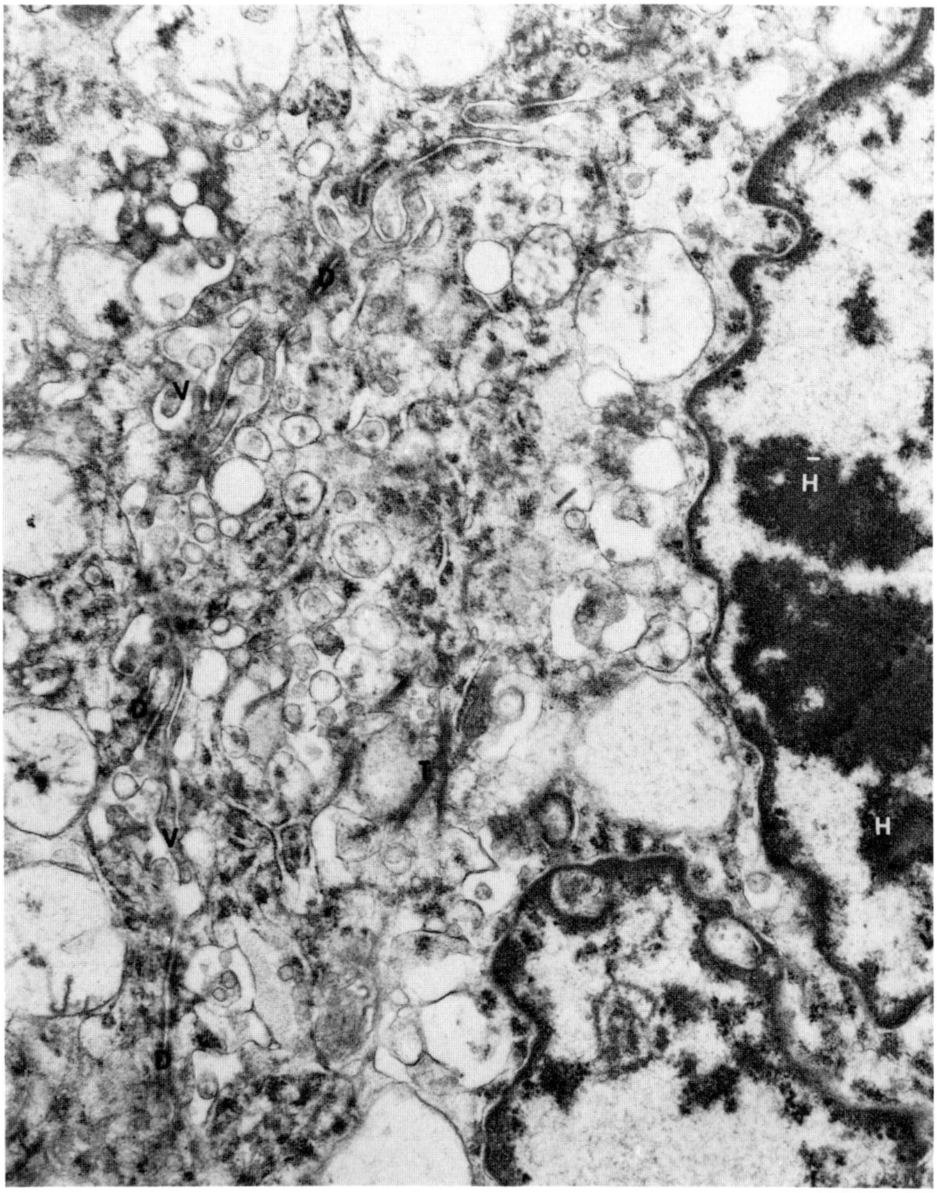

FIG. 4. Squamous cell carcinoma of lung, well differentiated. Large nucleus with clumped heterochromatin (*H*). There are numerous, well developed desmosomes (*D*), tonofibrils (*T*), and interdigitating microvilli (*V*). × 18,000.

The differentiation from metastatic adenocarcinoma may be difficult or impossible and is aided by the association with a scar or the origin from an area of atypical metaplasia of bronchial epithelium.

Bronchioloalveolar Carcinomas constitute 5% of all lung cancers and according to Liebow,[52] are well-differentiated, peripheral adenocarcinomas not arising in a cartilage containing bronchus and tending to use the walls of alveoli as supporting stroma without destroying the interstitial pulmonary framework. They are papillary and may produce mucus, sometimes in large amounts. These features are reproduced by their lymph node metastases.

Differentiation from metastatic ovarian and colonic carcinomas may be difficult. Bronchioloalveolar carcinomas spread slowly and metastasize outside the thoracic cavity in only 25% of cases. There is still a lack of precise knowledge about their origin, which accounts for the equivocal name.[52] Some tumors comprise cells that have cytoplasmic inclusions typical of type II alveolar cells (granular pneumocytes), others contain secretory bronchiolar cells of Clara type, and some include both. On the basis of ultrastructural studies some investigators have suggested a bronchiolar origin[27, 72] and others an alveolar[16, 53, 60] origin for these tumors. However, bronchioloalveolar carcinomas under the electron microscope are frequently indistinguishable from well-differentiated adenocarcinomas[8] (Fig. 6). The lack of a sharper definition for this tumor has made some authors[52] doubt the necessity of their inclusion in a separate category.

Small Cell Carcinomas represent 19% of all lung carcinomas and 43% of positive bronchial biopsies[94] which indicates their usual central location, arising in the lining epithelia of major bronchi. The male/female ratio is 19/1. It is one

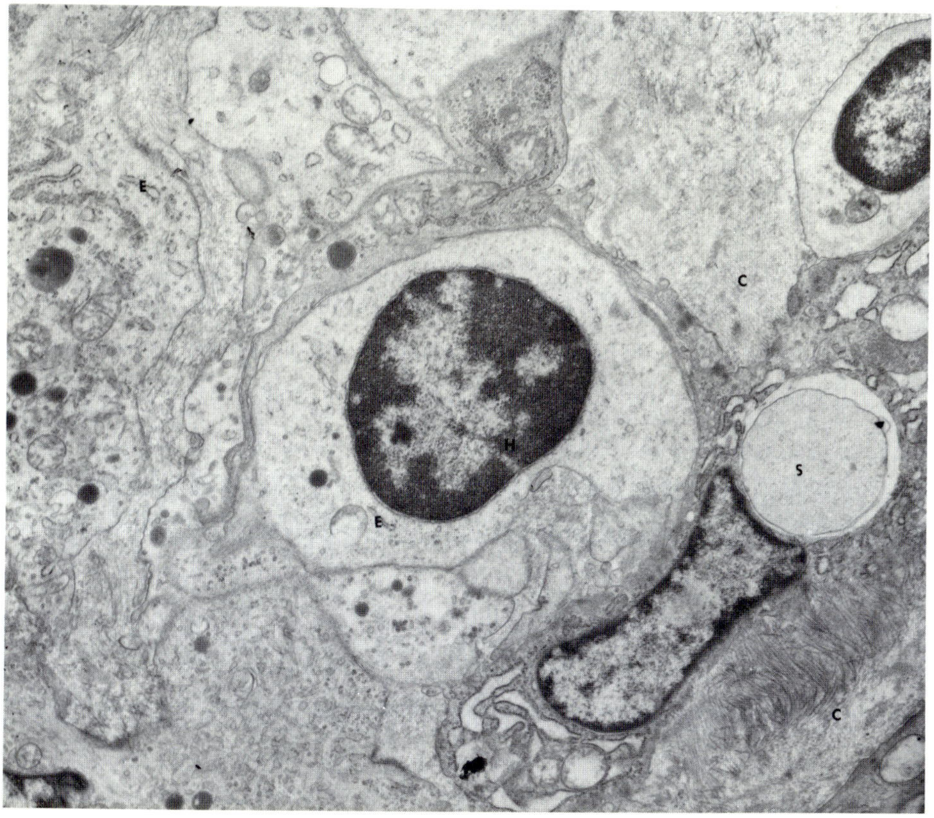

FIG. 5. Adenocarcinoma of lung, well differentiated. Cells with large nuclei comprising heterochromatin (*H*); cytoplasm with profiles of endoplasmic reticulum (*E*) and free ribosomes; secretory vacuole (*S*) with mucin-like content; intercellular collagen (*C*). × 15,000.

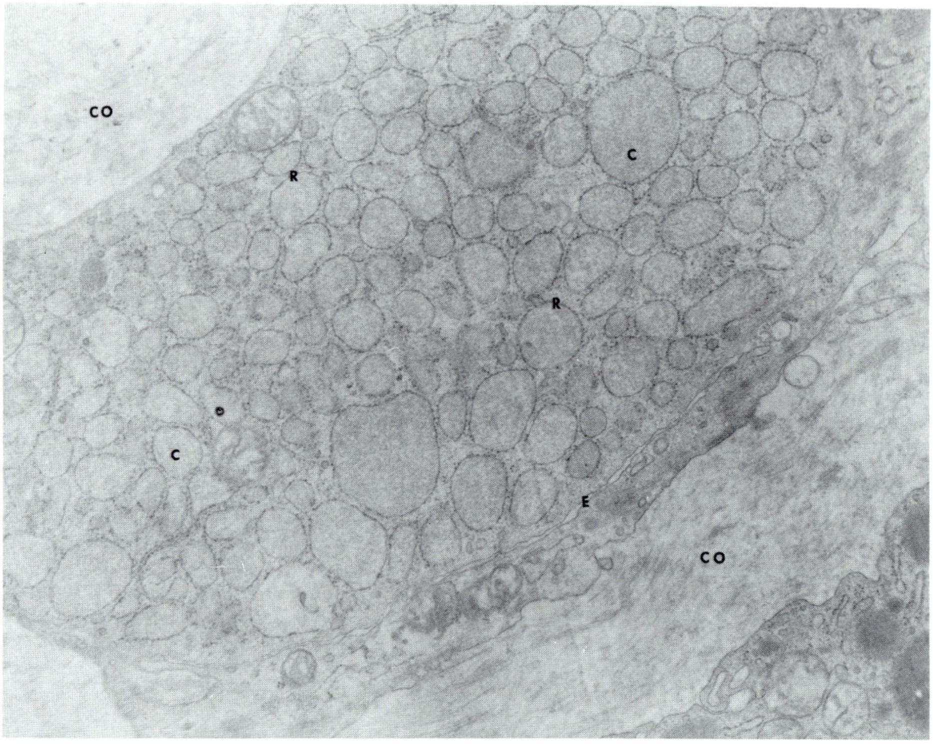

FIG. 6. Bronchioloalveolar mucinous carcinoma of lung. Cytoplasmic processes of cancer cells are packed with distended cisternae (*C*) studded with ribosomes (*R*) and filled with flocculent, mucinous material. Nondistended endoplasmic reticulum (*E*); intercellular collagen (*CO*). × 21,000.

of the most malignant tumors due to both its very high growth potential and its ability to metastasize early. These tumors have a short doubling time of about 45 days,[31] and a large growth fraction surpassed by few other tumors.[61] The tumor cells invade lymph and blood vessels early, and at the time of initial diagnosis, 84% of patients already have extrathoracic disease.[21] Due to this capacity for distant metastasis, the prognosis cannot be based on the size of the tumor, and survival at 5 years is not higher than 1–2%. Small cell carcinomas appear to be related to the effect of strong carcinogenic agents as shown by Saccomanno *et al.*[74] in the uranium miners in which this type of tumor occurred more frequently than in the general population. Histologically it exhibits distinctive patterns of ribbons, streamers, or rosettes very similar to the carcinoid tumors of the lung.[51] The tumor cells are delicate, prone to necrosis and to the characteristic crushing effect commonly observed in the biopsy specimens. In contrast to the abundant cellular stromal reaction of other lung cancers, notably squamous cell carcinoma, the small cell carcinomas are usually not accompanied by reactive cellular infiltrates.[43] The cells are often argentaffin-positive, another feature indicative of their origin from the Kulchitsky-like cells, normally present in the bronchial glands.[10, 33] According to cellular shape, the subtypes of polygonal, oat cell, and fusiform are distinguished by the WHO classification.[87] Under the electron microscope small cell carcinomas of the lung are characterized by the presence of intracellular neurosecretory granules initially described by Bensch *et al.*[10] and Hattori *et al.*[33] who also postulated the common origin of oat cell and carcinoid tumors of the lung. The granules have a diameter of 600–2000 Å, are enveloped in a limiting membrane and seem to be concentrated in the pseudopod-like cytoplasmic processes that these cells exhibit similar to those of nerve cells.[33] With the exception of carcinoid tumors, neurosecretory granules have not been observed in any other types of lung neoplasms.[10, 33] In 26% of cases, small cell carcinomas of the lung are associated with paraneoplastic syndromes,[21] most often produced by the secretion of abnormal peptides with endocrine activity.

Large Cell Carcinomas are most often peripheral and behave much like bronchogenic adenocarcinomas. The histology is undifferentiated, sometimes with focal mucin production and sometimes with clear cells that may contain glycogen. The nuclei are highly pleomorphic with giant cells and nuclear monstrosities. Phagocytosis of tumor cells by tumor cells is frequently observed. To some authors this group is a waste-basket collection[94] and, as expected, a low degree of diagnostic reproducibility is often the result.

Combined Carcinomas represent the coexistence of squamous as well as adenocarcinoma patterns. They occur in only 0.4–1.9% of all cases[92] and the term should not be used for tumors that are predominantly adenocarcinoma and show occasionally a small area of squamous metaplasia.

ECTOPIC PRODUCTION OF HORMONES BY LUNG CANCERS

The discovery of the production of polypeptide hormones by lung cancers has opened up a new chapter of human pathology. Among endocrine disorders of hormone excess, Cushing's syndrome in men, hypercalcemia, inappropriate antidiuresis, and organic hypoglycemia are due more often to non-endocrine tumors than to primary disorders of the respective endocrine systems.[67]

According to the derepression hypothesis, the release of negative gene controls or activation of specific genes that determine the synthesis of polypeptide hormones can occur during the process of neoplastic transformation. Thus hormones that are related evolutionarily may be derepressed together, giving rise to tumors that produce multiple hormones. It has also been noted that the association of ectopic hormones with particular tumors is not at random but occurs predictably.

A satisfactory explanation for the ectopic secretion of hormones by non-endocrine tissues and tumors, has been provided by the concept of the APUD system developed by Pearse.[70, 71] The system comprises a widely distributed number of endocrine cells, located in both endocrine and non-endocrine organs, that share a number of cytochemical and ultrastructural characteristics. These cells are thought to arise from the neural crest and have the capacity for amine precursor uptake and decarboxylation, being therefore designated by the term APUD.[70] The distribution of polypeptide hormone-producing APUD cells and the tumors to which they can give rise is shown in Figure 7.[63] APUD cells of the Kulchitsky type are present throughout the foregut, including the epithelium of the lung, a derivative of the former.[28]

Tumors of the lung, particularly small cell carcinomas and carcinoids, are frequently associated with the production of polypeptide hormones (Table 6).

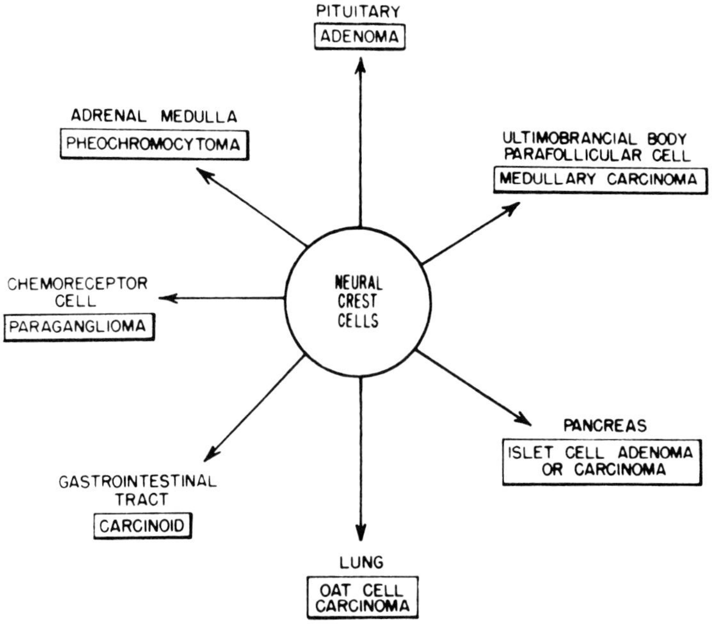

FIG. 7. Normal and tumoral derivatives of neural crest cells. (From the National Institutes of Health Conference on Islet Cell Tumors, *Ann. Int. Med. 79:* 239–257, 1973.)

TABLE 6. ECTOPIC HORMONES PRODUCED BY LUNG CARCINOMAS

ACTH[30, 50, 67]
ADH (antidiuretic)[22, 38, 50, 67]
β-MSH (melanin-stimulating)[29, 38]
HCS (somatomammotrophin)[7, 67]
HCG (gonadotrophin)[26]
PTH (parathormon)[66, 67]
Neurophysin[32]
Renin[34]
Insulin[85]
Glucagon[85]

Among these, ACTH secretion frequently, although not exclusively associated with small cell carcinomas,[38] produces hypercortisolism and very high levels of urinary hydroxycorticosteroids.[50, 67]

The syndrome of inappropriate antidiuretic hormone (ADH) secretion occurs more often in association with small cell carcinomas of the lung, the cells of which contain typical neurosecretory granules and secrete an arginine vasopressine hormone.[22, 38, 50, 67] Ectopic gonadotropin production causing gynecomastia was reported in 4 cases of large cell anaplastic carcinomas of the lung.[26] Production of somatomammotrophin (growth hormone) by the lung has been associated with acromegalic changes as well as with hypertrophic osteoarthropathy.[67] In other cases (7 of 18 lung carcinomas examined), growth hormone was detected by radioimmunoassay in the general circulation without being always coexistent with clinical symptoms. The lung tumors associated with it were more often of undifferentiated types.[7]

Parathyroid hormone, or a polypeptide similar to it, was synthesised in 20 bronchogenic carcinomas, 13 of which were of squamous cell type.[66, 67] The patients presented with hypercalcemia and hypophosphatemia without primary parathyroid disease or significant osseous metastases. Other ectopic hormones associated with lung cancer reported so far include β-melanin stimulating hormone (β-MSH) (two oat cell carcinomas[38] and one adenocarcinoma[29]), renin,[34] neurophysin,[32] insulin,[85] and glucagon.[85] In addition to hormones, as predicted from the derepression hypothesis, ectopic enzyme proteins such as amylase[29] and alkaline phosphatase,[67] as well as α-fetoprotein and carcino-embryonic antigen[66] have been identified in association with carcinomas of the lung.

The discovery by Yalow and Benson[91] that some of the ectopic hormones may circulate as a larger size precursor form that is nonfunctional yet immunoreactive, has brought the realization that the synthesis of hormones by tumors must be a more common occurrence than the clinical endocrine syndromes would indicate. In the case of ACTH produced by carcinoma of the lung, they[3, 91] identified a larger form of ACTH (big ACTH) that although not active endocrinologically can be detected by radioimmunoassay thus introducing a new, very efficient diagnostic tool. Of 24 patients with untreated carcinomas of lung of various histologic types, 21 had elevated plasma ACTH levels while the remaining 3 patients had detectable ACTH in tumor extracts and/or bronchial washings.[3] The predominant form of circulating hormone was the big ACTH that was present in all tumor tissues and metastases but in none of normal lung tissues or tissues of other tumors.

Thus the ACTH radioimmunoassay appears as a new diagnostic test, which can be helpful in the differential diagnosis of metastases with unknown primary as well as in monitoring the recurrence of lung cancer after the initial treatment.[3]

IMMUNOLOGY OF LUNG CANCER

Remarkable progress has been achieved in the detection, localization, and surgical treatment of pulmonary cancer, yet the total number of cures still falls short of our expectations. The significant reduction in the death rate of cervical carcinoma obtained by early diagnosis and treatment is not likely to occur in the management of lung cancer where still only 1 out of 3 patients diagnosed is operable and only 1 out of 9 is cured.[6] This very unsatisfactory situation provides a strong stimulus for research in other areas, notably in immunology, with hopes for the development of immunodiagnostic methods.

There is presently good evidence for the existence of tumor-associated antigens in both animals[24] and humans.[36] In lung cancer patients, various studies have indicated the existence of impaired immunity expressed by low counts of T-lymphocytes in the peripheral blood,[12, 41, 65] decrease in phytohemagglutinin-induced lymphocyte transformation,[4, 12, 41, 96] and depressed response to skin testing with various antigens.[12, 40, 41, 48, 96] However, histologic sections of lung carcinoma consistently show a strong cellular stromal reaction, expressed by abundant infiltrates of lymphocytes and plasma cells.[42, 43, 94]

To evaluate the morphology of the local cellular reaction to cancer of the lung we examined 50 lung carcinomas of different histologic types and grades and were able to recognize patterns of cellular reaction that were characteristic for the different histologic types.[43] The amount of cellular infiltration was highest in squamous cell carcinoma (Fig. 8) and lowest or nonexistent in small cell carcinoma (Fig. 9). Moreover, within the various histologic categories, the well-differentiated carcinomas appeared to be accompanied by more reactive cells than the poorly differentiated tumors. We have also found a consistent correlation between squamous cell carcinoma and plasma cells, which are characteristically present in these neoplasms, in numbers proportional to the degree of tumor differentiation and formation of keratin. To investigate the activity of such cellular infiltrates at the tumor site, we stained sections with fluorescein-labeled anti-immunoglobulin and showed that large amounts of Ig of different classes, and particularly of IgA, are locally produced by these cells (Fig. 10).

Some investigators have shown that immunoglobulins are present in larger amounts in the bronchial washings[54] and tissue eluates[84] of lung cancer than in those of normal lung while others[46] found decreased levels of IgG in malignant as compared to nonmalignant pleural effusions.

To investigate the presence of specific antigens in lung cancer, attempts have been made to immunize animals with various tissue fractions and then to use the heterologous antisera for the identification of tumor antigens.[25, 30, 54, 59, 64, 86] After exhaustive adsorption, such antisera were used with variable results in immunodiffusion, and immunofluorescence assays to identify proteins specific for lung cancer. This approach, similarly used in the investigation of other tumors, has

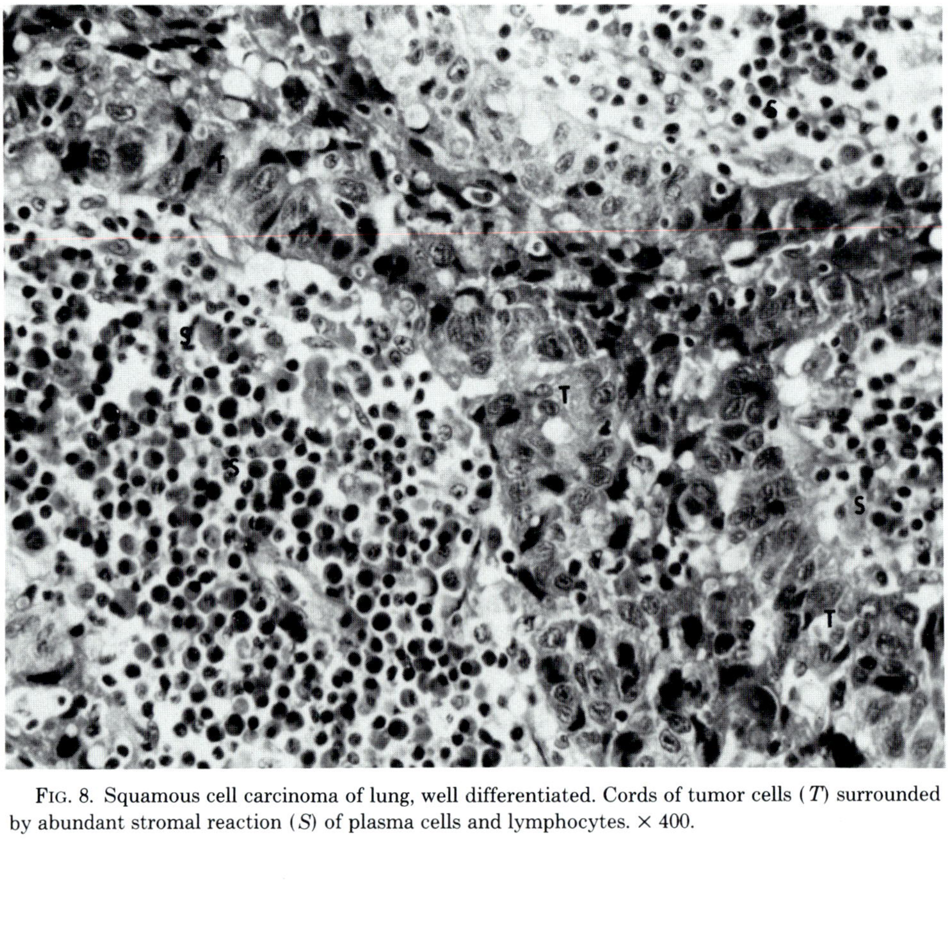

FIG. 8. Squamous cell carcinoma of lung, well differentiated. Cords of tumor cells (*T*) surrounded by abundant stromal reaction (*S*) of plasma cells and lymphocytes. × 400.

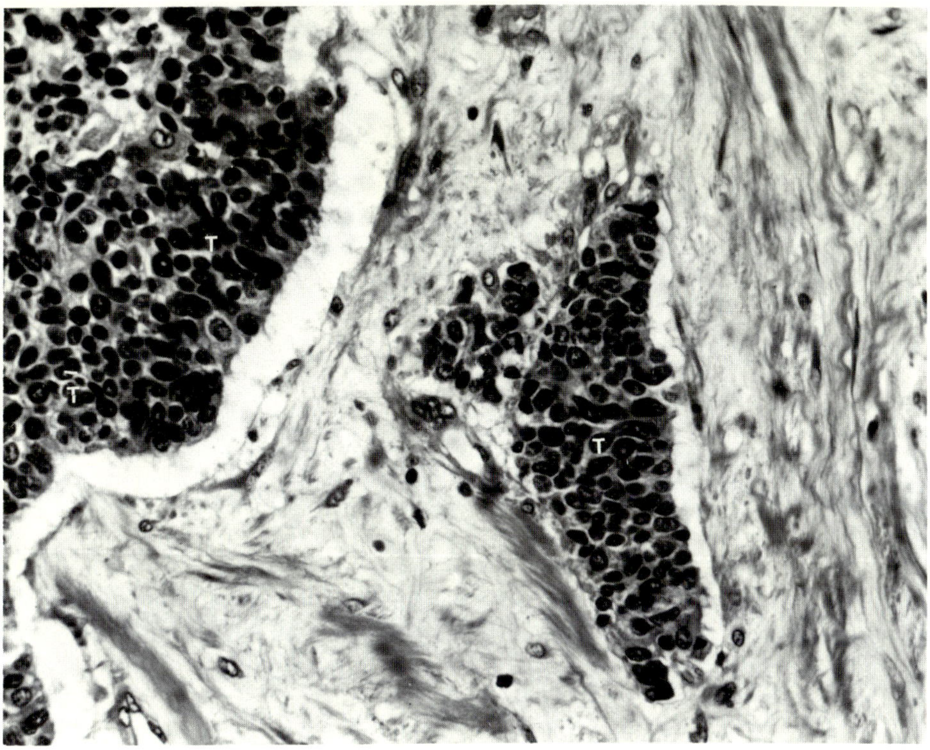

FIG. 9. Small cell carcinoma of lung, oat cell type. Cords of tumor cells (*T*) with no stromal reaction. × 400.

not produced consistent results due to the lack of specificity of antisera, raised against a multitude of unknown antigens.

Other workers have explored the humoral immunity to lung cancer by searching for tumor-specific antibodies in the patients' sera.[30, 42, 80, 97] We have shown that sera of individuals with squamous cell carcinoma have circulating antibodies against squamous cell components that can be detected in 87% of cases by immunofluorescence and complement fixation tests.[42] Zeromski *et al.*[97] and Smith *et al.*[80] have demonstrated by immunofluorescence and radioimmunoassays, respectively, the presence of serum antibodies to antigens present in lung cancer cells. However, the results of studies concerned with the detection of humoral immunity to lung cancer, as with other tumors in general, have not been very encouraging, probably because antigens and antibodies circulate freely in infinitesimal amounts and are mostly locked in antigen-antibody complexes.

Assuming that the host's response to tumor growth must be maximal at the site of the tumor, it appeared to us that this might be the optimal place to explore for the presence of tumor-reactive lymphoid cells as well as for tumor-associated antigens and antibodies. The abundant stromal reaction associated with some types of lung tumors is a strong indication that immune surveillance is operative against cancer of the lung.[44] Applying methods previously used in our laboratory in the detection and isolation of antibodies associated with ovarian carcinoma,[20] we searched for specific antibodies in the eluates of lung tumors and their

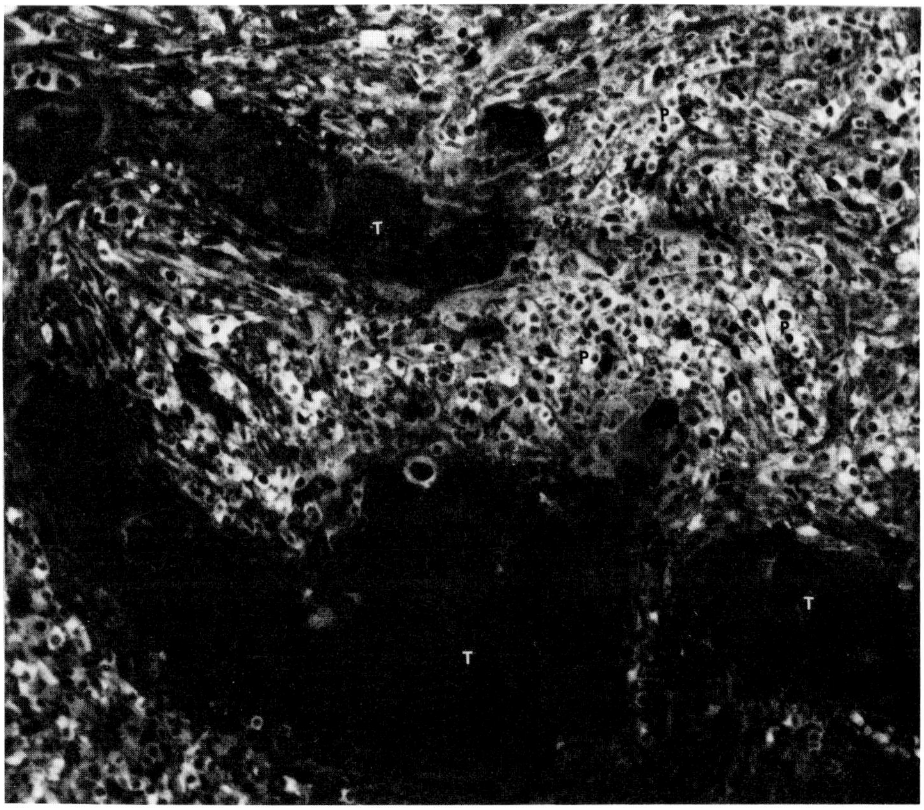

FIG. 10. Squamous cell carcinoma of lung, well differentiated, stained with fluorescein-isothiocynate (FITC)-labeled antihuman IgA serum. Cords of tumor cells (*dark areas*) (*T*) surrounded by numerous IgA positive plasma cells (*P*). × 400.

TABLE 7. INDIRECT IMMUNOFLUORESCENCE ASSAYS OF LUNG TUMOR ELUATES AND EFFUSIONS

Eluates and effusions	Cells tested		
Origin	Lung cancer (10)[b]	Normal lung (8)[c]	Nonpulmonary tumors (8)[d]
Squamous cell carcinoma of lung (7)[a] Pleural Effusions	47/53[e]	0/32	3/42
Adenocarcinoma of lung (9) Pleural Effusions	48/59	0/42	4/47
Lung cancer eluates (9)	46/58	0/35	0/45
Nonpulmonary tumors (6) Pleural and peritoneal effusions	1/37	0/24	4/30

[a] Numbers in parentheses indicate number of different eluates and effusions.
[b] Number of different cell suspensions of lung adeno and squamous cell carcinomas tested.
[c] Number of different cell suspensions of fetal and adult normal lungs tested.
[d] Number of different cell suspensions of nonpulmonary tumors (including carcinomas of breast, colon, uterine cervix, endometrium, larynx, hepatoma, and melanoma) tested.
[e] Number of positive tests per total number of cell suspensions tested (applies to all test results).

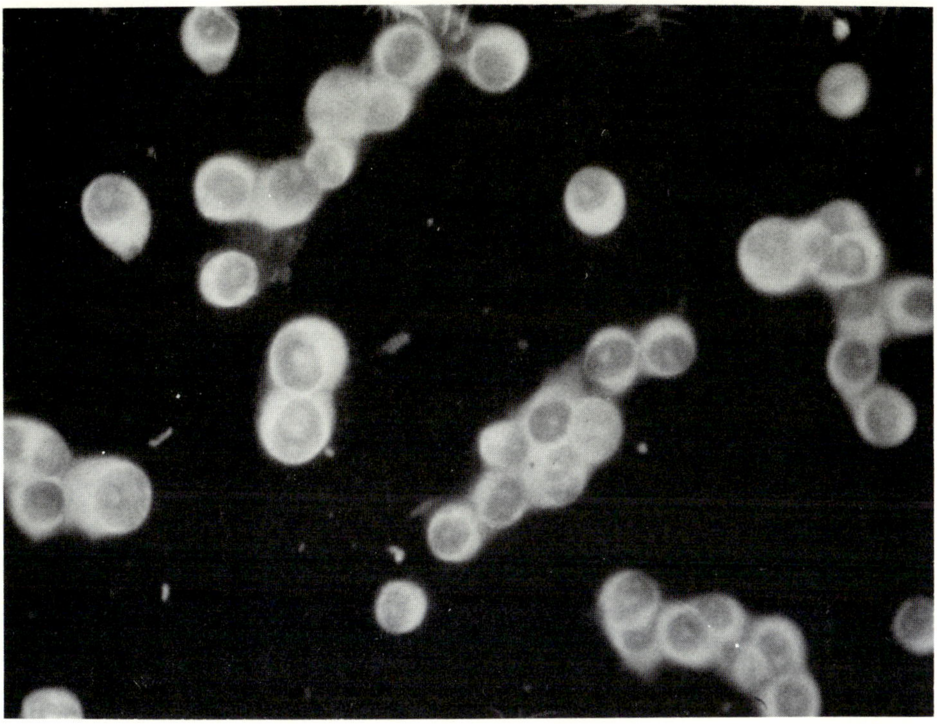

FIG. 11. Adenocarcinoma of lung, cultured *in vitro* for 4 days, reacted in indirect immunofluorescence with a pleural effusion fluid of adenocarcinoma of lung in dilution 1:16 and stained with FITC-labeled antihuman IgG serum, shows strong cytoplasmic fluorescence. × 250.

effusions.[43] Using these fluids, we disassociated the immune complexes at low pH and salt precipitated out the immunoglobulins which were then concentrated, purified and assayed in immunofluorescence against tissue cultured lung cancer cells. The latter included 17 lung tumors of various histologic types that were cultured for intervals of up to 92 days during which time they preserved their characteristic morphologic features as demonstrated by electron microscopic examination.

Tumor eluates prepared from 5 squamous cell carcinomas and 4 adenocarcinomas of the lung in dilutions of 1:8 to 1:64 reacted positively in indirect immunofluorescence with both tissue cultures and fresh cell suspensions of different lung carcinomas (Table 7). The stained cells exhibited bright granular fluorescence (Fig. 11), while cell suspensions and cultures of normal adult and fetal lung cells as well as of nonpulmonary tumors were consistently negative above dilutions of 1:4. Similarly prepared eluates of unaffected lung tissues, distal to the tumors, were also negative when tested in immunofluorescence.

The pleural effusions from patients with lung cancer yielded similar results when immunoglobulin fractions were assayed by immunofluorescence (Table 7). A total of 16 Ig preparations obtained from 9 pleural effusions from patients with squamous cell carcinoma and from 7 with adenocarcinoma showed positive cytoplasmic fluorescence with cell suspensions and cultures of carcinoma cells of similar types but not with those of normal adult or fetal lung. The same preparations also showed some reactivity against cell suspensions of carcinomas of ovary and colon but not at dilutions above 1:16. Immunoglobulin fractions similarly prepared from pleural and peritoneal effusions not associated with tumors were negative in the immunofluorescence assays. Recently,[68] we have tested fractions of bronchial washings from patients with lung cancer and from normal controls and obtained results comparable to those previously recorded for tumor eluates and effusions.

From the work presently under way in the field of lung tumor immunology, convincing evidence is available that patients with cancer of the lung are reacting to their tumors, mounting both cellular and humoral immune responses. For the study of the host reaction and the recovery of tumor specific antigens and antibodies, the author believes that the tumor site is preferable to the serum, offering more opportunities for investigation. The lung is suitable for obtaining fluids directly from the tumor site. Sputum and bronchial washings are easy to collect and can be used in routine screening procedures, once reliable immunologic assays have been developed.

The strategy that we propose, depends on the isolation and purification of specific antibodies as the first step in the identification of lung cancer antigens, the crucial discovery that can lead to the development of immunodiagnosis and immunotherapy.

Ten years or more from now at the Annual Meeting of the Academy another speaker will stand on the platform in the Grand Ballroom of an undetermined hotel and review the progress made in lung cancer during the past decade. What will he say? It is not likely that people will smoke less or that the air will be much cleaner. But perhaps by that time we will know what the active carcinogens are or what genetic makeup is particularly prone to carcinogenesis. And perhaps immunology will indeed turn out to be the great hope of modern medicine. If anything else is solved by 1987 our future speaker should rest assured that there will always be new tumor classifications to talk about.

ACKNOWLEDGMENTS

Grateful appreciations to my research associates B. Dorsett, E. Paluch, and M. Sabbath for their contributions to the immunologic and tissue culture work, to T. Bamberger for secretarial help, and to the Department of Photography of Lenox Hill Hospital for the technical work.

I am also thankful and deeply indebted to Drs. G. Saccomanno, R. Yesner, L. B. Woolner, M. Melamed, L. Sobin, and S. C. Sommers for sharing with me their expertise in this field.

REFERENCES

1. Abbey, Smith R., Nigam, B. K., and Thompson, J. M.: Second primary lung carcinoma. *Thorax 31:* 507–516. 1976.
2. Auerbach, O., Garfinkel, L., and Parks, V. R.: Histologic type of lung cancer in relation to smoking habits, year of diagnosis and sites of metastases. *Chest 67:* 382–387, 1975.
3. Ayvazian, L. F., Schneider, B., Gewirtz, G., and Yalow, R. S.: Ectopic production of big ACTH in carcinoma of the lung. Its clinical usefulness as a biologic marker. *Am. Rev. Resp. Dis. 111:* 279–287, 1975.

4. Barnes, E. W., Farmer, A., Penhale, W. J., Irvine, W. J., Roscoe, P., and Horne, N. W.: Phytohemagglutinin-induced lymphocyte transformation in newly presenting patients with primary carcinoma of the lung. *Cancer 36:* 187–193, 1975.
5. Beamis, J. F., Stein, A., and Andrews, J. L.: Changing epidemiology of lung cancer. Increasing incidence in women. *Med. Clin. N. Am. 59:* 315–325, 1975.
6. Beattie, E. J., Jr.: Lung cancer. *Ca-A Can. J. Clin. 24:* 96–99, 1974.
7. Beck, C., and Burger, H. G.: Evidence for the presence of immunoreactive growth hormone in cancers of the lung and stomach. *Cancer 30:* 75–79, 1972.
8. Bedrossian, C. W. M., Weilbaecher, D. G., Bentinck, D. C., and Greenberg, S. D.; Ultrastructure of human bronchiolo alveolar cell carcinoma. *Cancer 36:* 1399–1413, 1975.
9. Bennett, D. E., Sasser, W. F., and Ferguson, T. B.: Adenocarcinoma of the lung in men. A clinicopathologic study of 100 cases. *Cancer 23:* 431–439, 1969.
10. Bensch, K. G., Corrin, B., Pariente, R., and Spencer, H.: Oat-cell carcinoma of the lung. Its origin and relationship to bronchial carcinoid. *Cancer 22:* 1163–1172, 1968.
11. Berge, T., and Toremalm, N. G.: Bronchial cancer—a clinical and pathological study. I: Histopathology and metastases. *Scand. J. Resp Dis. 56:* 109–119, 1975.
12. Brugarolas, A., Han, T., Takita, H., and Minowada, J.: Immunologic assays in lung cancer. Skin tests, lymphocyte blastogenesis and rosette-forming cell count. *N.Y.S. J. Med. 73:* 747–750, 1973.
13. Carroll, R.: The influence of lung scars on primary lung cancer. *J. Pathol. Bacteriol. 83:* 293–297, 1962.
14. Carter, D., Marsh, B. R., Baker, R. R., Erozan, Y. S., and Frost, J. K.: Relationships of morphology to clinical presentation in ten cases of early squamous carcinoma of the lung. *Cancer 37:* 1389–1396, 1976.
15. Cihak, R. W., Ishimaru, T., Steer, A., and Yamada, A.: Lung cancer at autopsy in A-bomb survivors and controls, Hiroshima and Nagasaki 1961–1970. I. Autopsy findings and relation to radiation. *Cancer 33:* 1580–1588, 1974.
16. Coalson, J. J., Mohr, J. A., Pirtle, J. K., Dee, A. L., and Rhoades, E. R.: Electron microscopy of neoplasms in the lung with special emphasis on the alveolar cell carcinoma. *Am. Rev. Resp. Dis. 101:* 181–197, 1970.
17. Davies, D. F.: A review of detection methods for the early diagnosis of lung cancer. *J. Chronic Dis. 19:* 819–845, 1966.
18. Doll, R., and Pike, M. C.: Trends in mortality among British doctors in relation to their smoking habits. *J. Roy. Coll. Phys.* (London) *6:* 216–223, 1972.
19. Donné, A., and Faucault, L.: Cours de Microscopie complémentaire des études médicales, anatomie microscopique et physiologie des fluides de l'economie. Atlas exécuté d'aprés nature au microscope daugauerréptype. Paris, J. B. Baillière, 1844–1845.
20. Dorsett, B. H., Ioachim, H. L., Stolbach, L., Walker, J., and Barber, H. R. K.: Isolation of tumor-specific antibodies from effusions of ovarian carcinomas. *Int. J. Can. 16:* 779–786, 1975.
21. Eagan, R. T., Maurer, L. H., Forcier, R. J., and Tulloh, M.: Small cell carcinoma of the lung: Staging, paraneoplastic syndromes, treatment and survival. *Cancer 33:* 527–532, 1974.
22. Epstein, S., Ranchod, M., and Goldswain, P. R. T.: Pituitary insufficiency, inappropriate antidiuretic hormone (ADH) secretion, and carcinoma of the bronchus. *Cancer 32:* 476–481, 1973.
23. Feinstein, A. R., Gelfman, N. A., and Yesner, R.: Observer variability in the histopathologic diagnosis of lung cancer. *Am. Rev. Resp. Dis. 101:* 671–684, 1970.
24. Foley, E. J.: Antigenic properties of methylcholantrene-induced tumors in mice of the strain of origin. *Cancer Res. 13:* 835–837, 1953.
25. Frost, M. J., Rogers, G. T., Bagshawe, K. D.: Extraction and preliminary characterization of a human bronchogenic carcinoma antigen. *Br. J. Cancer 31:* 379–386, 1975.
26. Fusco, F. D., Rosen, S. W.: Gonadotropin-producing anaplastic large-cell carcinomas of the lung. *N. Engl. J. Med. 275:* 507–515, 1966.
27. Gellers, A., and Toker, C.: Pulmonary adenomatosis and peripheral adenocarcinoma of the lung. An ultrastructural demonstration of common morphologic findings. *Arch. Pathol. 88:* 148–154, 1969.
28. Gmelich, J. T., Bensch, K. G., and Liebow, A. A.: Cells of Kulchitzky type in bronchioles and their relation to the origin of peripheral carcinoid tumor. *Lab Invest. 17:* 88–98, 1967.
29. Gomi, K., Kameya, T., Tsumuraya, M., Shimosato, Y., Zeze., F., Abe, K., and Yoneyama, T.:

Ultrastructural, histochemical and biochemical studies of two cases with amylase, ACTH, and β-MSH producing tumor. *Cancer 38:* 1645–1654, 1976.

30. Granlund, D. J., and Ritts, R. E.: Soluble proteins of human bronchogenic carcinomas. *Mayo Clin. Proc. 51:* 19–27, 1976.
31. Green, R. A., Humphrey, E., Close, H., and Patno, M. E.: Alkylating agents in bronchogenic carcinoma. *Am. J. Med. 46:* 516–525, 1969.
32. Hamilton, B. P. M., Upton, G. V., Amatruda, T. T., Jr. Evidence for the presence of neurophysin in tumors producing the syndrome of inappropriate antidiuresis. *J. Clin. Endo. Metab. 35:* 764–767, 1972.
33. Hattori, S., Matsuda, M., Tateishi, R., Nishihara, H., and Horai, T.: Oat-cell carcinoma of the lung. Clinical and morphological studies in relation to its histogenesis. *Cancer 30:* 1014–1024, 1972.
34. Hauger-Klevene, J. H.: High plasma renin activity in an oat cell carcinoma: A renin-secreting carcinoma? *Cancer 26:* 1112–1114, 1970.
35. Harley, H. R. S.: Cancer of the lung in women. *Thorax 31:* 254–263, 1976.
36. Hellström, I., Hellström, K. E., Pierce, G. E., and Yang, J. P. S.: Cellular and humoral immunity to different types of human neoplasms. *Nature* (London) *220:* 1352–1354, 1968.
37. Hinson, K. F. W., Miller, A. B., and Tall, R.: An assessment of the world health organization classification of the histologic typing of lung tumors applied to biopsy and resected material. *Cancer 35:* 399–405, 1975.
38. Hirata, Y., Matsukura, S., Imura, H., Yakura, T., Ihjima, S., Nagase, C., and Itoh, M.: Two cases of multiple hormone-producing small cell carcinoma of the lung. Coexistence of tumor ADH, ACTH and β-MSH. *Cancer 38:* 2575–2582, 1976.
39. Hoffman, E. F., and Gilliam, A. G.: Lung cancer mortality. Geographic distribution in the United States for 1948–1949. *USPHS Report 69:* 1033–1042, 1954.
40. Hollinshead, A. C., Stewart, T. H. M., and Herberman, R. B.: Delayed-hypersensitivity reactions to soluble membrane antigens of human malignant lung cells. *J. Nat. Can. Inst. 52:* 327–338, 1974.
41. Holmes, E. C., and Golub, S. H.: Immunologic defects in lung cancer patients. *J. Thorac. Cardiovasc. Surg. 71:* 161–168, 1976.
42. Ioachim, H. L., Dorsett, B., Paluch, E.: Cellular and humoral reactions to squamous cell carcinoma of the lung. Proceedings of the XIth International Cancer Congress, Florence, Italy, *2:* 104, 1974.
43. Ioachim, H. L., Dorsett, B. H., and Paluch, E.: The immune response at the tumor site in lung carcinoma. *Cancer 38:* 2296–2309, 1976.
44. Ioachim, H. L.: The stromal reaction of tumors: An expression of immune surveillance. Guest Editorial. *J. Nat. Cancer Inst. 57:* 465–475, 1976.
45. Johnston, W. W., and Frable, W. J.: The cytopathology of the respiratory tract. A Review. Am. *J. Pathol. 84:* 372–424, 1976.
46. Kay, A. B., Smith, A. F., McGavin, C. R., and Tuft, S. B.: Immunoglobulins and complement in pleural effusions associated with bronchogenic carcinoma. *J. Clin. Pathol. 29:* 887–889, 1976.
47. Kennedy, A.: Relationship between cigarette smoking and histological type of lung cancer in women. *Thorax 28:* 204–208, 1973.
48. Krant, J. K., Manskopf, G., Brandrup, C., and Madoff, M. A.: Immunologic alterations in bronchogenic cancer. Sequential Study. *Cancer 21:* 623–631, 1968.
49. Kreyberg, L.: Histological lung cancer types. A morphological and biological correlation. *Acta Pathol. Microbiol. Scand.* (Suppl.) *157,* 1962.
50. Liddle, G. W., Nicholson, W. E., Island, D. P., *et al:* Clinical and laboratory studies of ectopic humoral syndromes. *Rec. Prog. Horm. Res. 25:* 283–314, 1969.
51. Liebow, A. A.: Tumors of the lower respiratory tract. Armed Forces Institute of Pathology *Atlas of Tumor Pathology,* Section 5, Fasc. 17, Washington, D. C.
52. Liebow, A. A.: In *Thoracic and Cardiovascular Surgery with related Pathology.* edited by Glenn, W. W. L., Liebow, A. A., and Lindskog, G. E. 3rd ed. New York, Appleton-Century-Crofts, 1975.
53. Lupulescu, A. P., and Brinkman, G. L.: Cytoplasmic inclusion bodies in pulmonary tumors: An electron microscopic study. *Am. J. Clin. Pathol. 56:* 553–557, 1971.
54. Mandel, M. A., Dvorak, K. J., Worman, L. W., and DeCosse, J. J.: Immunoglobulin content in the bronchial washings of patients with benign and malignant pulmonary disease. *N. Engl. J. Med. 295:* 694–698, 1976.

55. Marsh, B. R., Frost, J. K., Erozan, Y. S., and Carter, D.: Occult bronchogenic carcinoma. Endoscopic localization and television documentation. *Cancer 30:* 1348–1352, 1972.
56. Martini, N., Beattie, E. J., Cliffton, E. E., and Melamed, M. R.: Radiologically occult lung cancer. Report of 26 cases. *Symp. Surg. Oncol. Surg. Clin. N. Am. 54:* 811–823, 1974.
57. Martini, N., and Melamed, M. R.: Multiple primary lung cancers. *J. Thorac. Cardiovasc. Surg. 70:* 606–612, 1975.
58. Melamed, M. R., Flehinger, B., Miller, D., Osborne, R., Zaman, M., McGinnis, C., and Martini, N.: Preliminary report of the lung cancer detection program in New York, 1976.
59. Mohr, J. A., Nordquist, R. E., Rhoades, E. R., Coalson, R. E., and Coalson, J. J.: Alveolar cell carcinoma-like antigen and antibodies in patients with alveolar cell carcinoma and other cancers. *Cancer Res. 34:* 1904–1907, 1974.
60. Mollo, F., Canese, M. G., and Campobasso, O.: Human peripheral lung tumours: Light and electron microscopic correlation. *Br. J. Can. 27:* 173–182, 1973.
61. Muggia, F. M., Oster, S. K., Hansen, H. H.: Cell kinetic studies in patients with small-cell carcinoma of the lung. *Proc. Am. Assoc. Can. Res. 13:* 16, 1972 (abstr.).
62. Mulvihill, J. J.: Host factors in human lung tumors: An example of ecogenetics in oncology. *J. Nat. Can. Inst. 57:* 3–7, 1976.
63. NIH Conference on Islet Cell Tumors: Current concepts and management. *Ann. Int. Med. 79:* 239–257, 1973.
64. Nordquist, R. E.: Specific antigens in human alveolar cell carcinoma. *Cancer Res. 33:* 1790–1795, 1973.
65. Olkowski, Z. L., McLaren, J. R., and Mansour, K. A.: Immunocompetence of patients with bronchogenic carcinoma. *Ann. Thorac. Surg. 21:* 546–551, 1976.
66. Omenn, G. S., Roth, S. I., Baker, W. H.: Hyperparathyroidism associated with malignant tumors of nonparathyroid origin. *Cancer 24:* 1004–1012, 1969.
67. Omenn, G. S. Pathobiology of ectopic hormone production by neoplasms in man. *Pathobiol. Ann.* edited by Ioachim, H. L., New York, Appleton-Century-Crofts *3:* 177–216, 1973.
68. Paluch, E., Dorsett, B., and Ioachim, H. L.: Isolation of tumor-associated antibodies from lung carcinomas and their effusions. *Fed. Proc. 36:* 1327, 1977 (abstr. 5611).
69. Papanicolaou, G. N., Cromwell, H. A.: Diagnosis of cancer of the lung by the cytologic method. *Dis. Chest 15:* 412–421, 1949.
70. Pearse, A. G. E.: The cytochemistry and ultrastructure of polypeptide hormone-producing cells of the APUD series and the embryologic, physiologic and pathologic implications of the concept. *J. Histochem. Cytochem. 17:* 303–313, 1969.
71. Pearse, A. G. E.: The APUD cell concept and its implications in pathology. In *Pathology Annual 1974.* edited by Sommers, S. C. New York, Appleton-Century-Crofts, *9:* 27–41, 1974.
72. Razzuk, M. A., Race, G. J., Lynn, J. A., Martin, J. A., Urschel, H. C., and Paulson, D. L.: Observations on ultrastructural morphology of bronchogenic carcinoma. *J. Thorac. Cardiovasc. Surg. 59:* 581–586, 1970.
73. Saccomanno, G., Saunders, R. P., Archer, V. E., Auerbach, O., Kuschner, M., and Beckler, P. A.: Cancer of the lung: The cytology of sputum prior to the development of carcinoma. *Acta Cytol. 9:* 413–423, 1965.
74. Saccomanno, G., Archer, V. E., Auerbach, O., Kuschner, M., Saunders, R. P., and Klein, M. G.: Histologic types of lung cancer among uranium miners. *Cancer 27:* 515–523, 1971.
75. Saccomanno, G., Archer, V. E., Auerbach, O., and Saunders, R. P.: Susceptibility and resistance to environmental carcinogens in the development of carcinoma of the lung. *Human Pathol. 4:* 487–495, 1973.
76. Saccomanno, G., Archer, V. E., Auerbach, O., Saunders, R. P., and Brennan, L. M.: Development of carcinoma of the lung as reflected in exfoliated cells. *Cancer 33:* 256–270, 1974.
77. Schneiderman, M. A., and Levin, D. L.: Trends in lung cancer. Mortality, incidence, diagnosis, treatment, smoking, and urbanization. *Cancer 30:* 1320–1325, 1972.
78. Seidman, H., Silverberg, E., and Holleb, A. I.: Cancer statistics, 1976. A comparison of white and black populations. *Ca-A Can. J. Clin. 26:* 2–29, 1976.
79. Selikoff, I. J., Churg, J., Hammond, E. C.: Asbestos exposure and neoplasia. *JAMA 188:* 22–26, 1964.
80. Smith, K. O., Gehle, W. D., Newman, J. T., Standley, D. L., and Voltz, P. W.: An approach to the serodiagnosis of human lung cancer. Cell culture lines reactive as antigens with tumor patients' sera. *Cancer 38:* 157–165, 1976.

81. Sobin, L. H.: Multiplicity of lung tumour classifications. *Rec. Results Can. Res. 39:* 29–35, 1972.
82. Steele, J. D., Kleitsch, W. P., Dunn, J. E., Jr., and Buell, P.: Survival in males with bronchogenic carcinomas resected as asymptomatic solitary pulmonary nodules. *Ann. Thorac. Surg. 2:* 368–376, 1966.
83. Surgeon General Advisory Committee Report: Smoking and Health. HEW-PHS Publ. 1103, 1964.
84. Thunold, S., Tönder, O., and Larsen, O.: Immunoglobulins in eluates of malignant human tumours. *Acta Pathol. Microbiol. Scand.* Sect. (A) (Suppl.) *236:* 97–100, 1973.
85. Unger, R. H., Lochner, J. de V., Eisentraut, A. M.: Identification of insulin and glucagon in a bronchogenic metastasis. *J. Clin. Endo. Metab. 24:* 823–831, 1964.
86. Watson, R. D., Smith, A. G., and Levy, J. G.: The use of immunoadsorbent columns for the isolation of antibodies specific for antigens associated with human bronchogenic carcinoma. *Br. J. Can. 29:* 183–188, 1974.
87. WHO: International histological classification of tumours: Histological typing of lung tumours. edited by Kreyberg, L., Liebow, A. A., and Uehlingen, E. A. W.H.O., Geneva, 1967.
88. Woolner, L. B., and McDonald, J. R.: Diagnosis of carcinoma of the lung. The value of cytologic study of sputum and bronchial secretions. *JAMA 139:* 497–502, 1949.
89. Woolner, L. B.: Pathology of early lung cancer, In *Mayo Lung Cancer Project—Atlas* (in preparation), 1977.
90. Wynder, E. L.: Etiology of lung cancer. Reflections on two decades of research. *Cancer 30:* 1332–1339, 1972.
91. Yalow, R. S., and Benson, S. A.: Characteristics of "big ACTH" in human plasma and pituitary extracts. *J. Clin. Endo. Metab. 36:* 415–423, 1973.
92. Yesner, R., Gerstl, B., and Auerbach, O.: Application of the world health organization classification of lung carcinoma to biopsy material. *Ann. Thorac. Surg. 1:* 33–49, 1965.
93. Yesner, R.: Observer variability and reliability in lung cancer diagnosis. *Can. Chemother. Rep.* (Suppl) *4:* 55–57, 1973.
94. Yesner, R.: Histologic typing of lung cancer with clinical implications. *Front. Rad. Ther. Oncol. 9:* 140–150, 1974.
95. Yoneyama, T., Naruke, T., Suemasu, K., and Ishikawa, S.: Bronchial carcinoma in patients with pre-existing unilateral lung disease. *Thorax 31:* 650–651, 1976.
96. Zeromski, J.: Immunologic studies in bronchogenic carcinoma. *Ann. Med. Sect. Pol. Acad. Sci. 19:* 197-236, 1974.
97. Zeromski, J., Gorny, M. K., Wruk, M., and Sapua, J.: Behaviour of local and systemic immunoglobulins in patients with lung cancer. *Int. Arch. Allergy Appl. Immunol. 49:* 548-563, 1975.

Chapter 12

The Basis of Pulmonary Edema, with Emphasis on Ultrastructure*

GIUSEPPE G. PIETRA

In the early 19th century, Laennec[16] defined edema of the lung as "an infiltration of serum into the substance of this organ, in such a degree as evidently to diminish its permeability to air, in respiration." He further added "although very common, this disease is very little known." Almost two centuries later pulmonary edema is still one of the most common lesions seen at the autopsy table and is often the immediate cause of death, but is rarely a primary pulmonary disease. However, the introduction of the electron microscope to the study of this problem has greatly contributed to a clearer understanding of its pathogenesis.

It is the purpose of this report to review current views on the ultrastructure of the lung that are relevant to liquid balance. The reader is referred to recent reviews,[11, 28, 36, 37] for a more comprehensive discussion of the pathophysiologic mechanisms.

CAUSES AND CLASSIFICATION OF PULMONARY EDEMA

Pulmonary edema has been defined as a pathologic state in which there is abnormal accumulation of water and solutes in the pulmonary extravascular space.[28] In the healthy subject, daily fluctuations in intra- and extravascular liquids in the lungs are kept within narrow limits by a complex interplay of physicochemical forces and structural devices. Physiologists generally assume that the microvascular endothelium behaves passively with regard to liquid exchange. This is probably an oversimplification since the endothelium of certain microvascular beds contains microfilaments which give the cell the capacity to change shape when it comes in contact with certain humoral substances.[23] Nevertheless, a useful starting point for a discussion of edema formation is Starling's law of capillary exchange[35] which described net flow of water across the capillary wall in terms of gradients of hydrostatic and oncotic pressures. Thus:

$$\dot{Q}f = k(Pc - Pi + \pi_i - \pi_c)$$

where $\dot{Q}f$ is the net rate of filtration, k represents the permeability coefficient, P and π are the hydrostatic and colloid osmotic pressures of plasma (c) and interstitial fluid (i), respectively. Accordingly, the net transcapillary pressure

---

* Supported in part by Grant No. HL-08805 from the National Heart and Lung Institute.

gradient determines bulk flow of liquids across the capillary wall, whereas the transcapillary concentration gradient determines net movement of solutes. Edema may result from an imbalance between hemodynamic and osmotic forces (hemodynamic edema) or from a greater porosity of the microvascular endothelium (permeability edema). Under normal conditions, the balance of hemodynamic forces in the lung tends to favor reabsorption of water. The capillary hydrostatic pressure is low, between 5 and 15 mm Hg, well below the oncotic effect of the plasma proteins, which is 28 mm Hg. The value of the interstitial forces has not been established with certainty, but the hydrostatic pressure is believed to be subatmospheric, as low as −16 mm Hg and the oncotic pressure of the interstitial fluid has been estimated to be −6 mm Hg.[13] In the lung, transcapillary movement of liquids is also influenced by alveolar and lymphatic forces.

Thus alveolar inflation has been found to affect the permeability coefficient of the alveolar wall to solutes, high inflation enhancing the porosity of the alveolar-capillary membrane to solutes.[10] On the other hand, the surfactant that coats the alveolar walls counters the transudation of liquids into the alveolar spaces at low alveolar volumes.

Liquids and proteins that escape into the interstitial space are removed by an elaborate system of lymphatic vessels, located in the extra-alveolar interstitium, and returned to the systemic veins. Drainage of liquids by the lymphatic system is favored by the rhythmic changes in lung volume during respiration. Lymph flow from the lungs increases during hyperventilation and decreases with hypoventilation. In general, pulmonary edema develops whenever the rate of liquid accumulation exceeds the reabsorptive capacity of the lymphatic vessels.

Hemodynamic edema. The intracapillary hydrostatic pressure can change rapidly and is by far the most important cause of this type of edema. Under most circumstances, the intracapillary hydrostatic pressure is dependent on the venous pressure which is transmitted passively to the capillaries. Thus, acute left heart failure or mitral valve disease most often causes this form of pulmonary edema. However, hemodynamic edema may also result from marked hypoalbuminemia or from a sudden increase in the negativity of the interstitial pressure, *i.e.,* during sudden re-expansion of a collapsed lung by too rapid removal of a pleural effusion. Finally, it may be associated with mechanical blockage of lymphatic vessels by neoplasms or scarring.

Permeability edema. This form usually reflects injury of the endothelium of pulmonary microvessels and/or the alveolar capillary membrane. Accordingly, the edema fluid frequently contains high concentrations of plasma proteins, including fibrinogen. Fibrin and necrotic cells from the damaged respiratory membrane give rise to the formation of hyaline membranes, one of the anatomic hallmarks of permeability edema. In some cases, *i.e.,* extensive viral infections, inhalation or aspiration of corrosive chemical substances, metal fumes or oxidizing agents, and high doses of X-rays, the cause of diffuse lung injury is known, but in most cases it is not. Thus, widespread microemboli may increase capillary permeability either by releasing chemical mediators of permeability or by obstructing a large portion of the pulmonary capillary bed forcing the entire cardiac output into fewer vessels. The increase linear velocity of blood flow through perfused vessels may physically damage the capillary endothelium.

Not all forms of edema can be easily categorized in the two varieties of hemodynamic and permeability edema. In clinical conditions it is likely that multiple factors may play a role. Pulmonary edema of uncertain pathogenesis includes neurogenic edema, "shock" lung, high altitude edema, and edema associated with overdosage of narcotics (heroin pulmonary edema). As will be discussed later in more detail (see "Stretched Pores"), there is no sharp distinction between hemodynamic and permeability edema since the porosity of the capillary wall, *i.e.*, the permeability coefficient, changes when the capillary hydrostatic pressure rises. Hemodynamic overload and leaky alveolar-capillary membrane probably account for the occurrence of edema in certain traumatic and vascular disorders of the central nervous system (neurogenic edema) and during successful recovery from prolonged systemic hypotension (shock lung).[11, 14, 28, 38] In neurogenic edema, massive hemodynamic overload of the left ventricle results from massive sympathetic discharge from the hypothalamic centers. This initial phase of hemodynamic edema is followed by a second phase in which leaky capillaries allow escape of plasma proteins into the extravascular compartment, even though the hemodynamics have returned to normal.[38] In shock lung, pulmonary edema that develops after recovery from the hypotensive state has been attributed to a combination of damaged respiratory membrane and therapeutic overhydration.[11] Damage to the alveolar-capillary membrane apparently results from the liberation of kinins and bacterial toxins from the ischemic gut, pulmonary arterial vasoconstriction, and the formation of platelet microthrombi.[1, 28]

The pathogenesis of high altitude pulmonary edema is uncertain. The disease develops in young, healthy native residents of high altitude who return home after a few days' sojourn at sea level. It may also affect the healthy but unacclimatized individual several hours after a rapid climb to elevations of over 3000 m. Edema formation has been attributed to an inordinate degree of hypoxic pulmonary arterial hypertension generated by a constitutionally predisposed person when exposed to tolerable levels of hypoxia.[11] Nonuniform precapillary vasoconstriction would then force the entire cardiac output through a smaller portion of the pulmonary capillary bed. Capillary hypertension in the overperfused areas will cause pulmonary edema.[39]

Even more mysterious is the pathogenesis of pulmonary edema that is associated with overdosage of heroin, methadone, and barbiturates. In these circumstances, the patient, frequently a drug addict, is comatose, hypoventilating, hypoxemic, and acidotic. Edema, which on chest X-ray has a patchy distribution, has been attributed either to left heart failure from hypoxic myocardial damage or to a direct toxic effect of the drug (or contaminants injected with the drug). Since edema occurs not only with "street" heroin but with overdosage of methadone and barbiturates, a direct toxic effect seems unlikely.[11]

DISTRIBUTION OF PULMONARY EDEMA

The distribution of edema fluid within the lung varies according to the type and duration of pulmonary edema. Edema fluid may remain confined to the interstitial space or extend into the alveoli and airways. On chest X-rays, early edema may cause blurring of vascular shadows, clouding of lung fields and Kerley's B lines reflecting liquid accumulation in the interlobular septa. Sometimes, it may have a "butterfly" distribution sparing the lung periphery. Interstitial edema is the earliest and most common variety of pulmonary edema. Yet, it remains frequently undetected. Rales are absent. Tachypnea, presumably due to stimulation of stretch receptors[21] by swelling of the interstitial connective tissue, is often the only clinical clue that signals interstitial edema. Pulmonary edema recognized at necropsy, usually refers to alveolar edema. While it is easy to recognize frank pulmonary edema at necropsy, difficulties arise in detecting early pulmonary edema even at microscopic examination. Pulmonary congestion often blurs the boundaries between vascular and extravascular compartments, and edema fluid can only be identified histologically on the basis of its protein content or the distortion it may cause in the interstitial space. Moreover, the distribution of edema fluid is altered by the effects of gravity and the time that has elapsed between death and the postmortem examination. The assessment of edema in the lungs fixed by inflation with formalin is totally unreliable due to displacement of edema fluid in the alveolar spaces by the fixative and artifactual widening of the peribronchial spaces. Theoretically, rapid freezing of the lungs in liquid freon or liquid nitrogen and embedding in paraffin by freeze-drying methods should allow the histologic evaluation of pulmonary edema, regardless of the protein content of the edema fluid. Unfortunately, the technique has limited applications since only very small pieces of tissue (1–2 mm) can be reliably processed. Determination of wet/dry lung weight ratios do not allow the distinction between increased intravascular and extravascular lung water. Fixation of the lung by intravascular perfusion with glutaraldehyde or paraformaldehyde-glutaraldehyde mixtures is limited in practice to experimental studies. At autopsy, satisfactory results can be obtained by transthoracic fixation of the lungs with paraformaldehyde-glutaraldehyde mixtures. Although ultrastructural studies are feasible only in lungs that are fixed immediately after death, material fixed in this manner can be used for light microscopy after embedding in plastic (Epon-Araldite mixtures or Methachrylate) and thin sectioning (1–2 μm) with excellent resolution of histologic details.

From the foregoing discussion it is obvious that the frequency of pulmonary edema at necropsy is underestimated. In our institution, pulmonary edema is detected in about 25% of all necropsies, but the frequency of pulmonary edema is influenced by the type of disease processes that comes to necropsy. It is extremely high in necropsies of patients with atherosclerotic or hypertensive heart disease or cerebrovascular accident.[4]

STRUCTURAL ASPECTS OF PULMONARY EDEMA

Pulmonary Extravascular Space

The pulmonary extravascular space consists of two compartments separated by an epithelial membrane: the interstitial space and the air space.

The Interstitial Space. This space varies from place to place within the lungs. In the alveolar septa, over the convexities of the capillaries the interstitium is reduced to a basement membrane 50 nm thick (Figs. 1 and 3), interposed between the capillary endothelium and the alveolar epithelium. The thinness of the alveolar-capillary barrier in these regions appears ideally suited for rapid gas exchange. On the opposite side and in portions of the septum devoid of capillaries,

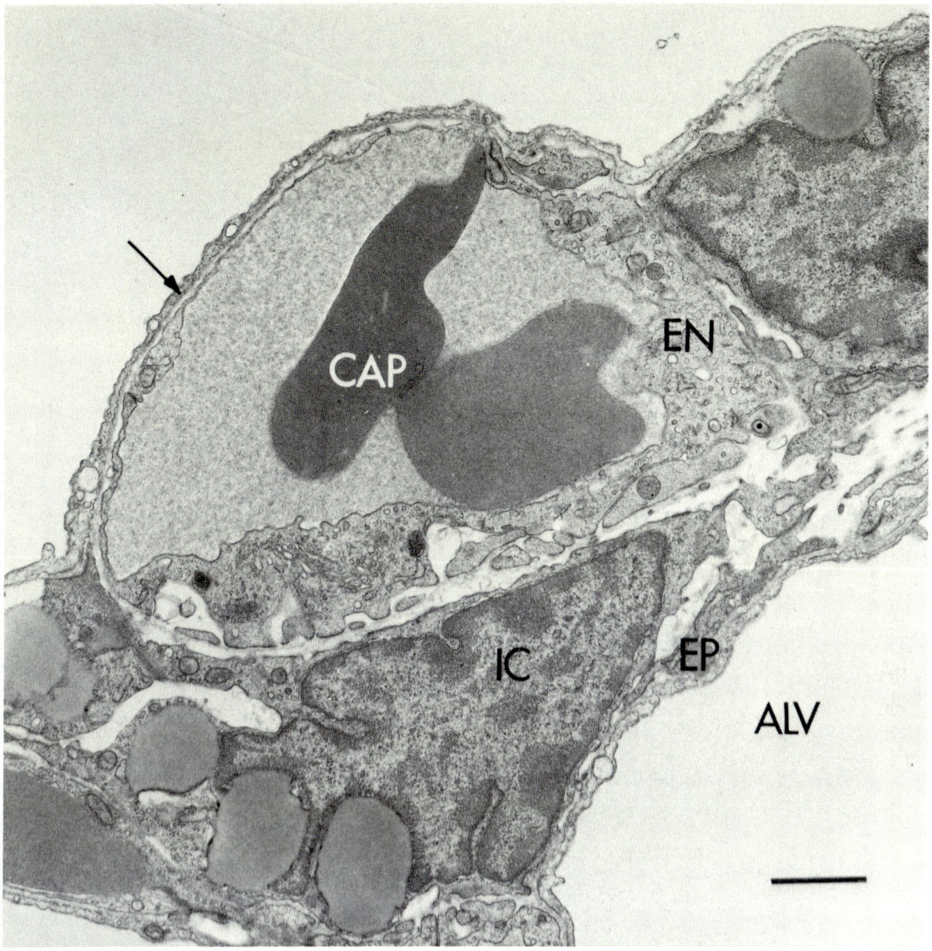

FIG. 1. Edge-on view of an alveolar septum of a mouse lung showing a septal capillary (*CAP*). The thin region of the septum is indicated by an *arrow*. On the opposite side, is the thick region of the septal interstitium containing connective tissue and an interstitial cell (*IC*). In small rodents interstitial cells frequently contain homogeneous osmiophilic cytoplasmic bodies. *EP*, squamous pneumocyte; *ALV*, alveolus. Uranyl acetate-lead hydroxide, × 13,000. The *bar* represents 1 μm.

the interstitial space is more abundant. Endothelial and epithelial cells with their basement membranes are separated by collagen and elastic fibers, various interstitial cells, and a ground substance composed of hydrophilic glycosoaminoglycans. Owing to their great capacity to bind water, glycosoaminoglycans function as "sumps," temporarily storing excessive amounts of water that have leaked from the alveolar capillaries as a result of daily fluctuation in cardiac activity.[11] In this way, water-logging of the thin, gas-exchanging regions is prevented. Swelling of the collagenous portions of the alveolar septum is the earliest and most constant ultrastructural sign of interstitial edema (Fig. 2) regardless of the mechanism by which edema formation occurs.

Between blood and interstitial space is the capillary endothelium composed of "continuous" endothelial cells. These extremely flattened cells contain few organ-

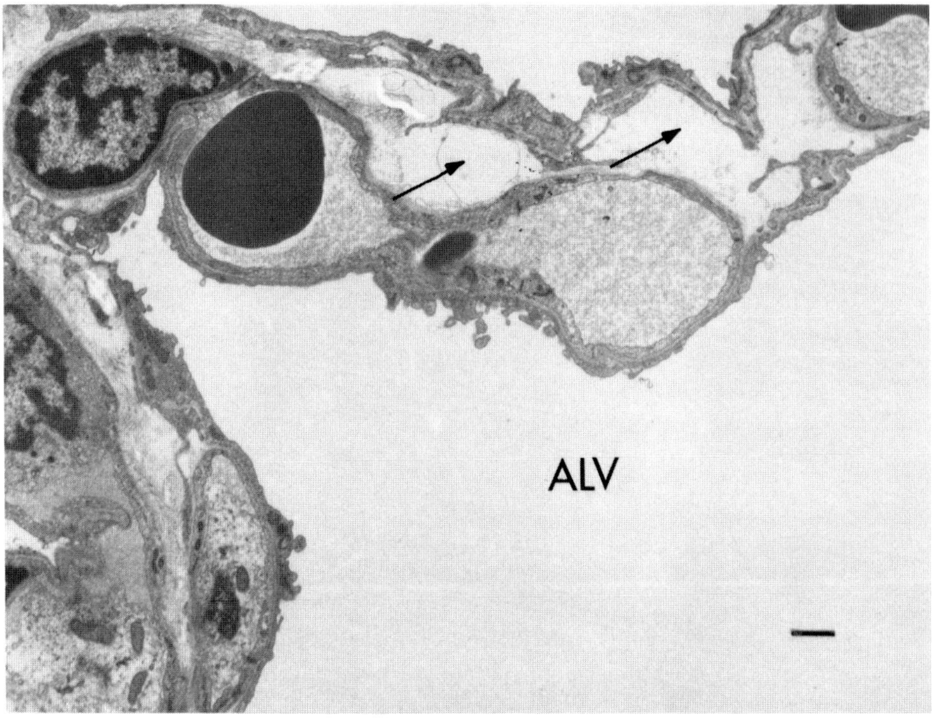

FIG. 2. View of an alveolar septum of an edematous dog lung. The *arrows* indicate swelling and electrolucency of the thick region of the septal interstitium. Note the absence of ultrastructural changes of the capillary endothelium or epithelium. Swelling of the septal interstitium is the first anatomic sign of pulmonary edema. Uranyl acetate-lead citrate, × 5,000. The *bar* represents 1 μm.

elles in their cytoplasm except for vesicles 50–80 nm in diameter which frequently open onto the luminal or abluminal endothelial surface (Fig. 3). Endothelial cells are held together by partial fusion of the outer leaflets of their bounding unit membranes (junctions). Between points of fusion are narrow slits, about 4 nm in width, that connect the intra- and extravascular compartments (Fig. 3).

Toward the alveoli, the interstitium is bound by the alveolar epithelium, composed mostly of type I (squamous) and type II (granular) pneumocytes. Although the two cell types are present in about equal number, the extremely flattened squamous cells line most of the alveolar surface. Hence, these cells represent the major barrier to the movement of liquids (and cells) from the interstitium to the alveoli, and vice versa. In many ways, the squamous pneumocyte resembles an endothelial cell since it has few organelles and many vesicles (Fig. 4) but, in contrast to the endothelial cells, the epithelial cells are held together by complete fusion of the outer leaflets of the bounding unit membranes forming "tight" junctions (Fig. 4).

The type II cells have been extensively discussed in this monograph; they will be only briefly mentioned here. In the normal lung their contribution to liquid exchange is related to the secretion of surface-active phospholipids. In pathologic conditions these cells may proliferate and line the entire alveolar surface. The effect of this type II cell hyperplasia on the permeability of the epithelium has not been explored.

The septal interstitium is in direct continuity with the peribronchial connective tissue that accompanies the bronchi and the extra-alveolar blood vessels. This peribronchial space contains abundant collagen and elastic fibers, lymphoid aggregates, nerves and mast cells. Two important structures distinguish the extra-alveolar interstitium from the septal interstitium; the lymphatic drainage and blood supply from the systemic circulation via the bronchial arteries of the extra-alveolar interstitium. As described by Miller,[19] the bronchial arteries give rise to a twin plexus of submucosal and adventitial microvessels that course the entire length of the bronchi, down to the terminal bronchioles. Perforating radicles cross the bronchial muscular layer and connect the two plexuses. The extent of the bronchial microcirculation varies in different species[18, 19, 23] but it is particularly well developed in large animals and man. In addition to providing the bronchi with nutrients and oxygen, the bronchial circulation may serve as a heat exchanger during respiration.

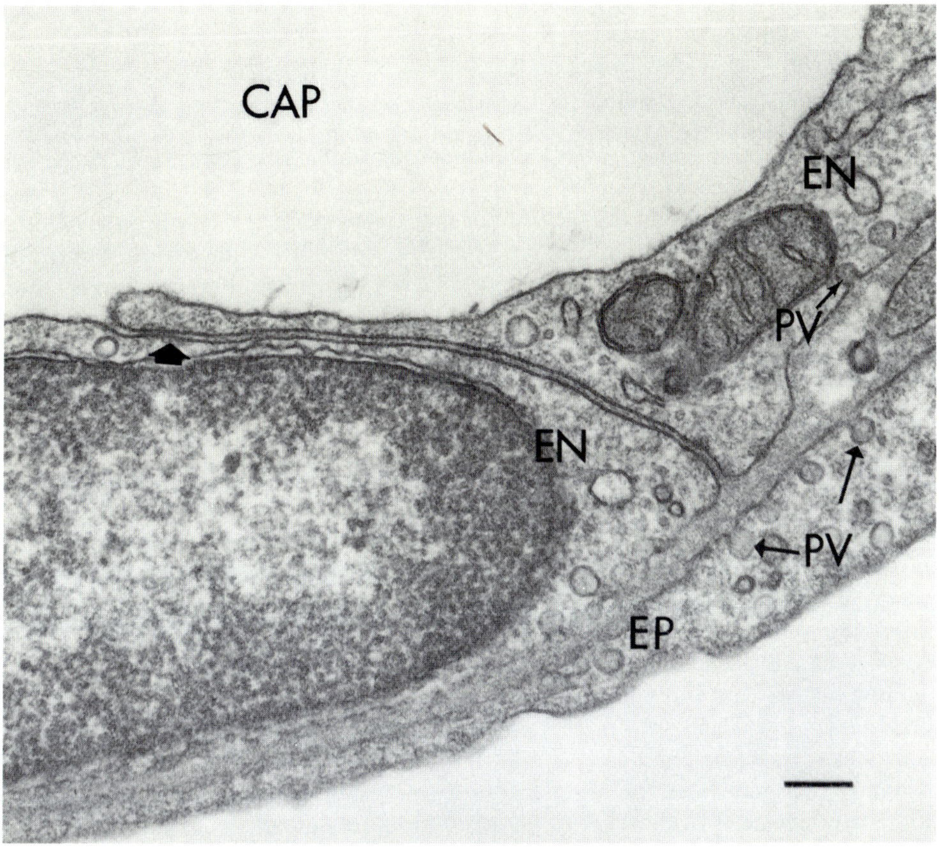

FIG. 3. Higher power view of the alveolar-capillary barrier showing an endothelial junction. The *arrow* points to an area of close approximation but no fusion of the cytoplasmic membranes of the two endothelial cells. *PV*, plasmalemmal vesicles of endothelium and squamous pneumocyte. Uranyl acetate-lead hydroxide, × 90,000. The *bar* represents 90 nm.

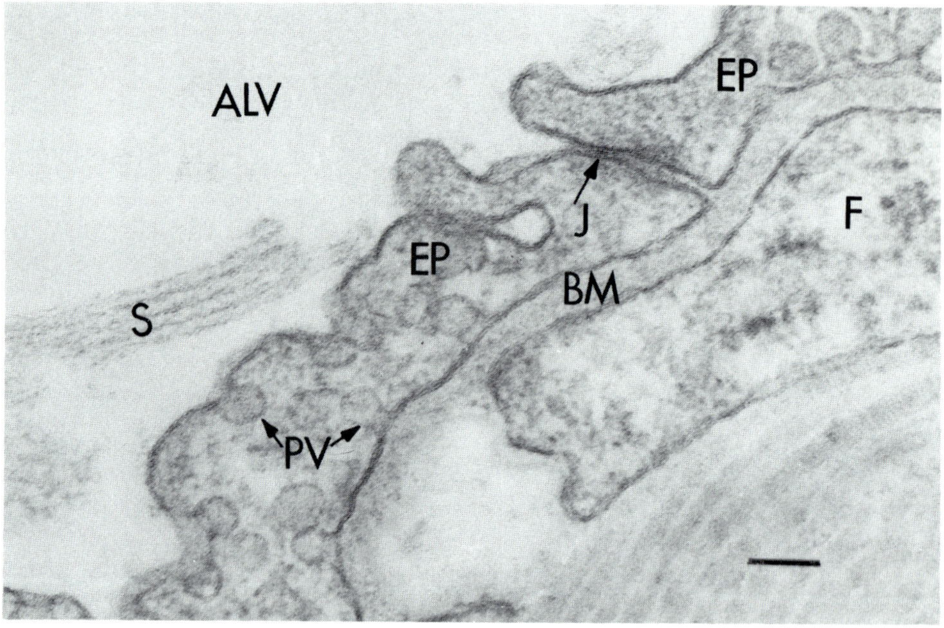

FIG. 4. An epithelial cell junction (*J*) between two squamous pneumocytes showing fusion of bounding unit membranes in the area indicated with the arrow. *S*, tubular myelin; *BM*, basement membrane; *F*, fibroblast. Uranyl acetate-lead citrate, × 100,000. *Bar* represents 100 nm.

The lymphatic vessels form an extensive network in the peribronchial (and interlobar) connective tissue. Immersed in the ground substance of the bronchial interstitium are numerous lymphatic capillaries, which are characterized by their relatively large lumens, extremely attenuated endothelial cells and discontinuous basement membrane. Contact between endothelial cells are made through extremely overlapping cytoplasmic processes forming interendothelial clefts of variable width.[17] Junctions are poorly developed. The endothelial cells are attached to bundles of collagen fibers radially arranged at the periphery of the lymphatic vessels. These "anchoring filaments"[17] may play an important role in maintaining the patency of the lymphatic vessels. Swelling of the interstitium, as a result of liquid accumulation, tends to stretch these anchoring filaments. The tension so generated is transmitted to the lymphatic endothelial cells pulling them away from the axis of the vessels. Moreover, it causes partial separation of adjoining cells and opening of the interendothelial clefts, thus favoring rapid passage of solutes and proteins into the lymphatic lumen.[17]

How liquids that have escaped from the septal capillaries reach the peribronchial space is still uncertain. Physiologic data indicate that gradients of subatmospheric pressure between septal and peribronchial interstitium favor the drainage of liquids from the septal interstitium to a more compliant extra-alveolar interstitial space.[13] Under the influence of gradients of subatmospheric pressure liquids move from the septal interstitium into the peribronchial space where they are reabsorbed by the lymphatic vessels.[11, 28, 36]

Since accumulation of liquids in the septal interstitium escapes detection by light microscopy, early studies on the sequence of events in pulmonary edema, using this technique, have led to the notion that peribronchial edema may precede septal edema in certain experimental conditions. Ultrastructural observations, however, indicate that in most forms of pulmonary edema swelling of the septal interstitium is the primary event.

The second component of the extravascular space, the air space, has a volume 5–10 times that of the interstitium[36] and offers no resistance to movement of liquids.

Structural Basis for Transcapillary Exchange

Movement of substances across the capillary wall can take place through the entire capillary surface or through "pores." Lipophilic molecules and water are thought to use the entire capillary surface. Hydrophilic molecules diffuse through pores according to transcapillary gradients of concentration. Two sets of pores have been proposed[27] to account for the movement of hydrophilic substances across capillaries lined by continuous endothelium. "Small" pores, 8-9 nm in diameter, that occupy about 0.2% of the entire capillary surface, allow rapid diffusion of small solutes less than 1,000 daltons. As the size of the molecules becomes larger they will meet increasing resistance in traversing the pore, until resistance will become infinite for molecules of diameter equal to that of the pores, *i.e.*, 90,000 daltons. Since most plasma proteins are larger than 90,000 daltons a second set of a few "large" pores, about 50 nm in diameter, has been proposed to account for the transcapillary movement of such large molecules.[27]

In an attempt to verify the existence of anatomic pores in the capillary endothelium, electron microscopists have utilized protein tracers of various size and followed their location in the capillary wall, at various time intervals after their injection intravenously.[14, 22, 29, 32] Of great popularity have been peroxidative enzymes, that can be localized ultrastructurally by cytochemical techniques.[12] Difficulties have arisen in extrapolating dynamic processes from static pictures and in discerning physiologic processes from artifacts introduced by the observer. Accordingly, there is not yet unanimity regarding the existence of anatomic pores. Palade and co-workers[32] have presented evidence indicating the existance of transendothelial channels resulting from transitory fusion of vesicles. These channels correspond to both sets of pores, "small" and "large." Others[14, 22, 29] have presented evidence in support of the notion that the junctions are the anatomic equivalent of the "small" pores, and pinocytotic vesicles that of the "large" pores. It is likely that the two theories are not mutually exclusive and that factors other than molecular size determine the routes taken by proteins and other macromolecules across the capillary endothelium.

In the lung, ultrastructural studies have revealed great differences in the permeability of endothelial and epithelial junctions to proteins. Thus, at normal capillary pressures, cytochrome *c* (mol. wt. 12,000) rapidly reaches the pulmonary interstitium crossing the interendothelial junctions, but is prevented from reaching the alveolar space by the junctions between both types of alveolar epithelial cells.[29] Under physiologic conditions, proteins cross the epithelial barrier exclusively by pinocytosis.[2, 29] These morphologic observations are consistent with physiologic studies indicating that the pulmonary endothelial pores have a radius of 4–5.8 nm, while epithelial pores have a radius of 0.6–1 nm, and the latter represent the major barrier to the passage of water-soluble substances from blood to the alveolar space.[10]

In thin sections, stained with heavy metals, the intercellular junctions can be recognized by partial or complete fusion of the outer leaflets of the bounding unit membrane of two adjacent cells (Fig. 4). The intercellular space contains osmiophilic material presumably glycoproteins. But these images provide little information on the organization of the cell membrane in the junctional region. (A three-dimensional view of cell membranes is provided by fracturing and frozen-etching unfixed or aldehyde-fixed (−150°C) specimens.) Freeze-fracturing cleaves the tissue along natural planes of weakness. In frozen membranes these planes pass preferentially along the hydrophobic plane of the lipid bilayer.[34] Thus, two inner faces of the membrane are exposed. By convention,[3] the half membrane close to the cytoplasm has been designated A or PF, the outer half of the membrane is called B or EF (Fig. 5*A*). Freeze-etching involves the sublimation of ice over the rapidly-frozen specimen and reveals the true surface of the membrane.[34] The fractured surfaces are then coated with an extremely thin layer of platinum and carbon. The tissue is digested away with mild alkali and the replica is mounted on grids for examination in the electron microscope. The cleaved surfaces reveal small particles (4–16 nm) distributed over smooth surfaces. It is generally agreed that the particles correspond to globular proteins and glycoproteins embedded within the membrane lipids[34] owing to the inherent asymmetry

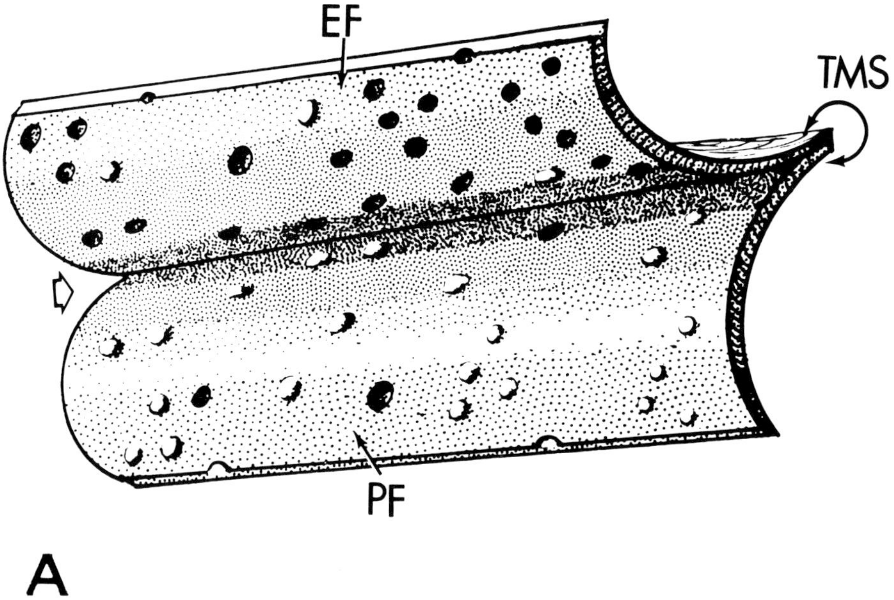

FIG. 5A: Diagrammatic representation of a freeze-fractured, nonjunctional, plasma membrane. The frozen membrane is fractured along the central, hydrophobic plane of the bilayer region. The exposed faces represent the inner aspects of the plasma membrane, not visible by scanning or transmission electron microscopy. By convention, the inner half of the split membrane proximal to the cell cytoplasm has been referred to as the A or PF face. The complementary outer half of the split membrane has been designated B or EF face. The cleaved membranes exhibit small particles, shown in the diagram as *white spheres*, which probably correspond to globular proteins embedded within the membrane lipids. *TMS*, true membrane surface, *large arrow* indicates the direction of the plane of fracture.

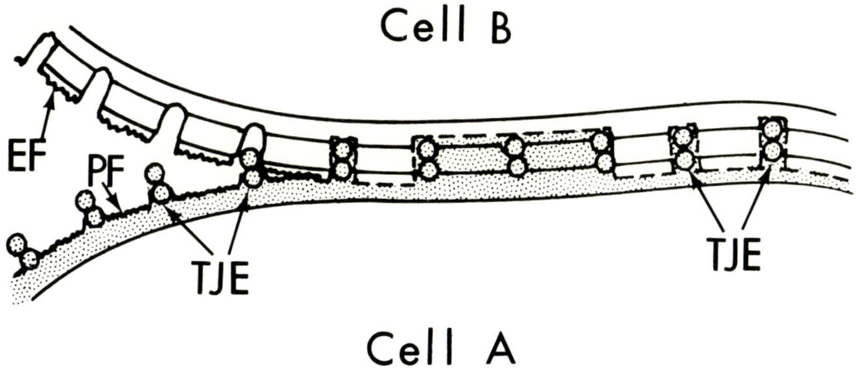

B

FIG. 5B: Diagrammatic interpretation of the fracture process in a junction between two cells, A and B. The plane of fracture is deflected from the central plane of the plasma membrane of cell A, moves around tight junctional elements (*TJE*), which held cells A and B together, into the membrane of cell B and then returns to the central plane of cell A. This fracturing behavior results in the formation of ridges or rows of particles on the PF face of cell A (*dotted area*) or in grooves in the EF face.

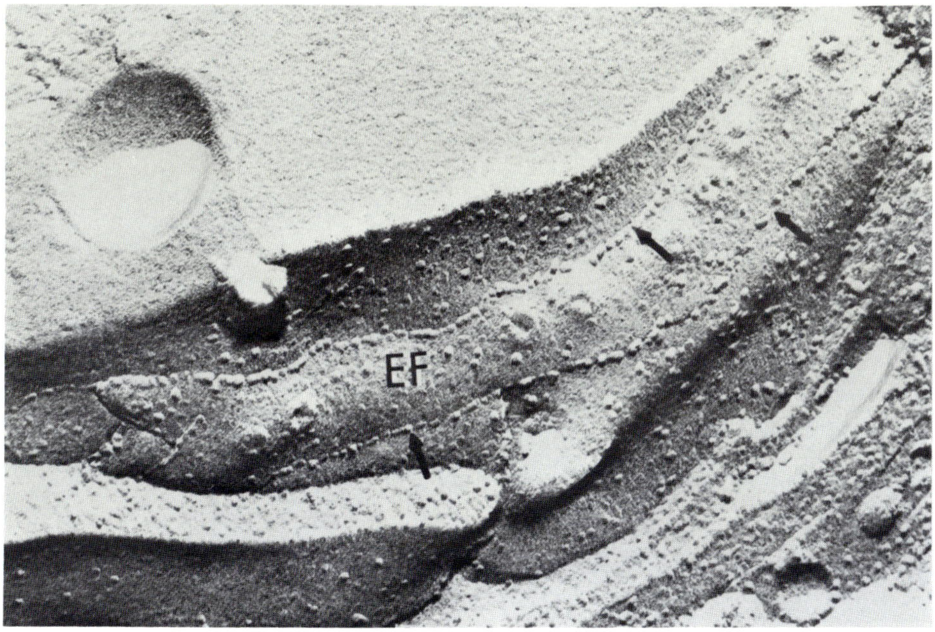

FIG. 6. Freeze-fracture replica of an endothelial junction of a capillary of the rabbit lung. Rows of particles (*arrows*) in shallow grooves over the exoplasmic face (*EF*). The openings of plasmalemmal vesicles appear as small craters. × 100,000.

of cell membranes, particles will tend to remain attached preferentially to one of the two membrane faces. The smooth background seen in freeze-fracture preparations corresponds to the membrane lipids. In the junctions, the plane of fracture skips from one cell to the other, moving around the points of fusion of cell membranes of adjacent cells (Fig. 5*B*). These fused elements will remain preferentially attached to one of the fracture faces, usually the PF face, forming ridges or rows of particles (Fig. 5*B*). On the opposite face, grooves are formed where the fused elements have been torn away from the fracture face.

Freeze-fracture studies of junctions of the capillary endothelium and alveolar epithelium of the mouse,[30] dog,[15] and rabbit[26] lung, have revealed structural differences that are consistent with the tracer studies. The junctions of the capillary endothelium reveal one to three, almost parallel rows of particles on grooves over the exoplasmic (EF) face (Fig. 6). Instead the epithelial junctions, of type I and II pneumocytes, consist of a complex network of solid strands on the PF face (Fig. 7) with complementary grooves on the EF face. Originally, permeability of intercellular junctions to ions, was believed to correlate with the number of strands that form a junction since it was observed that impermeable

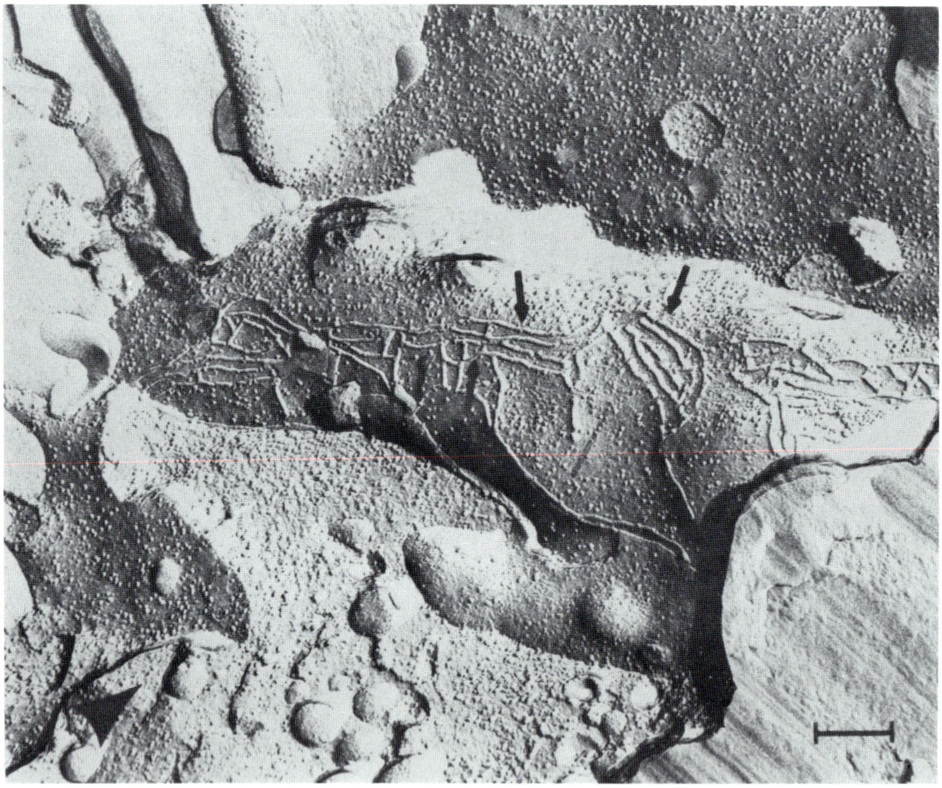

FIG. 7. Freeze-fracture replica of the PF face of an epithelial junction of a type II pneumocyte of the rabbit lung. The junction is composed of anastomosing solid fibers (*arrows*). The solid ridges seen in the epithelial junctions indicate sites of complete fusion of membrane proteins of two adjacent cells that bridge, and presumably completely seal, the intercellular space. The beaded appearance of the endothelial junction, depicted in Figure 6, indicates weaker interaction between interconnecting junctional elements. Moreover, the presence of only one or two strands and their discontinuous structure is consistent with the picture seen by transmission electron microscopy of narrow slits within the endothelial junctions that connect intra- and extravascular spaces. × 60,000. *Large arrow* indicates direction of shadowing. *Bar* indicates 60 nm.

epithelia had junctions composed of multiple anastomosing ridges whereas "leaky" epithelia had junctions composed of one or two rows of particles.[5] However, recent observations[20] on the permeability of the developing choroid plexus have failed to reveal a direct correlation between the structure of the junctions and their porosity to solutes. There is still uncertainty on the exact nature of the structures seen by freeze-fracturing since freeze-fracturing does not reveal the true cell surface of adjacent cells at the level of the junction. Moreover, the number of ridges seen by this technique is greater than the points of fusion seen in thin sectioning.[33] Indeed, it has been suggested that some of the components seen by freeze-fracturing may not be involved in anchoring two cells together but perform some other function.[33] Accordingly, no definite correlation can yet be made between the type of structures seen on fractured membrane faces and the degree of porosity of the junctions.

Stretched Pores

Our own experience[22, 24] indicates that the permeability of capillary endothelial and alveolar epithelial junctions to proteins is markedly influenced by the capillary hydrostatic pressure. At normal capillary pressure the endothelial junctions are impermeable to myoglobin (17,000 daltons), horseradish peroxidase (40,000 daltons), and hemoglobin (64,500 daltons) (Fig. 8). At a capillary pressure of 30 mm Hg the endothelial junctions become permeable to myoglobin and horseradish peroxidase but not to hemoglobin. At higher pressure (>50 mm Hg)

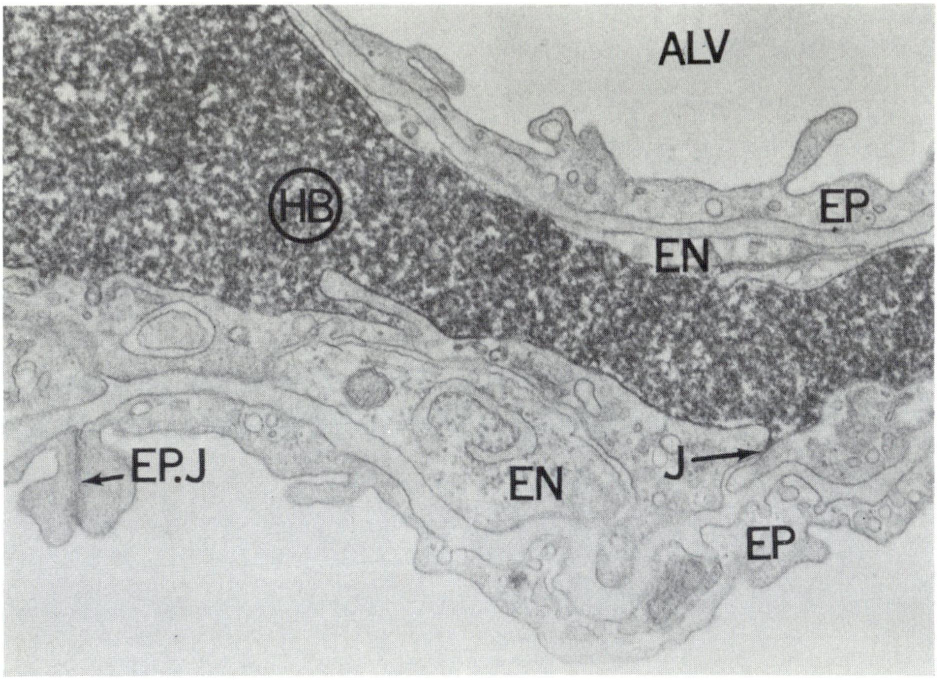

FIG. 8. Pulmonary capillaries of a dog lung after perfusion of a solution of hemoglobin (*Hb*) at normal perfusing pressure for 30 min. The osmiophilic reaction product is confined to the intravascular compartment. Lead hydroxide, × 9,000.

the endothelial junctions become permeable even to hemoglobin (Fig. 9), but the junctions of the alveolar and bronchiolar epithelium prevent escape of the tracer into the alveoli (Figs. 9 and 10). Only at capillary pressures greater than 50 mm Hg do the epithelial junctions become leaky with the development of alveolar edema (Fig. 11).

These data are consistent with physiologic observations[31] indicating that the size of the small pores is not fixed and tend to obscure the distinction between hemodynamic and permeability edema. Since the alveolar epithelium appears to be the major barrier to leakage of proteins from blood to alveoli, in the presence of damaged epithelium relative modest elevation of the capillary pressure may result in catastrophic alveolar flooding. Figure 12 depicts the alveolar-capillary membrane of a 61-year-old man who died of pulmonary edema three days after perforation of a peptic ulcer and development of *Escherichia coli* septicemia. The lungs were fixed transthoracically immediately after death. The picture shows alveolar edema and fibrin masses over a denuded basement membrane in the presence of a slightly damaged capillary endothelium. It is tempting to speculate that loss of squamous epithelial lining caused flooding of the alveoli with edema fluid.

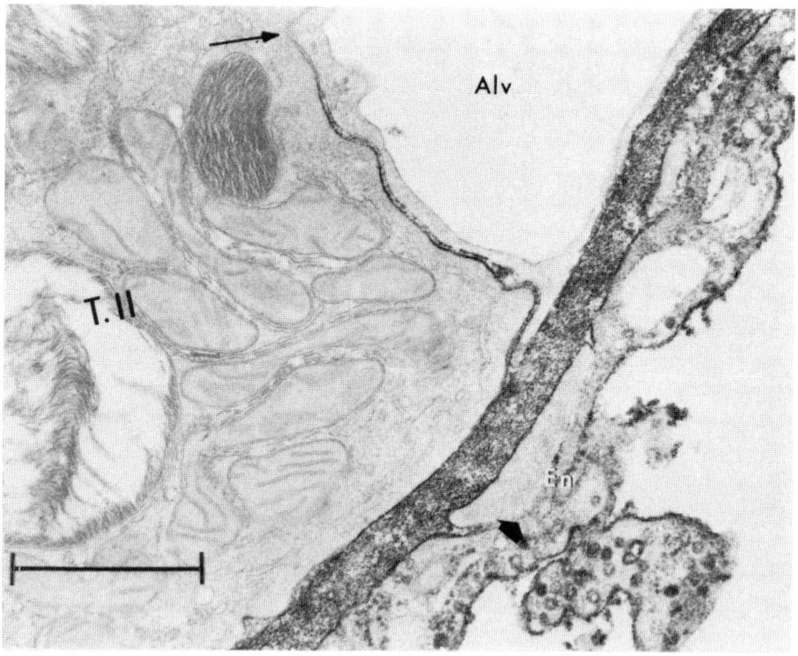

FIG. 9. Pulmonary capillary of a dog lung after perfusion of a solution of hemoglobin at a pressure of 45–50 mm Hg for 5 min. The reaction product stains the endothelial cleft (*thick arrow*), the basement membrane, the interstitial space, and a cleft between type II (*T.II*) and type I pneumocytes. The portion of the epithelial cleft near the air space is, however, unstained (*arrow*). Lead hydroxide, × 30,000. *Bar* is 1 μm.

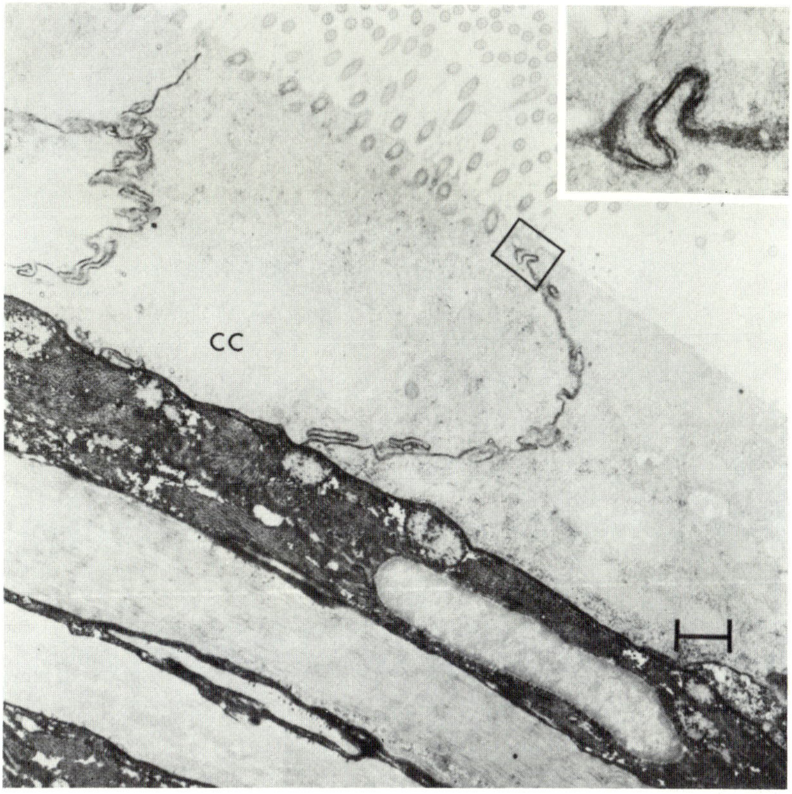

FIG. 10. Bronchial epithelium of a dog lung perfused with a solution of hemoglobin at high perfusing pressure. The reaction product stains the ground substance of the bronchial interstitial space and the clefts between the epithelial cells (*CC*) but it does not stain the luminal portions of the cleft (*inset*). The collagen fibers appear as electron-lucent fibers surrounded by the osmiophilic reaction product. Unstained section, × 10,000; *inset*, × 36,000. *Bar* indicates 1 μm.

ENDOTHELIAL DAMAGE

The pulmonary microvascular endothelium can be damaged in a variety of ways by circulating toxins,[7, 8] bacterial products,[6] pulmonary infections, drugs, or inhaled gases.[28] Most types of noncardiogenic edema fall into this group of endothelial injury. However, in clinical conditions it may be difficult to rule out the concomitant effect of capillary hypertension secondary to left heart failure or overzealous liquid administration. Conversely, patients with capillary hypertension may develop secondary alterations of the capillary endothelium.[28] Ultrastructural studies in experimental animals[6, 7] and in man[37] have emphasized swelling and necrosis of the endothelium, and frequently associated damage of the squamous pneumocytes. Widespread endothelial damage has been found in patients with advanced respiratory insufficiency that had become refractory to treatment.[37] In these instances, the alveolar liquids contain high concentrations of plasma proteins, including fibrinogen.[37] Organization of extravascular fibrinogen may be responsible for the development of severe interstitial fibrosis in patients

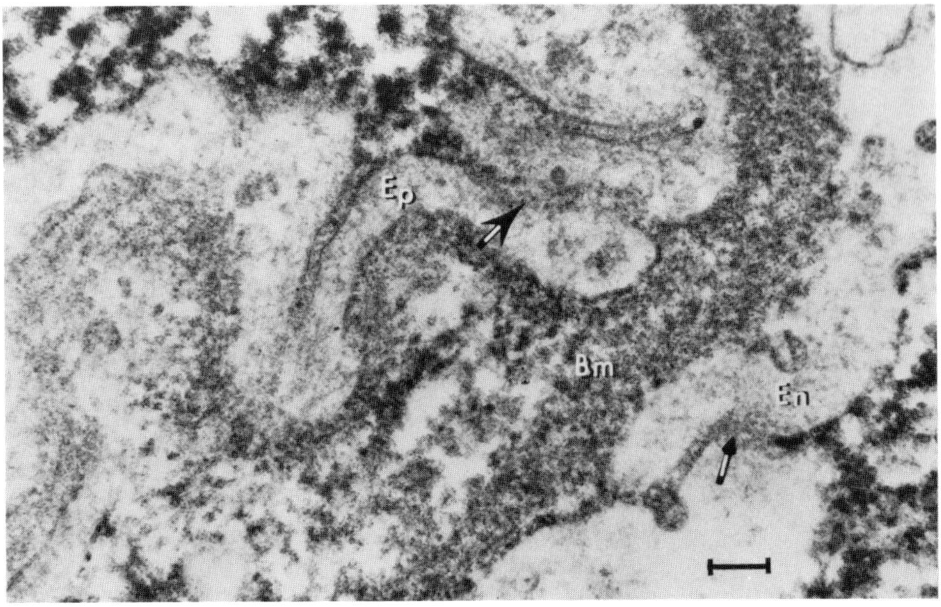

FIG. 11. Reaction product stains an endothelial junction (*small arrow*), the basement membrane, an epithelial junction (*thick arrow*), and extends into the alveolar space. The section is from the lung of a dog perfused with a solution of hemoglobin at a pressure of 50 mm Hg for 20 min. Diffuse osmiophilia of the epithelial cell (*EP*) suggests injury. Unstained section, × 80,000. *Bar* indicates 80 nm.

with severe endothelial damage maintained alive by extraordinary therapeutic measures, such as extracorporeal membrane oxygenation.

BRONCHIAL EDEMA

Changes in pulmonary hemodynamics and permeability are certainly the most important determinants of pulmonary edema. However, we have recently called attention to leaky bronchial microvessels as a potential cause of interstitial edema. The permeability of the bronchial venular plexus appears to be selectively influenced by endotoxin[25] or by chemical mediators of permeability, such as histamine and bradykinin.[23] The anatomic basis for this effect appears to be transient "stretching" of interendothelial junctions of bronchial venules, so that plasma or even blood escape into the bronchial interstitium (Figs. 13 and 14). There are two important consequences of leaky bronchial microvessels. Proteins that escape from these blood vessels in the proximity of the lymphatic vessels may alter the oncotic pressure in the interstitial space and interfere with the ability of the lymphatic system to drain interstitial fluid. Secondly, agents that cause bronchial venules to leak are also potent arterial vasoconstrictors and bronchoconstrictors. Peribronchial edema and bronchoconstriction both contribute to alteration of $\mathring{V}/\mathring{Q}$ ratios in individual respiratory units. It is conceivable that this may initiate the sequence of events leading to "congestive micro-atelectasis" one of the earliest anatomic manifestations of shock lung. Indeed appreciable amounts of kinins are released into the circulation during hemor-

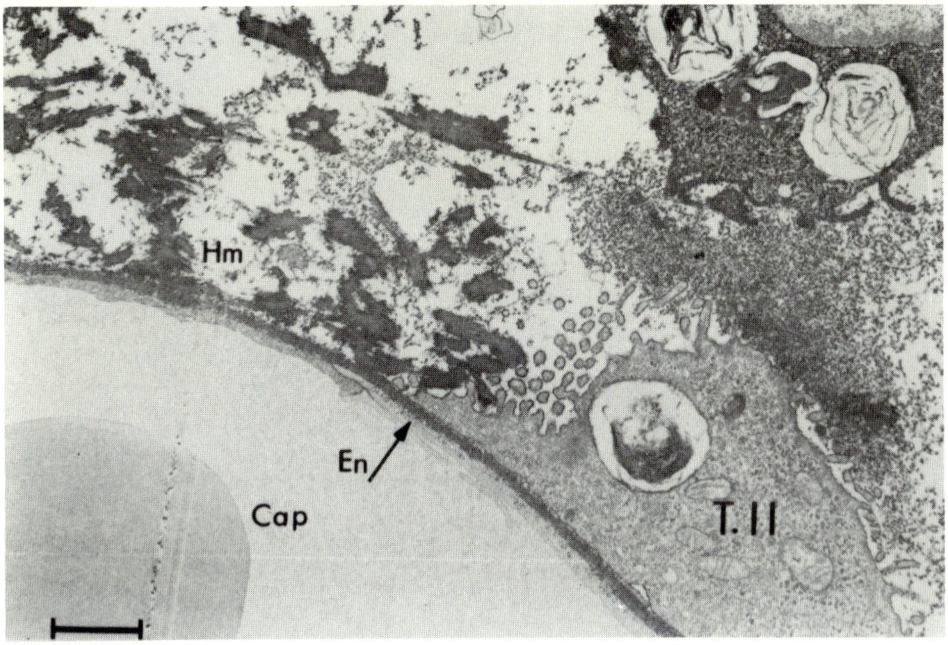

FIG. 12. Electron micrograph from a lung of a 61-year-old man who died of massive pulmonary edema following hypovolemic shock and *E. coli* septicemia. The tissue was fixed transthoracically immediately after death. There is alveolar edema and hyaline membrane formation (*HM*) over a denuded portion of the alveolar septum. A type II cell nearby appears well preserved. The capillary endothelium is relatively normal (*arrow*). Uranyl acetate-lead hydroxide, × 8,000. *Bar* indicates 1 μm.

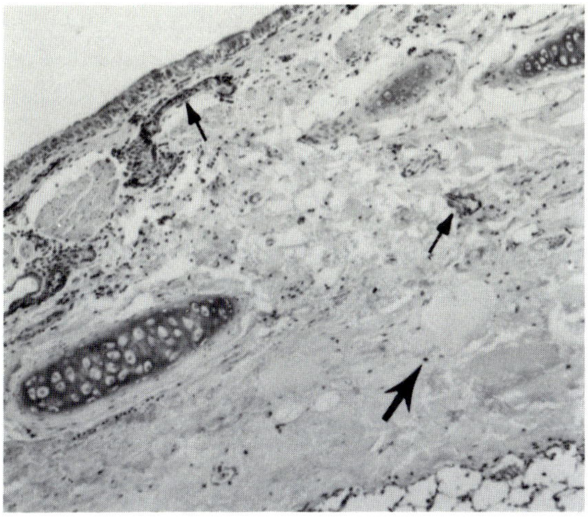

FIG. 13. Dog killed 1 hour after the onset of profound systemic hypotension as a result of the injection of 5 mg/kg body weight of *E. coli* lipopolysaccharide intravenously. Colloidal carbon was injected intravenously to identify sites of leakage. Marked peribronchial edema (*thick arrow*) and leaky venules (*fine arrows*) can be seen. H.E., × 150.

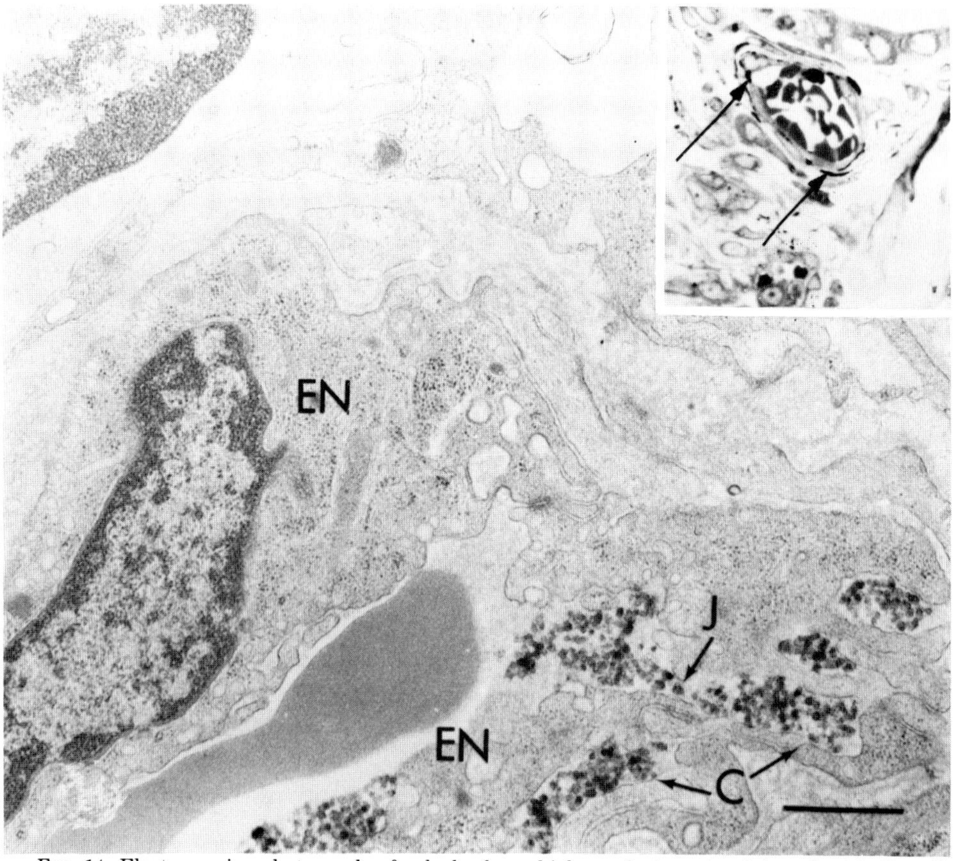

FIG. 14. Electron microphotograph of a leaky bronchial venule in a dog injected with *E. coli* lipopolysaccharide. Carbon particles (*C*) are seen within an opened endothelial junction (*J*) and in the perivascular space. Uranyl acetate-lead citrate, × 12,000. *Bar* indicates 1 μm. *Inset*: 1-μ section of Epon embedded lung tissue of a leaky bronchial venule showing deposits of carbon (*arrows*) in the adventitia.

rhagic or septic shock.[1] Leaky bronchial vessels are undoubtedly responsible for the edematous bronchial mucosa in extrinsic asthma and various inflammatory reactions of the lungs. The bronchial circulation is greatly expanded in pulmonary hypertension, mitral stenosis, cyanotic heart disease, and in some patients with chronic obstructive lung disease, but the significance of this expanded microvascular bed in water balance of the lungs is unknown and I will conclude with Dr. De Burgh Daly: "Concerning the significance of the bronchial arterial system in health and disease we are still largely in the dark, but that this may be a fruitful field for investigation is unquestionable."[9]

SUMMARY

In the normal lung, a delicate interplay of physical forces and structural devices maintains the gas-exchanging membranes hydrated but unflooded. Liquids leaking from the alveolar capillaries are prevented from interfering with gas-exchange by a combination of mechanisms: the alveolar epithelium prevents easy access of liquids into the alveolar space; glycosoaminoglycan "sumps" in the thick portion of the septum bind excess liquid, thereby protecting the gas-exchanging thin portions of the alveolar-capillary barrier from water-logging; gradients of subatmospheric pressure promote the rapid transfer of liquids from the septal "sumps" into a compliant peribronchial space for further disposal by the lymphatic vessels. "Leaky" pulmonary and bronchial microvessels upset the osmotic forces in the interstitial space and interfere with the capacity of the lymphatic system to reabsorb liquids. Accumulation of excess liquids is limited initially to the interstitium. When the capacity of this space to bind liquids is overcome alveolar edema develops.

ACKNOWLEDGMENT

The constant encouragement, advice, and criticism of Dr. Alfred P. Fishman is gratefully acknowledged. J. M. Minda, Marianne Yachinsky, and Lew Johns have provided skillful technical assistance.

REFERENCES

1. Berry, H. E., Collier, J. G., and Vane, J. R.: The generation of kinins in the blood of dogs during hypotension due to hemorrhage. *Clin. Sci. 39:* 349–365, 1970.
2. Bignon, J., Chahinian, P., Feldmann, G., and Sapin, C.: Ultrastructural immunoperoxidase demonstration of autologous albumin in the alveolar capillary membrane and in the alveolar lining material in normal rats. *J. Cell Biol. 64:* 503–509, 1975.
3. Branton, D., Bullivant, S., Gilula, N. B., Karnovsky, M. J., Moor, H., Muhlethaler, K., Northcote, D. H., Packer, L., Satir, B., Satir, P., Speth, V., Staehlin, L. A., Steere, R. L., and Weinstein, R. S.: Freeze-etching nomenclature. *Science 190:* 54–56, 1975.
4. Cameron, G. R.: Pulmonary oedema. *Br. Med. J. 1:* 965–972, 1948.
5. Claude, P., and Goodenough, D. A.: Fracture faces of zonulae occludentes from "tight" and "leaky" epithelia. *J. Cell Biol. 58:* 390–400, 1973.
6. Coalson, J. J., Hinshaw, L. B., Guenter, C. A., Berrell, E. L., and Greenfield, L. J.: Pathophysiologic responses of the subhuman primate in experimental septic shock. *Lab. Invest. 32:* 561–569, 1975.
7. Cottrell, T. S., Levine, O. R., Senior, R. M., Wiener, J., Spiro, D., and Fishman, A. P.: Electron microscopic alterations at the alveolar level in pulmonary edema. *Circ. Res. 21:* 783–797, 1967.
8. Cunningham, A. L., and Hurley, J. V.: Alpha-napthyl-thiourea-induced pulmonary oedema in the rat: A topographical and electron-microscope study. *J. Pathol. 106:* 25–35, 1972.
9. Daly, I. DeBurgh: The physiology of the bronchial vascular system. *Harvey Lectures 31:* 235–255, 1936.
10. Egan, E. A.: Effect of lung inflation on alveolar permeability to solutes. In *Lung Liquids.* Ciba Foundation Symposium 38 (New Series), pp. 101–114. Elsevier-Excerpta Medica, North Holland, Amsterdam, Oxford, New York, 1976.
11. Fishman, A. P.: Pulmonary edema. The water-exchanging function of the lung. *Circulation 46:* 390–408, 1972.
12. Graham, R. C., and Karnovsky, M. J.: The early stages of absorption of injected horseradish peroxidase in the proximal tubules of mouse kidney. Ultrastructural cytochemistry by a new technique. *J. Histochem. Cytochem. 14:* 291–302, 1966.
13. Guyton, A. C., Taylor, A. E., Drake, R. E., and Parker, I. E.: Dynamics of subatmospheric pressure in the pulmonary interstitial fluid. In *Lung Liquids.* Ciba Foundation Symposium 38 (New Series), pp. 77–100. Elsevier-Excerpta Medica, North Holland, Amsterdam, Oxford, New York, 1976.
14. Hücker, H., Frenzel, H., Kremer, B., and Richter, J. E.: Time sequence and site of fluid accumulation in experimental neurogenic pulmonary edema. *Res. Exp. Med. 168:* 219–227, 1976.
15. Inoue, S., Michel, R. P., and Hogg, J. C.: Zonulae occludentes in alveolar epithelium and capillary endothelium of dog lungs studied with the freeze-fracture technique. *J. Ultrastruct. Res. 56:* 215–225, 1976.

16. Laennec, R. T. H.: *A Treatise on the Diseases of the Chest and on Mediate Auscultation.* Translation by J. Forbes, Philadelphia, Desilver, Thomas & Co., 1835.
17. Leak, L. V., and Kato, F.: Electron microscopic studies of lymphatic capillaries during early inflammation. I: Mild and severe thermal injuries. *Lab. Invest. 26:* 572–588, 1972.
18. McLaughlin, R. F., Jr., Tyler, W. S., and Canada, R. O.: Subgross pulmonary anatomy in various mammals and man. *JAMA 175:* 694–697, 1961.
19. Miller, W. S.: *The Lung.* Springfield, Ill., Charles C Thomas, pp. 74–83, 1937.
20. Mollgard, K., Malinowska, D. H., and Saunders, N. R.: Lack of correlation between tight junction morphology and permeability properties in developing choroid plexus. *Nature 264:* 293–294, 1976.
21. Paintal, A. S.: Mechanism of stimulation of type J pulmonary receptors. *J. Physiol. 203:* 511–532, 1969.
22. Pietra, G. G., Szidon, J. P., Leventhal, M. M., and Fishman, A. P.: Hemoglobin as a tracer in hemodynamic pulmonary edema. *Science* (Washington) *166:* 1643–1646, 1969.
23. Pietra, G. G., Szidon, J. P., Leventhal, M. M., and Fishman, A. P.: Histamine and interstitial pulmonary edema in the dog. *Circ. Res. 29:* 323–337, 1971.
24. Pietra, G. G., Szidon, J. P., and Fishman, A. P.: Leaky pulmonary vessels. *Trans. Assoc. Am. Phys. 85:* 369–376, 1972.
25. Pietra, G. G., Szidon, J. P., Carpenter, H. A., and Fishman, A. P.: Bronchial venular leakage during endotoxin shock. *Am. J. Pathol. 77:* 387–406, 1974.
26. Pietra, G. G.: Unpublished observations.
27. Renkin, E. M.: Transport of large molecules across capillary walls. *Physiologist 7:* 13–28, 1964.
28. Robin, E. D., Gross, C. E., and Zelis, R.: Pulmonary edema. *N. Engl. J. Med. 288:* 239–246, 292–304, 1973.
29. Schneeberger, E. E., and Karnovsky, M. J.: The influence of intravascular fluid volume on the permeability of newborn and adult mouse lungs to ultrastructural protein tracers. *J. Cell Biol. 49:* 319–334, 1971.
30. Schneeberger, E. E., and Karnovsky, M. J.: Substructure of intercellular junctions in freeze-fractured alveolar-capillary membranes of mouse lung. *Circ Res. 38:* 404–411, 1976.
31. Shirley, H. H., Wolfram, C. G., Wasserman, K., and Mayerson, H. S.: Capillary permeability to macromolecules: Stretched pore phenomenon. *Am. J. Physiol. 190:* 189–193, 1957.
32. Simionescu, N., Simionescu, M., and Palade, G. E.: Permeability of muscle capillaries to small heme-peptides. Evidence for the existence of patent transendothelial channels. *J. Cell Biol. 64:* 586–607, 1975.
33. Simionescu, M., Simionescu, N., and Palade, G. E.: Segmental differentiations of cell junctions in the vasculature endothelium. The microvasculature. *J. Cell Biol. 67:* 863–885, 1975.
34. Staehelin, L. A.: Structure and function of intercellular junctions. *Int. Rev. Cytol. 39:* 191–283, 1974.
35. Starling, E. H.: On the absorption of fluids from the connective tissue spaces. *J. Physiol. 19:* 312–326, 1896.
36. Staub, N. C.: Pulmonary edema. *Physiol Rev. 54:* 678–811, 1974.
37. Teplitz, C.: The core pathobiology and integrated medical science of adult acute respiratory insufficiency. *Surg. Clin. N. Am. 56:* 1091–1133, 1976.
38. Theodore, J., and Robin, E. D.: Pathogenesis of neurogenic pulmonary oedema. *Lancet 2:* 749–751, 1975.
39. Viswanathan, R., Jain, S. K., and Subramanian, S.: Pulmonary edema of high altitude. III: Pathogenesis. *Am. Rev. Resp. Dis. 100:* 342–349, 1969.

Chapter 13

Recent Advances in the Pathology of the Pulmonary Vasculature*

WILLIAM D. EDWARDS AND JESSE E. EDWARDS

While the pathology of the pulmonary vascular bed has been a subject of interest for over a century, only in the past three decades has this area been extensively studied. The common factor associated with both the functional and the structural alterations of the pulmonary vascular bed is abnormally high pulmonary arterial pressure, a phenomenon usually called pulmonary hypertension. Once pulmonary hypertension is established, right ventricular hypertrophy is a constant finding.

It is important to recognize that pulmonary arterial pressure is regulated by two factors, namely the volume of pulmonary blood flow per unit of time and the resistance to this flow. Thus, pulmonary hypertension may occur in the presence of normal or near normal resistance if the pulmonary flow is excessive, or may occur in the presence of normal or even subnormal flow if the pulmonary vascular resistance is elevated.

This discussion will approach the subject from three aspects, namely (1) the effects of alveolar hypoxia, (2) clinical primary pulmonary hypertension, and (3) the responses of the pulmonary vasculature to corrective or palliative surgical procedures for cardiac disease. Two recent publications which deal with the subject of pulmonary hypertension and from which much of the information in this chapter was gathered include the forthcoming book by the Wagenvoorts[111] on the pathology of the pulmonary vasculature and the presentation by Naeye before the Academy in 1973 and published a year later.[75]

ALVEOLAR HYPOXIA

In 1946, Von Euler and Liljestrand[101] demonstrated in cats that breathing low oxygen tension air caused an elevation of pulmonary arterial pressure on the basis of precapillary arterial vasoconstriction. This observation was then confirmed experimentally in humans[115] and has practical implications in humans.

Hypoxia is one of the most potent pulmonary arterial vasoconstrictors known. Therefore, pulmonary hypertension may result from long-standing hypoxia of any cause, including high altitude, diminished minute ventilation, chronic upper

---

* This study was supported by USPHS Research Grant No. 5 RO1 HL05694 and Research Training Grant No. 5 TO1 HL05570 from the National Heart, Lung and Blood Institute, and by the Bremer Foundation and the Saint Paul Foundation, St. Paul, Minnesota.

airway obstruction, and chronic diffuse pulmonary parenchymal diseases. In these conditions, pulmonary vascular resistance is elevated while pulmonary blood flow is normal or subnormal.

High Altitude Residence

In high altitude residents, the prevailing pulmonary arterial pressure is higher than in residents at sea level. The level of pulmonary arterial pressure is directly related to the altitude of residence.[22] Thus, compared to an average normal mean pulmonary arterial pressure at sea level of about 12 mm Hg, the average resting mean pressure at Denver, Colorado (5,000 feet; 1,600 m) was 15 mm Hg, at Leadville, Colorado (10,000 feet; 3,100 m) was 25 mm Hg,[11, 99] and in the Peruvian Andes (14,000 feet; 4,500 m) was 28 mm Hg[79] (Fig. 1).

Moreover, at elevations of 10,000 and 14,000 feet, the mean pulmonary arterial pressures with exercise, rose to 54 and 60 mm Hg, respectively.[99] That the pulmonary vascular resistance in high altitude residents is labile is supported by the observation that pulmonary arterial pressures fall when subjects are brought to sea level and rise again when they return to their high altitude environment.[94]

The lability of pulmonary hypertension in the average high altitude resident is consistent with the histologic appearance of the pulmonary vascular bed. Intimal fibrosis is uncommon, and the plexiform lesions of fixed irreversible pulmonary hypertension are not present.

The pulmonary trunk exhibits medial thickening, and the fetal aortic pattern of elastic lamellae is usually maintained in the pulmonary trunk until approximately nine years of age.[86, 87] Atherosclerotic plaques are often present in the pulmonary trunk and major pulmonary arteries, and the amount is roughly proportional to the elevation of pulmonary arterial pressure.

Although the small elastic and large muscular pulmonary arteries have normal or mildly hypertrophied media, the small muscular arteries are characteristically involved and exhibit distinct medial hypertrophy (Fig. 2*a*). The arterioles show development of a well-defined muscular layer.[6, 108] There is an apparent increase in the number of small pulmonary arteries.[14]

The intima of the small muscular pulmonary arteries is often involved by the development of a smooth muscle layer with longitudinal orientation.[45, 47, 108] Al-

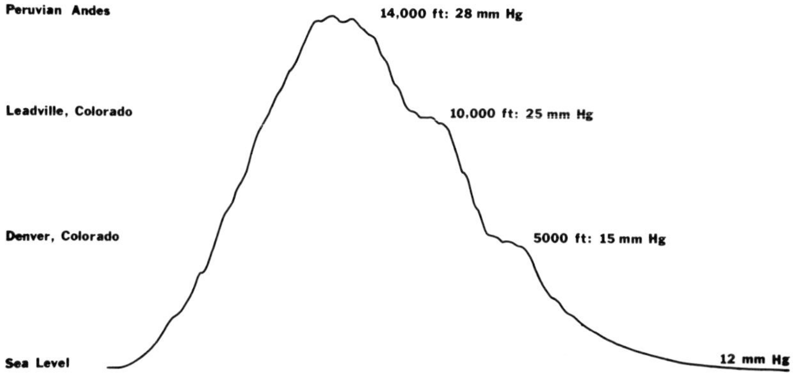

FIG. 1. Average normal mean pulmonary arterial pressure as a function of altitude.

though this muscle layer rarely causes functional luminal narrowing, it is fairly characteristic of pulmonary hypertension of chronic hypoxic origin (Fig. 2, *b* and *c*). The pulmonary capillaries are normal. The pulmonary veins and venules may develop medial hypertrophy and arterialization, as well as intimal fibrosis and longitudinal smooth muscle layers.

Hypoxia with Normal Lungs

Chronic alveolar hypoxia may occur in a variety of conditions in which the pulmonary parenchyma and the oxygen tension of the inspired air are normal. The structural changes in the small muscular pulmonary arteries and the arterioles are similar to those in high altitude residents.[45, 47, 74] Similarly, if the cause of hypoxia is removed, a reversal of the structural changes occurs, and the pulmonary arterial pressure decreases toward normal values.[45]

Such cases include hypoxia due to decreased minute ventilation and due to chronic upper airway obstruction. Inadequate respiratory excursion may be present in extreme obesity (Pickwickian syndrome)[15, 45, 47, 74, 93] and in various musculoskeletal disorders such as kyphoscoliosis, chronic poliomyelitis, and progressive muscular dystrophy.[48, 69, 73] Chronic upper airway obstruction may result from enlarged tonsils, and removal of the tonsils has been shown to be followed by regression of pulmonary hypertension.[70, 71]

Chronic Diffuse Pulmonary Parenchymal Disease

Chronic alveolar hypoxia may occur in several conditions in which the pulmonary blood flow and the oxygen tension of the inspired air are normal but in which chronic diffuse pulmonary parenchymal disease is present. Chronic hypoxia stimulates pulmonary arterial vasoconstriction, resulting in elevated pulmonary vascular resistance and in the development of pulmonary hypertension.[1, 2, 27, 44] However, factors other than hypoxia may also contribute to the increased pulmonary vascular resistance. In instances of extensive loss of normal pulmonary structure, the vascular bed is reduced in capacity, and resistance may increase. Air trapping and elevated alveolar pressure may also result in increased pulmonary vascular resistance.[43]

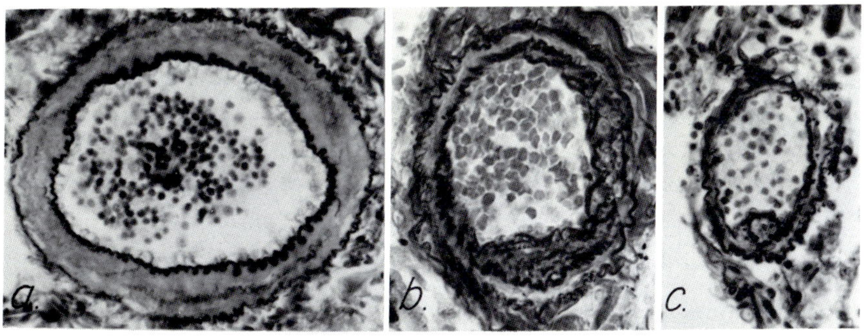

FIG. 2. Hypoxic pulmonary hypertension in high altitude residents. Elastic-van Gieson. *a*, Medial hypertrophy of muscular pulmonary artery. × 230. *b* and *c*, Longitudinal smooth muscle cells in the intima of small muscular pulmonary arteries. *b*, × 350; *c*, × 230. (Reproduced by permission, see Ref. 11.)

The chronic diffuse pulmonary parenchymal diseases which may be associated with pulmonary hypertension include chronic obstructive pulmonary disease (emphysema and chronic bronchitis), bronchial asthma, bronchiectasis, interstitial pulmonary fibrosis and the pneumoconioses.

The structural changes in the pulmonary blood vessels are similar to those in high altitude residents. Although the media of the pulmonary trunk is thickened, its elastic pattern is of the adult type.[46] Intrapulmonary elastic arteries may exhibit medial hypertrophy and intimal atheromas. Large muscular arteries have normal media, while small muscular arteries and arterioles have medial hypertrophy.[54] Longitudinal smooth muscle bundles are also frequently present in the intima of these smaller arteries.[108, 52]

The pulmonary alveolar capillaries are often quite diminished in number. Pulmonary veins and venules may exhibit medial hypertrophy, intimal fibrosis, and longitudinal intimal smooth muscle bundles. Bronchial arteries may be large and may form large bronchopulmonary arterial anastomoses.[66, 67] Bronchial veins may likewise form large dilated bronchopulmonary venous anastomoses.[65] An increase in the bronchial circulation is often quite prominent in bronchiectasis.[36]

CLINICAL PRIMARY PULMONARY HYPERTENSION

Clinically, the term primary pulmonary hypertension has been used to denote several distinct pathologic entities. A 1973 report of the World Health Organization (WHO) deals with this subject, defining primary pulmonary hypertension as a condition in which pulmonary hypertension is clinically present for no known reason.[116] Therefore, pulmonary hypertension associated with cardiac or pulmonary disease is excluded, as is hypoxic pulmonary hypertension.

Three morphologic types of primary pulmonary hypertension are proposed in the WHO report, namely (1) plexogenic pulmonary arteriopathy, (2) recurrent pulmonary thromboembolism, and (3) pulmonary veno-occlusive disease.[116] Although these three diseases are histologically distinct, their clinical presentations may be so similar that they may frequently only be distinguished by lung biopsy or at necropsy.

Clinically, each of these three diseases is characterized by progressive dyspnea, and fatigue and dyspnea on exertion are the presenting symptoms in most cases. Syncope, chest pain, hemoptysis, and cyanosis may also be present. Right heart failure and sudden death are not uncommon.

By chest roentgenography, the pulmonary trunk is seen to be enlarged, and the peripheral pulmonary vascular markings are usually diminished. By electrocardiography, right ventricular hypertrophy is demonstrated. By hemodynamic studies, elevated pulmonary arterial pressure and a normal pulmonary arterial wedge or left atrial pressure are characteristic.

Plexogenic Pulmonary Arteriopathy

Plexogenic pulmonary arteriopathy involves the muscular pulmonary arteries and arterioles, resulting in high levels of pulmonary vascular resistance and pulmonary hypertension with normal or subnormal pulmonary blood flow.

Although in children the sex incidence of plexogenic pulmonary arteriopathy is equal,[102, 107] in adults, females are affected four to five times as frequently as males.[92, 102, 107, 113] In one large series, the condition was uncommon in children so that most patients were 16–40 years old (mean age of 23 years; range of four days to 69 years).[107] Death usually occurs two to three years after the onset of symptoms, although survivals as briefly as one month and as long as 29 years have been reported.[92, 107, 113]

The initial structural change is medial hypertrophy of the muscular pulmonary arteries (Fig. 3*a*) and muscularization of the arterioles (Fig. 3*b*). Intimal cellular proliferation may be present, but more common is the development of obstructive concentric intimal fibrosis in large muscular arteries (Fig. 4). One should bear in mind that an artery which is normal at one level may have an obstructive lesion at another level so that the number of obstructed arteries is greater than may be apparent.[92]

In the small muscular arteries, characteristic plexiform lesions develop (Fig. 5), and are the basis for the designation of plexogenic pulmonary arteriopathy. Other changes include dilatation lesions and pulmonary arteritis in various stages (Figs. 6 and 7). The pulmonary vascular lesions are identical to those in congenital cardiac shunts with pulmonary hypertension. However, morphometric microangiographic studies have demonstrated selective "loss" of arteriolar segments 100–280 μm in internal diameter.[82]

The pulmonary trunk has an adult elastic pattern unless pulmonary hypertension develops within the first year of life, in which case a fetal aortic pattern of elastic lamellae may persist. Atheromas of the elastic pulmonary arteries are common. The alveolar capillaries are normal. Pulmonary veins and venules are characteristically normal. Pulmonary hemosiderosis is often present but mild.

The etiology of plexogenic pulmonary arteriopathy is unknown, but most

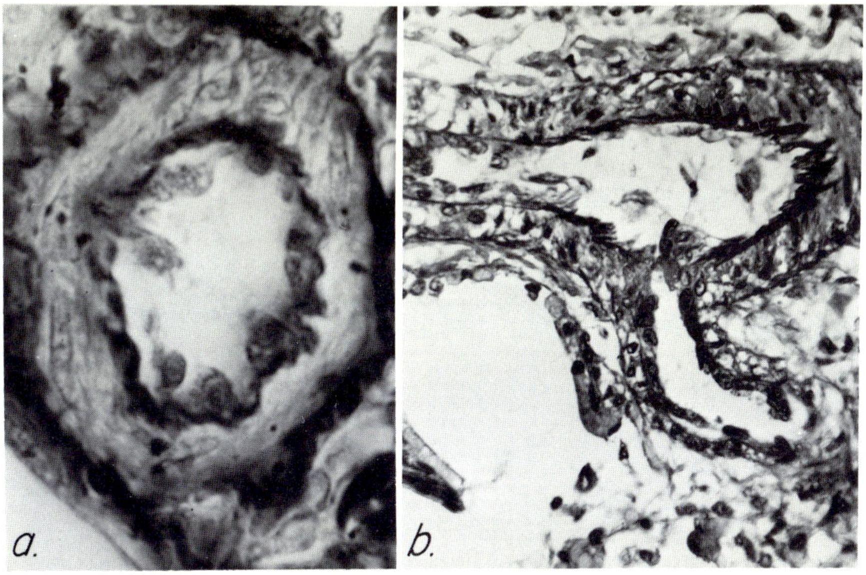

FIG. 3. Plexogenic pulmonary arteriopathy in early stage. *a*, Medial hypertrophy of small muscular pulmonary artery. Elastic-van Gieson, × 500. *b*, Medial hypertrophy of small muscular artery with muscularization of an arteriolar branch. Elastic-van Gieson, × 300.

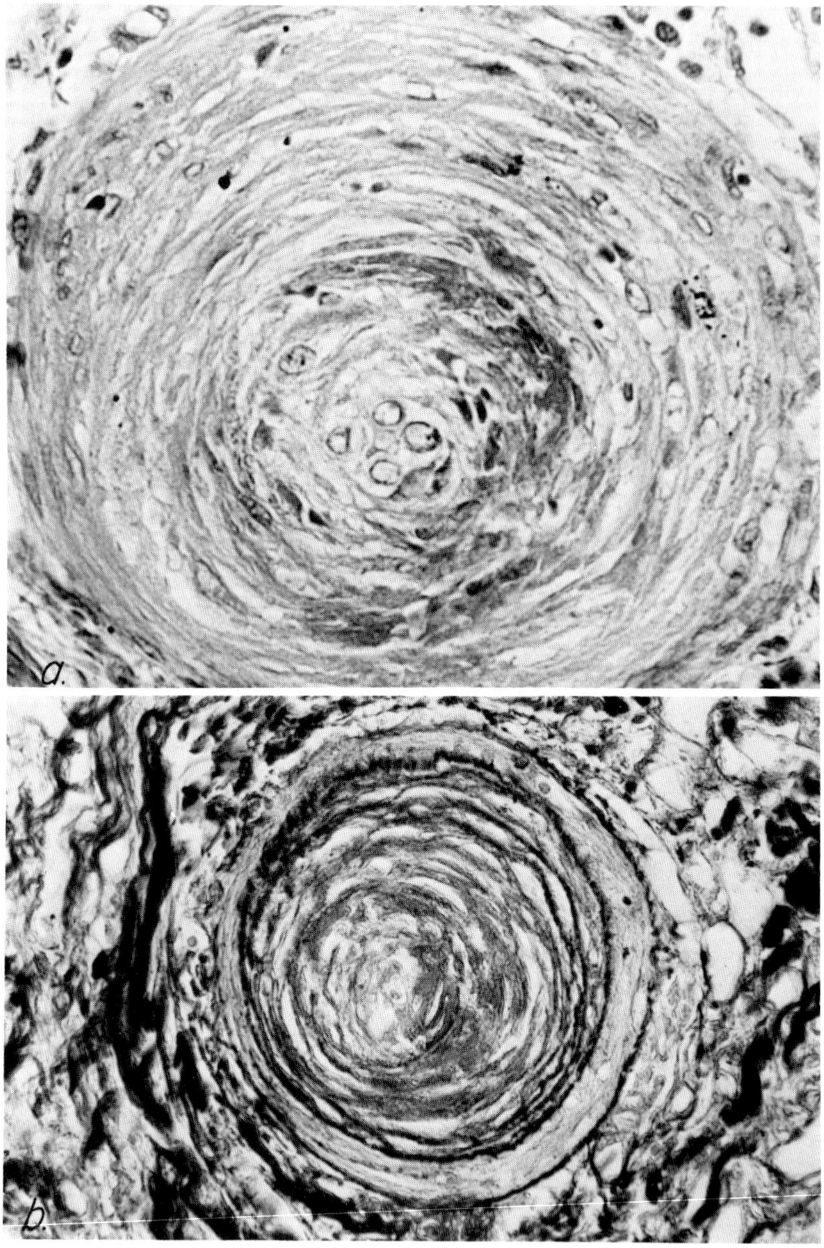

FIG. 4. Plexogenic pulmonary arteriopathy in late stage. Obstructive concentric intimal fibrosis of muscular pulmonary arteries. *a*, Hematoxylin and eosin, × 380. *b*, elastic-van Gieson, × 300.

evidence supports a vasospastic origin of the disease.[107, 109, 116] Although the vasoconstriction is not initiated by hypoxia, low alveolar oxygen tension may accentuate the vasospasm.[107] It is of interest that plexogenic pulmonary arteriopathy is more common at high altitude than at sea level.[7, 59]

Intense vasospasm of the muscular pulmonary arteries may lead to fibrinoid necrosis and pulmonary arteritis, and organization of these lesions may lead to

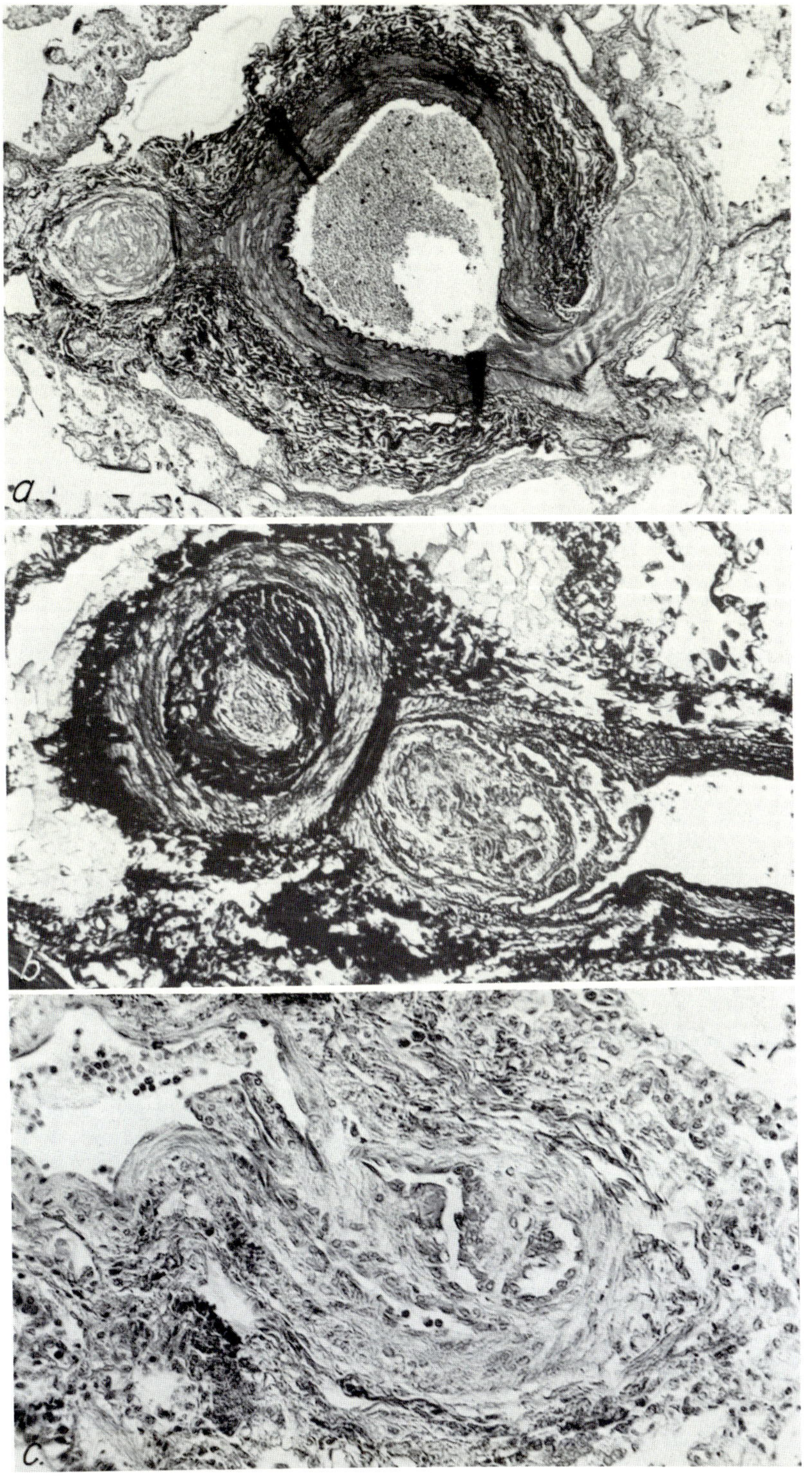

FIG. 5. Plexogenic pulmonary arteriopathy in late stage. Plexiform lesion in muscular pulmonary arteries. *a* and *b*, Elastic-van Gieson, × 45 and × 90, respectively. *c*, Hematoxylin and eosin, × 180.

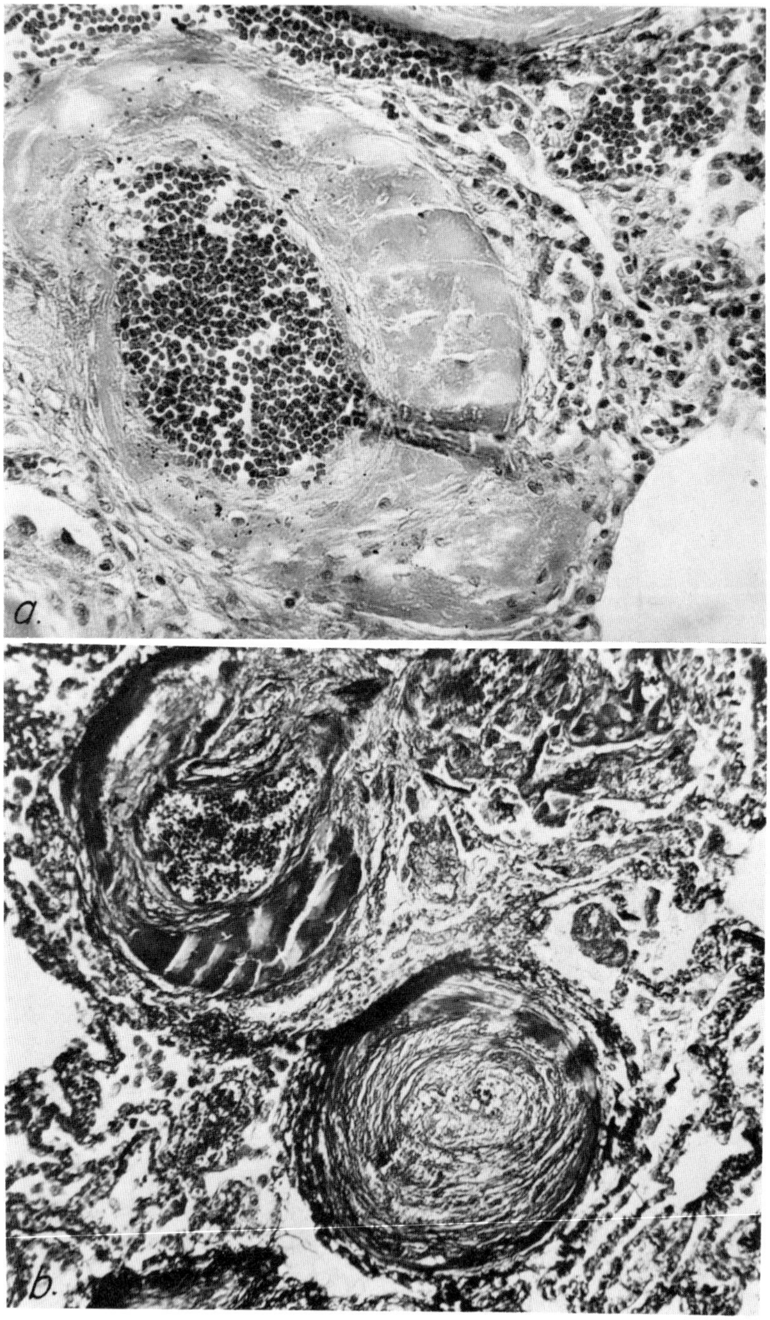

FIG. 6. Plexogenic pulmonary arteriopathy in late stage. Fibrinoid necrosis of muscular pulmonary arteries, with concentric intimal fibrosis of adjacent artery in *b*. *a*, Hematoxylin and eosin, × 180. *b*, Elastic-van Gieson, × 80.

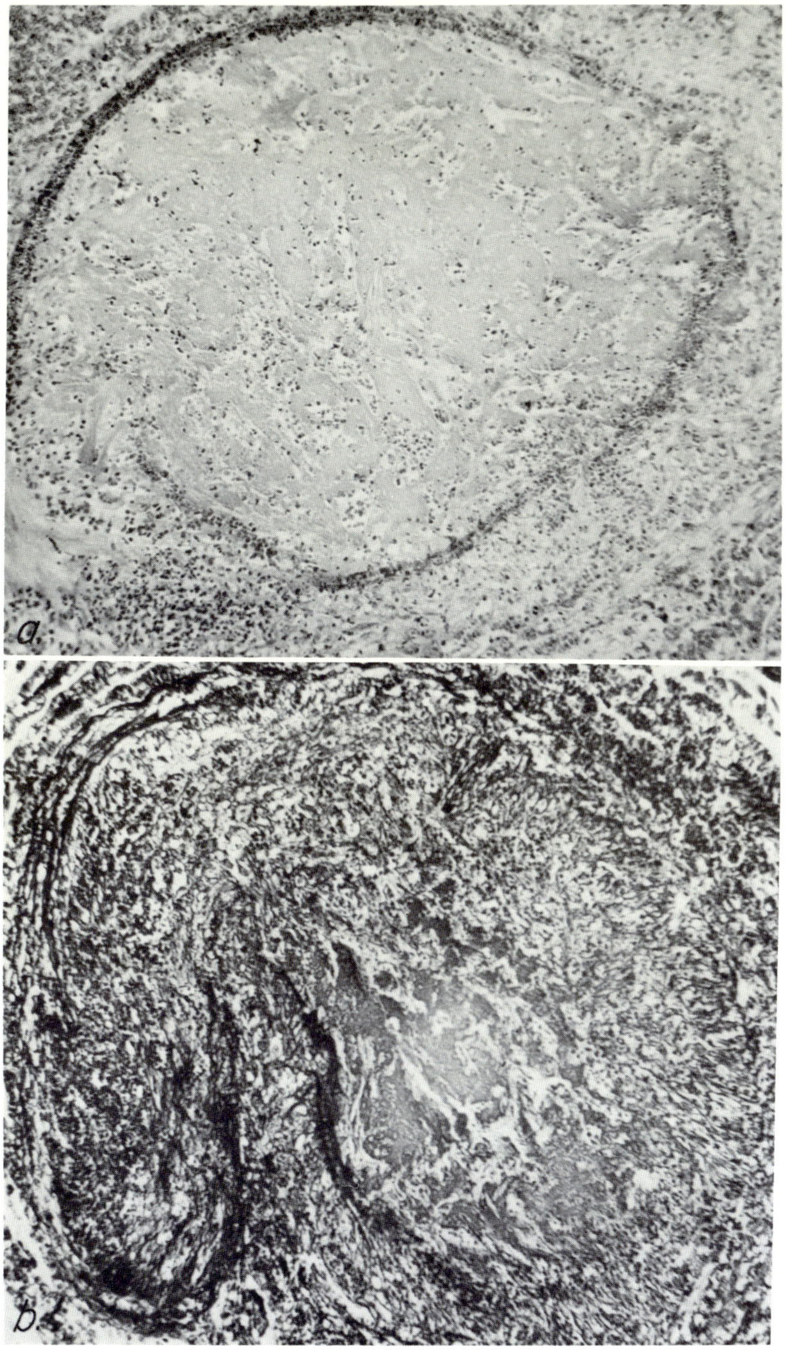

FIG. 7. Plexogenic pulmonary arteriopathy in late stage. Pulmonary arteritis with luminal obstruction. *a*, Leukocytic infiltration of wall and thrombosis. Hematoxylin and eosin, × 90. *b*, Destruction of elements of wall and thrombosis. Elastic-van Gieson, × 80.

the formation of the plexiform lesions.[107, 109] In rats, the drug fulvine causes marked vasoconstriction of pulmonary arteries, followed by medial hypertrophy and fibrinoid necrosis.[57, 58, 61, 112]

In light of the proposed vasospastic origin of plexogenic pulmonary arteriopathy, the coexistence of Raynaud's phenomenon is of interest. Digital vasospasm has been reported in 7–30% of patients with this form of pulmonary hypertension.[107, 113, 116] Various autoimmune connective tissue diseases may also be present.[107, 116]

Plexogenic pulmonary arteriopathy probably represents the result of prolonged pulmonary arterial vasoconstriction due to individual hyperreactivity of these vessels to various stimuli.[107, 116] The initial response by the pulmonary vascular bed is arterial medial hypertrophy. The more advanced intimal lesions develop at some later time.

While the aforementioned report of WHO[116] does not include simple medial hypertrophy, without known cause, as part of the spectrum of plexogenic pulmonary arteriopathy, in the authors' view, this change should be considered the initial one, with the plexiform lesion being one of the complications of the vasospastic pulmonary hypertension.

The changes observed histologically in the plexogenic type of primary pulmonary hypertension are the same as those observed in cases of cardiac septal defects. Therefore, it is histologically impossible to separate a case of septal defect complicated by hypertensive pulmonary vascular disease from a case of septal defect complicated by the fortuitous presence of the plexogenic type of primary pulmonary hypertension.[8]

Also recognized is the fact that in some instances of hepatic cirrhosis, pulmonary hypertension with plexogenic pulmonary arteriopathy may be observed. The pulmonary vascular lesions are usually not thrombotic in origin.[64, 89, 90] The favored hypothesis is that intestinal metabolites may escape inactivation by the liver and cause pulmonary arterial vasoconstriction,[32, 51, 89] particularly in hyperreactive vessels.[42]

Similarly, various dietary substances may induce pulmonary arterial vasospasm and result in plexogenic pulmonary arteriopathy. Although the pyrrolizidine alkaloids, such as fulvine, which are present in Crotalaria plants, may cause pulmonary vascular disease in rats[57, 58, 61, 112] and in nonhuman primates[3, 18] and may cause hepatic veno-occlusive disease in humans,[13] these chemicals apparently do not cause pulmonary hypertension in humans. On the other hand, anorexigenic drugs such as aminorex fumarate have been implicated in the epidemic of plexogenic pulmonary arteriopathy in Switzerland, West Germany, and Austria.[41] Although the incidence of primary pulmonary hypertension fell to pre-epidemic levels following discontinuation of the use of the drug,[41] the induction of pulmonary vascular lesions by the administration of aminorex fumarate to experimental animals has not yet been accomplished.[16, 95, 120]

Recurrent Pulmonary Thromboembolism

Multiple recurrent pulmonary thromboemboli, in various stages of organization within the pulmonary arterial system, may result in high levels of pulmonary vascular resistance and pulmonary hypertension with normal or subnormal pulmonary blood flow.

Clinically, two groups of patients may be identified, namely (1) those with a step-like clinical course characterized by acute episodes of dyspnea and chest pain alternating with relatively symptom-free periods, and (2) those with an insidious onset and a clinical course characterized by progressive dyspnea.[33, 40, 119] The latter group consists primarily of females,[40] and a history of phlebitis, leg trauma, or recent pregnancy can often be elicited.[33]

It is the view of the authors that clinical evidence of thrombosis or embolization is neither necessary nor sufficient to establish the diagnosis of thromboembolic pulmonary hypertension. In our view, this diagnosis should be made only when thromboembolic occlusive lesions of the pulmonary arterial system are present which do not resemble those of plexogenic pulmonary arteriopathy. Diagnosis is established by lung biopsy or at necropsy.

In the vast majority of cases, the source of the emboli is thrombosis of the veins of the lower extremities,[117] although in some reports no source of emboli could be found in most patients.[34] Other recognized sources of pulmonary emboli include thrombosis of the pelvic veins and long-standing indwelling venous catheters. *In situ* pulmonary thrombosis may occur in hypercoagulable states such as polycythemia and may occur in obstruction to flow such as follows carcinomatous embolism to small pulmonary arteries and arterioles.

In thromboembolic pulmonary hypertension, obstructive lesions involve the muscular pulmonary arteries and arterioles far more frequently than the elastic pulmonary arteries. Although involvement is functionally widespread, one must bear in mind that such lesions are focal and that by serial sections, long segments of any one particular artery may be uninvolved before an obstructive area is encountered.

Since these lesions are of varying age, the histologic picture is variable and includes vascular connective tissue resembling a classical organized and recanalized thrombus (Fig. 8*a*), eccentric intimal fibrous thickening (Fig. 8, *b* and *c*), intimal fibroelastic pads from old organized mural thrombi (Fig. 8*d*), and fibrous septa crossing arterial lumens (Fig. 9*a*). Favoring the diagnosis is the observation of recent thrombi undergoing organization (Fig. 9*b*). Since the pulmonary arterial pressure is elevated, medial hypertrophy of muscular pulmonary arteries is present, but is usually less pronounced than in the plexogenic type. The pulmonary capillaries and veins are normal. Collateral circulation from the bronchial arteries and from the diaphragm and thoracic cage becomes prominent.

Patients with thromboembolic pulmonary hypertension are often asymptomatic until the disease is well advanced. Compensation by the remaining uninvolved pulmonary circulation may allow relatively normal pulmonary vascular function in spite of extensive thromboembolism.[12] Other compensatory mechanisms include thrombolysis and organization with recanalization of thrombi.[88, 118]

The tremendous capacity of the pulmonary vascular bed to compensate in the presence of extensive obstructive lesions may help to explain why animal models often fail to demonstrate chronic elevations of pulmonary arterial pressure. Although the morphologic lesions in the pulmonary arteries of experimental

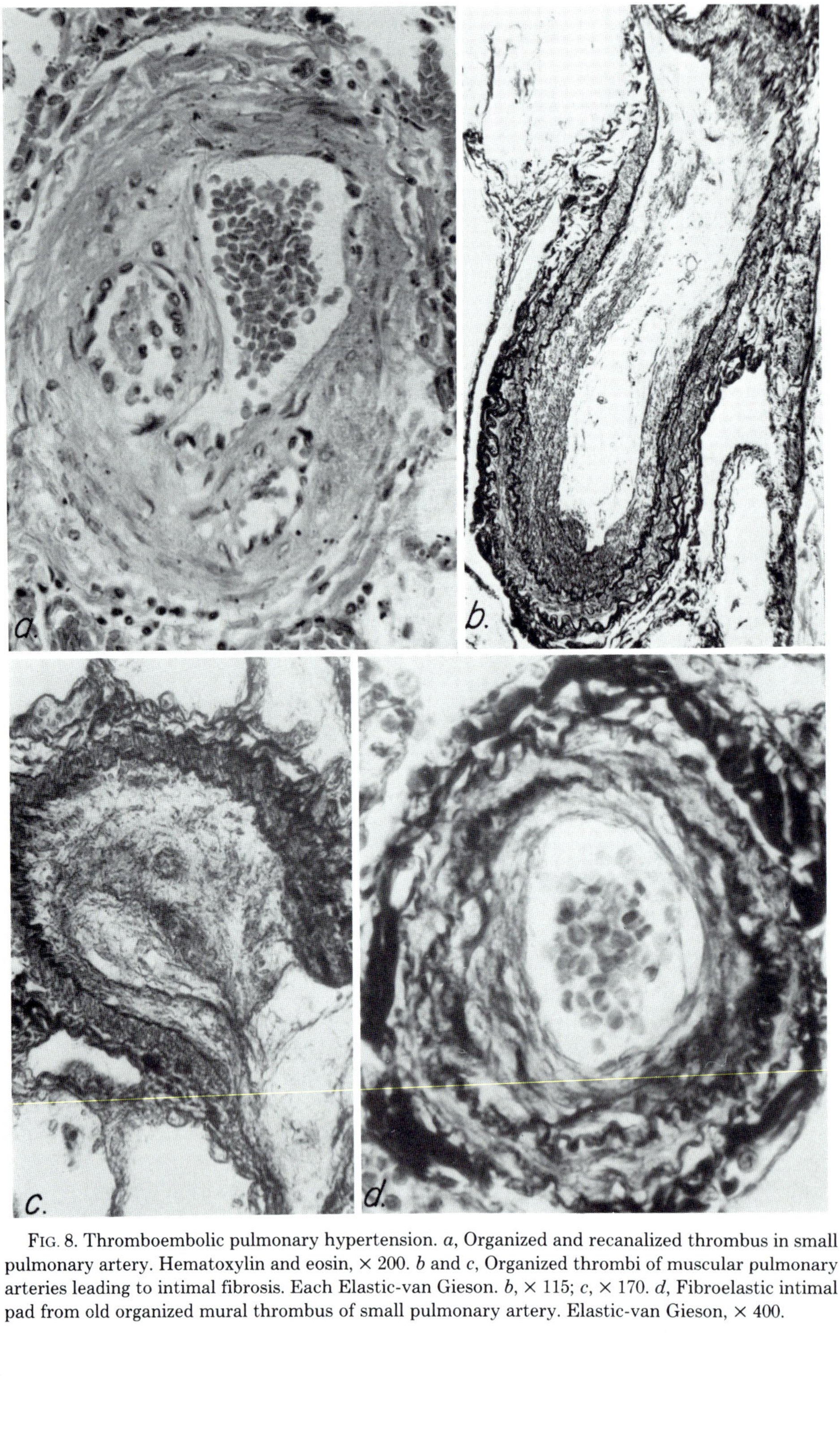

FIG. 8. Thromboembolic pulmonary hypertension. *a*, Organized and recanalized thrombus in small pulmonary artery. Hematoxylin and eosin, × 200. *b* and *c*, Organized thrombi of muscular pulmonary arteries leading to intimal fibrosis. Each Elastic-van Gieson. *b*, × 115; *c*, × 170. *d*, Fibroelastic intimal pad from old organized mural thrombus of small pulmonary artery. Elastic-van Gieson, × 400.

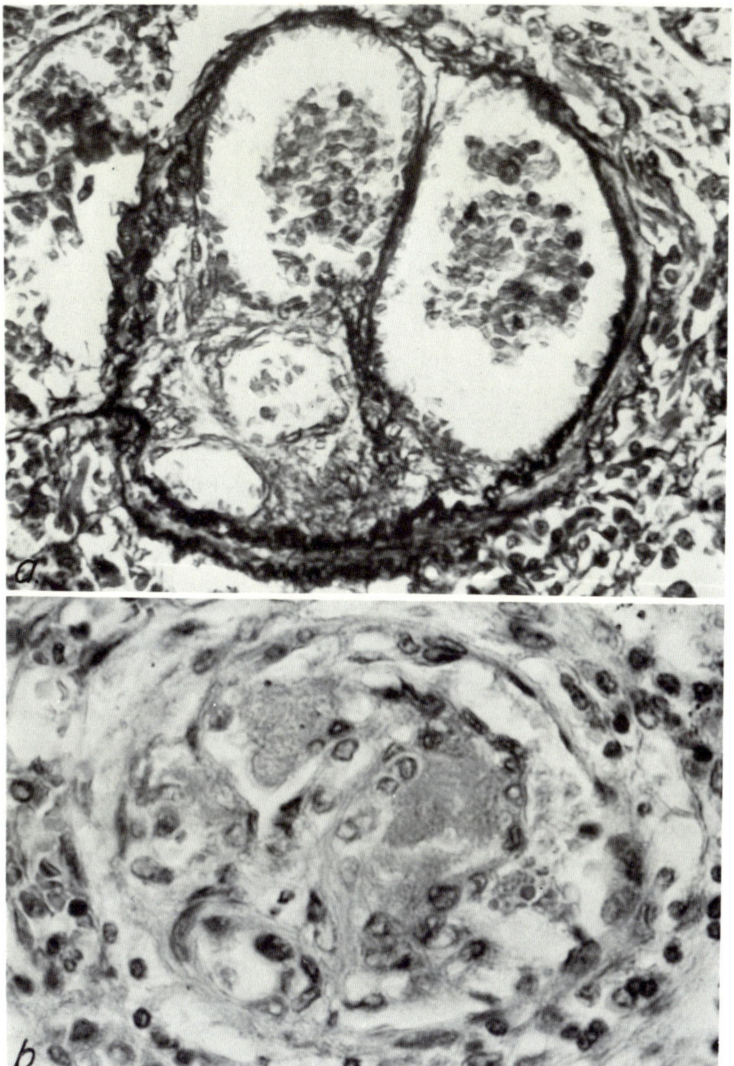

FIG. 9. Thromboembolic pulmonary hypertension. *a*, Organized and recanalized pulmonary arterial thrombus with fibrous septa crossing the lumen. Elastic-van Gieson, × 250. *b*, Organizing thrombus in small pulmonary artery. Hematoxylin and eosin, × 400.

animals are similar to those in humans, the intravenous administration of small fragments of autogenous clots resulted in only transient pulmonary hypertension in dogs[37] and only mild pulmonary hypertension in rabbits.[77]

Pulmonary Veno-occlusive Disease

Pulmonary veno-occlusive disease involves the pulmonary venules and veins, resulting in high levels of pulmonary vascular resistance and pulmonary arterial and capillary hypertension with normal or subnormal pulmonary blood flow.

Pulmonary congestion is common, and septal and alveolar pulmonary edema may often be observed radiographically. Of the three entities which comprise clinical primary pulmonary hypertension, pulmonary veno-occlusive disease has received the most recent emphasis and is also the most rare. By 1975, only 31 cases of this disease had been reported.[103]

Pulmonary veno-occlusive disease primarily affects children and young adults. In the 31 reported cases, the mean age was 19 years, and the age range was 8 weeks to 48 years.[103] Males and females are equally affected. The disease is usually fatal, and the average duration from onset of symptoms to death is 1–2 years, although survivals range from a few weeks to 7 years.[103] This form of pulmonary hypertension is an acquired rather than a congenital condition. The structural lesion is at the level of the small pulmonary veins and venules and appears to be of thrombotic origin.[17, 68, 83, 96, 103, 110]

The pulmonary intimal fibrous tissue is partially or totally occlusive and may involve 30–95% of the veins and venules.[49, 110] The intimal fibrous lesions range from being edematous and relatively acellular to densely fibrotic, causing either partially obstructive intimal pads or severe degrees of luminal occlusion (Figs. 10 and 11*a*). Fibrous tissue yielding cavernous spaces within venous lumens is a sign of recanalized thrombi (Fig. 11 *a–c*). The media of the pulmonary veins is usually normal. However, occasionally medial hypertrophy and "arterialization" occur as a response to distal focal obstruction.

Secondary to the pulmonary hypertension, medial hypertrophy of the muscular pulmonary arteries commonly develops. Arterial thrombi and patchy eccentric fibrosis are often present. Concentric intimal fibrosis, arteritis, and plexiform lesions are absent.

Distension and tortuosity of capillaries is seen in this condition as in other situations in which obstruction to egress of blood from the lung is present, as in mitral stenosis. Other effects of the pulmonary venous obstructive nature of the condition include extensive pulmonary hemosiderosis (Fig. 11*d*), dilatation of visceral pleural and pulmonary lymphatic vessels and edema of interlobular septa.

In this condition, as in others wherein obstruction to pulmonary venous flow exists, pleural adhesions tend to develop (Fig. 12). These may result from the organization of high protein transudates in the pleural cavity. Within the adhesions are blood and lymphatic vessels which, perhaps, form collaterals to allow flow of blood or fluid components of blood out of the pulmonary vascular bed.

The lungs often contain focal patchy areas of interstitial fibrosis or interstitial pneumonia,[14, 102] and an infectious etiology for pulmonary veno-occlusive disease is often proposed because of these findings.[68, 102, 105] It has been postulated that pulmonary viral infections could account both for the *in situ* venous thrombosis and for the interstitial pneumonia or fibrosis.[68, 102, 105] A viral infection could initiate pulmonary venous thrombosis by at least two mechanisms, namely (1) depletion of plasminogen activator from the venous endothelium[4] and (2) immune complexes in the capillary basement membranes which activate clotting factors or platelets.[21] However attractive these hypotheses may be, viruses have not been isolated or serologically implicated in any case of pulmonary veno-occlusive disease, and the stimulus for pulmonary venous thrombosis is still unknown. The disease may possibly be initiated by a variety of agents.[103]

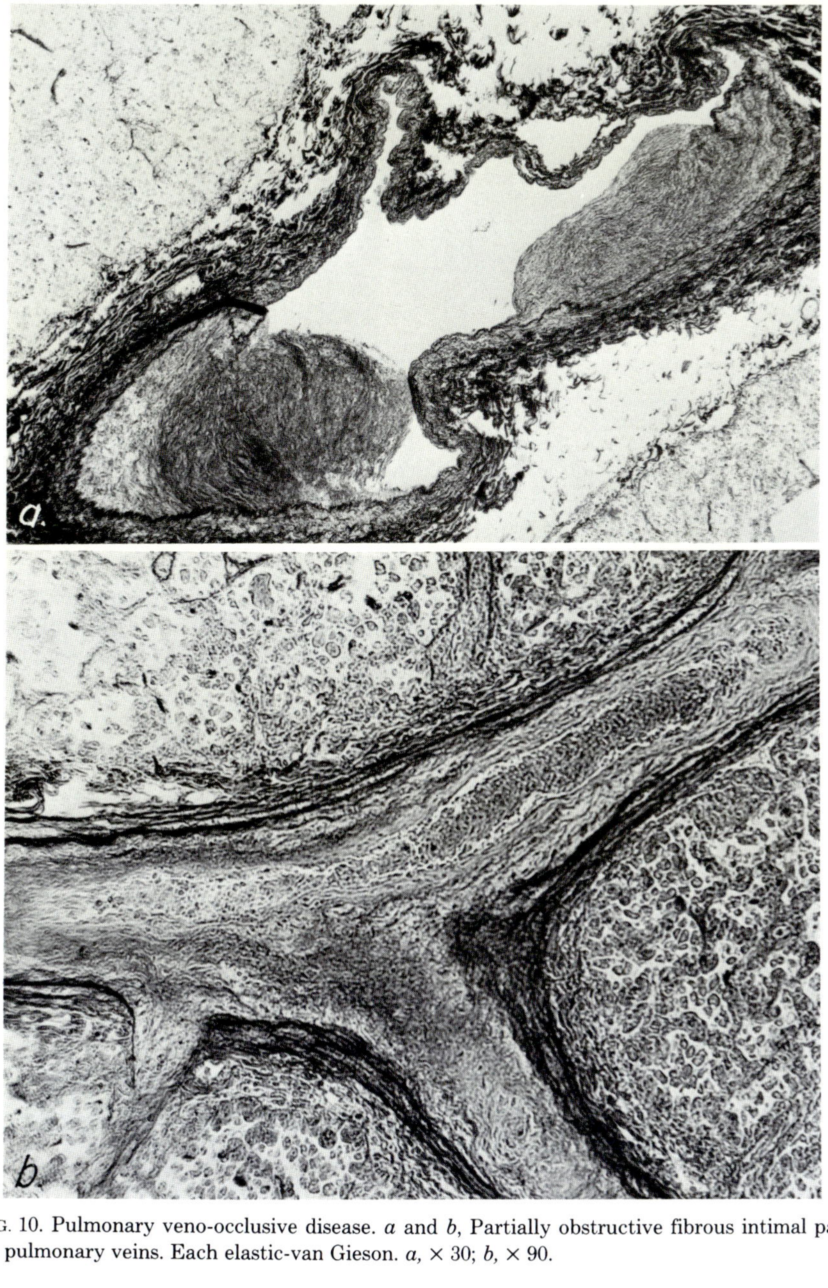

FIG. 10. Pulmonary veno-occlusive disease. *a* and *b*, Partially obstructive fibrous intimal pads of small pulmonary veins. Each elastic-van Gieson. *a*, × 30; *b*, × 90.

PULMONARY VASCULAR RESPONSES TO SURGICAL TREATMENT OF CARDIAC DISEASES

The pulmonary vascular bed is often greatly affected by specific types of cardiac disease, and the secondary pulmonary vascular lesions in some cases may dictate the patient's clinical course and management. Similarly, either palliative

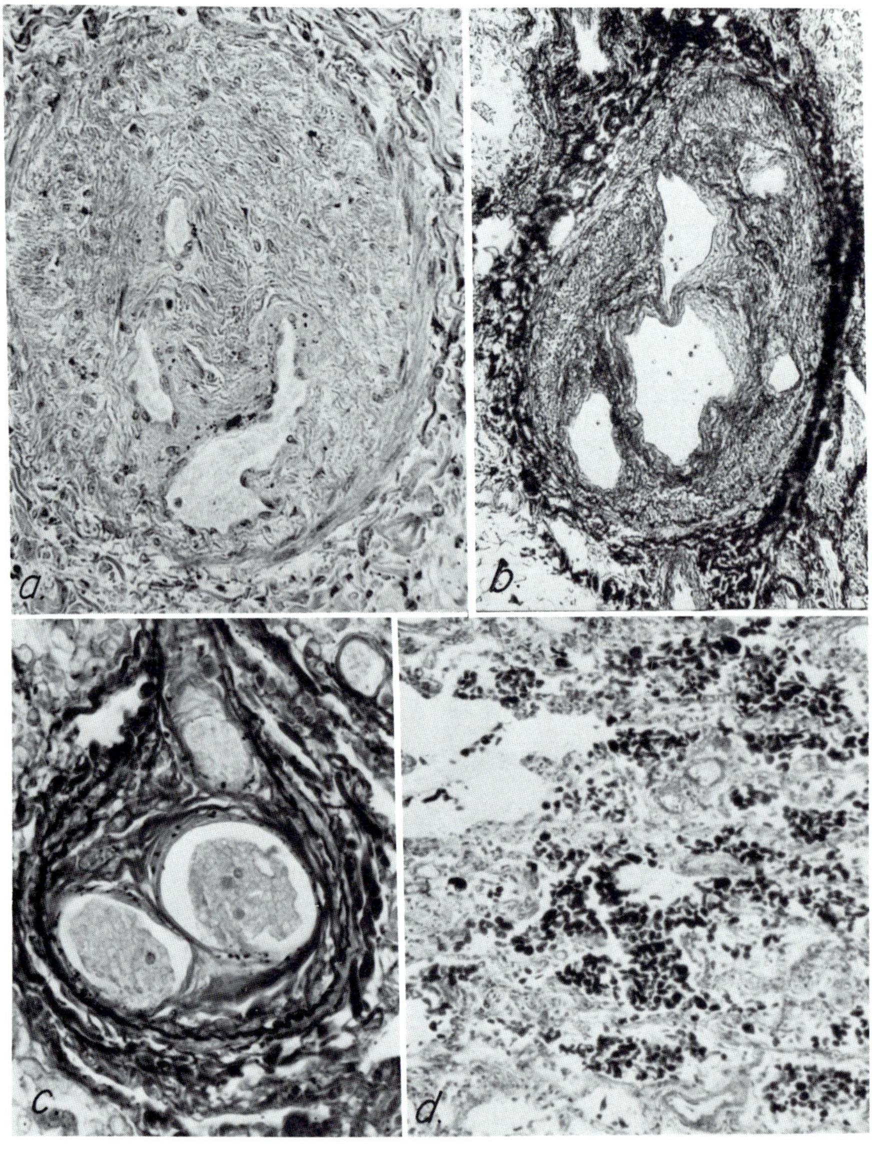

FIG. 11. Pulmonary veno-occlusive disease. *a–c*, Recanalized pulmonary venous thrombi. *a*, Hematoxylin and eosin, × 180. *b* and *c*, Elastic-van Gieson, × 90 and 240, respectively. *d*, Pulmonary hemosiderosis. Iron stain, × 90.

or corrective surgical procedures for the primary cardiac disease may significantly alter the pulmonary hemodynamics.

The postoperative changes in the pulmonary vascular bed will be considered in three specific forms of congenital heart disease and one type of acquired valvular heart disease, namely (1) ventricular septal defect, (2) tetralogy of Fallot, (3) complete transposition of the great arteries and (4) mitral stenosis.

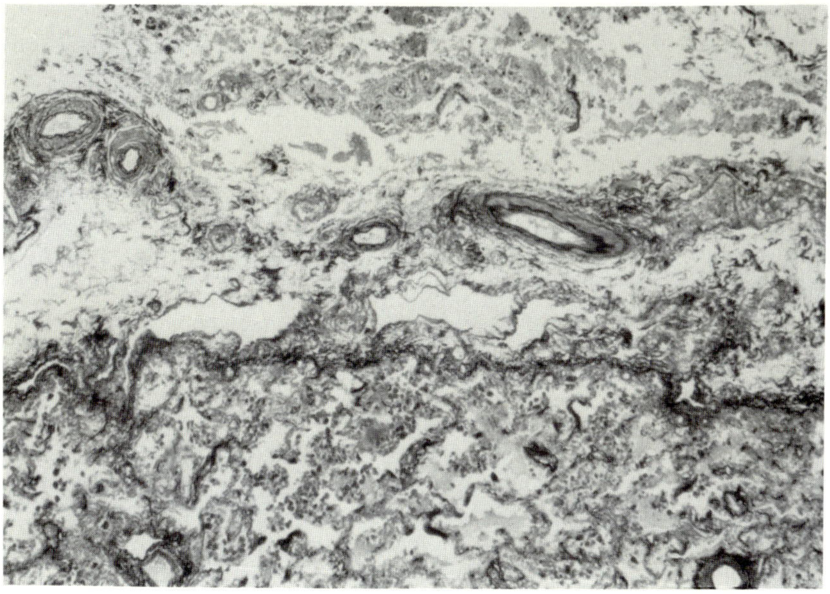

FIG. 12. Pulmonary veno-occlusive disease. Pleural adhesions, dilated pleural lymphatic vessels and pleural blood vascular anastomoses. Elastic-van Gieson, × 45.

VENTRICULAR SEPTAL DEFECT

Large ventricular septal defects have certain hemodynamic features which are shared by other forms of congenital heart disease, including wide patent ductus arteriosus, persistent truncus arteriosus, and single ventricle without pulmonary stenosis. The early stage of large ventricular septal defect is characterized by a large left-to-right shunt and labile pulmonary vascular resistance. Initially, the muscular pulmonary arteries and arterioles respond with medial hypertrophy and later with intimal cellular proliferation. The medial component of these changes is considered reversible.[25, 50]

The late stage of large ventricular septal defect is characterized by a right-to-left shunt and a fixed high level of pulmonary vascular resistance.[86] Progressive pulmonary vascular lesions include obstructive concentric intimal fibrosis in large muscular arteries and plexiform lesions, as well as "dilation lesions" and arteritis. The latter changes are the same as those of plexogenic pulmonary arteriopathy and are considered to be irreversible.[26, 50] They usually do not develop before two years of age and often develop even later.

In the early stage of the disease, when a left-to-right shunt exists, either a palliative or a corrective surgical procedure may be performed. The palliative procedure consists of the creation of pulmonary stenosis to protect the pulmonary vasculature (so-called pulmonary arterial banding). The corrective procedure consists of surgical closure of the ventricular septal defect.

In patients with large left-to-right shunts, comparison of lung biopsies obtained at the time of pulmonary arterial banding with those obtained several years later shows that medial hypertrophy regresses (Fig. 13*a*).[24] Additionally, minor degrees of intimal fibrosis, if present, have a tendency to become more fibrous (Fig. 13*b*). These observations correlate well with various animal models.[9, 10, 31, 38] Until data are available, one must assume that similar changes in the pulmonary vessels occur following surgical closure of defects.

When intimal lesions including the plexiform lesion occur, there is a tendency for the left-to-right shunt to fall in volume, and a right-to-left shunt usually develops. At the present time, patients who have reached this late stage in their disease are not subjected to operation since the pulmonary arterial lesions are considered irreversible.

However, a transitional stage exists between the early stage with a large left-to-right shunt and the late stage with a right-to-left shunt. Such patients have bidirectional shunting with only a small left-to-right shunt or no such shunt. Surgical closure of defects in such patients is followed by variable alterations in pulmonary pressure and pulmonary vascular resistance. In some patients the pulmonary arterial pressure falls toward normal, while in others it remains significantly elevated. In those patients with near-normal pressure at rest postoperatively, there is some indication that, with normal activity and its associated rise in pulmonary blood flow, the pulmonary pressure rises inappropriately. This would tend to accentuate existing obstructive lesions and to be followed by the appearance of new ones (Fig. 13, *b–d*). In essence, some patients in this transitional stage may benefit from operation, but many will have persistent elevation of pulmonary vascular resistance and chronic persistent, or even progressive, pulmonary hypertension.[5, 19, 35, 56, 84, 91, 109, 114]

One must bear in mind that the fall in pulmonary arterial pressure immediately after surgical closure of a ventricular septal defect is due to decreased pulmonary blood flow[98] and a fall in pressure is most evident in patients with the early stages of pulmonary vascular disease and absent in those with the late stages of pulmonary vascular disease. Only the more gradual delayed fall in pressure is due to regression of morphologic lesions with a concomitant fall in pulmonary vascular resistance.[62, 81, 98] If the vascular lesions fail to regress, resistance will remain unchanged, and if the vascular lesions progressively develop, resistance and pressure will increase.

Tetralogy of Fallot

In the natural state of tetralogy of Fallot, small muscular pulmonary arteries are thin-walled and have a tendency to develop *in situ* thrombi due to polycythemia and decreased pulmonary blood flow. The thrombi are of different ages and may exhibit various stages of organization, recanalization, focal mural thickening, and luminal fibrous septa (Fig. 14*a*). The occurrence of such lesions, though bearing a direct relationship to the degree of pulmonary stenosis, usually is not sufficiently widespread to cause a significant increase in total pulmonary vascular resistance. Hence, there is no recognizable defect in the pulmonary vascular bed at the time of operation.

The palliative operation for tetralogy of Fallot consists of creating an anastomosis between a systemic artery and a pulmonary artery to increase pulmonary blood flow. Usually, such an operation does not become complicated by secondary

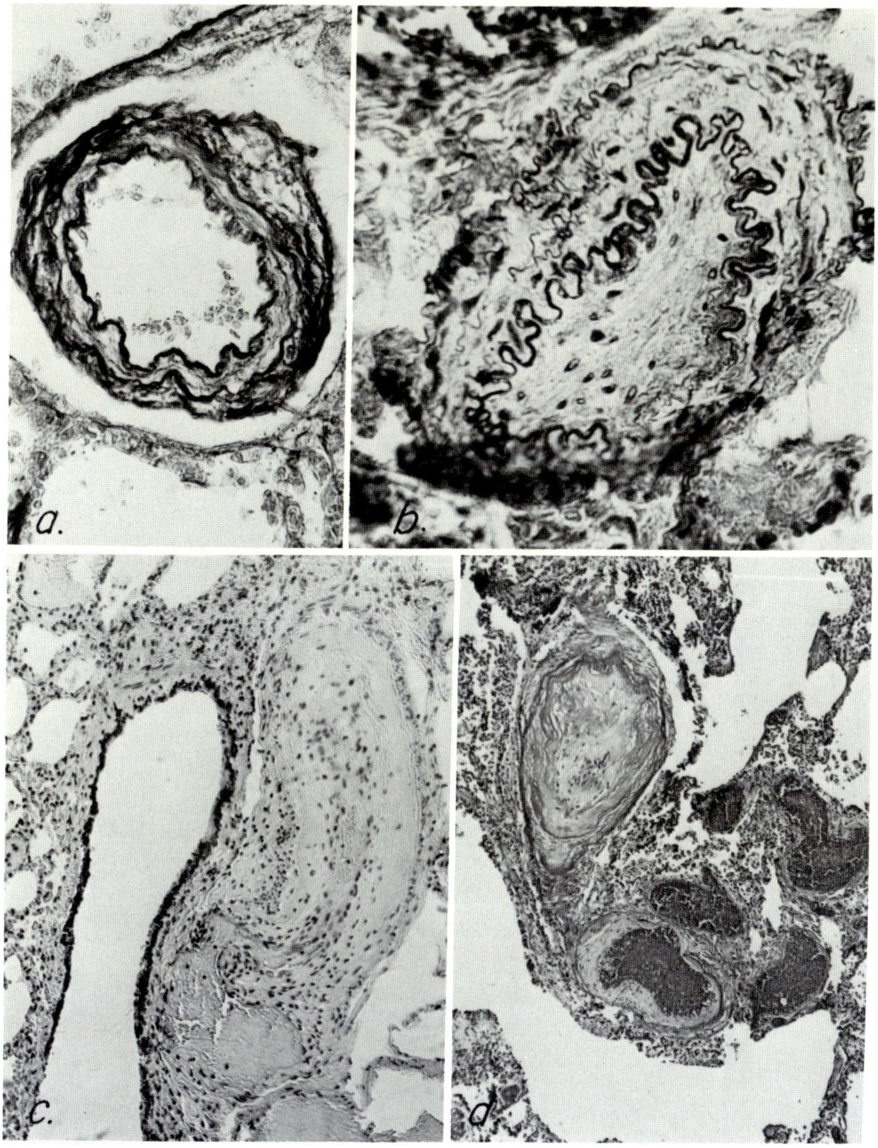

FIG. 13. Muscular pulmonary arteries in two cases of large ventricular septal defect. *a*, Three years after pulmonary arterial banding. Although mild residual medial hypertrophy is present in a small muscular artery, the picture suggests some resolution of medial hypertrophy. Elastic-van Gieson, × 240. *b–d*, A second case four years after closure of defect suggesting progression in severity of disease. *b*, Large muscular artery occluded by intimal fibrosis. Elastic-van Gieson, × 300. *c*, Plexiform lesion. Hematoxylin and eosin, × 100. *d*, Dilation lesions. Elastic-van Gieson, × 50.

changes in the pulmonary vasculature. However, complicating obstructive lesions have been observed (Fig. 14). These usually take the form of nonspecific intimal fibrous thickening, although plexiform lesions have been reported.[85, 104] The incidence of cases having significant secondary lesions depends upon time (usually 2–10 years) and upon the size of the orifice of the anastomosis.

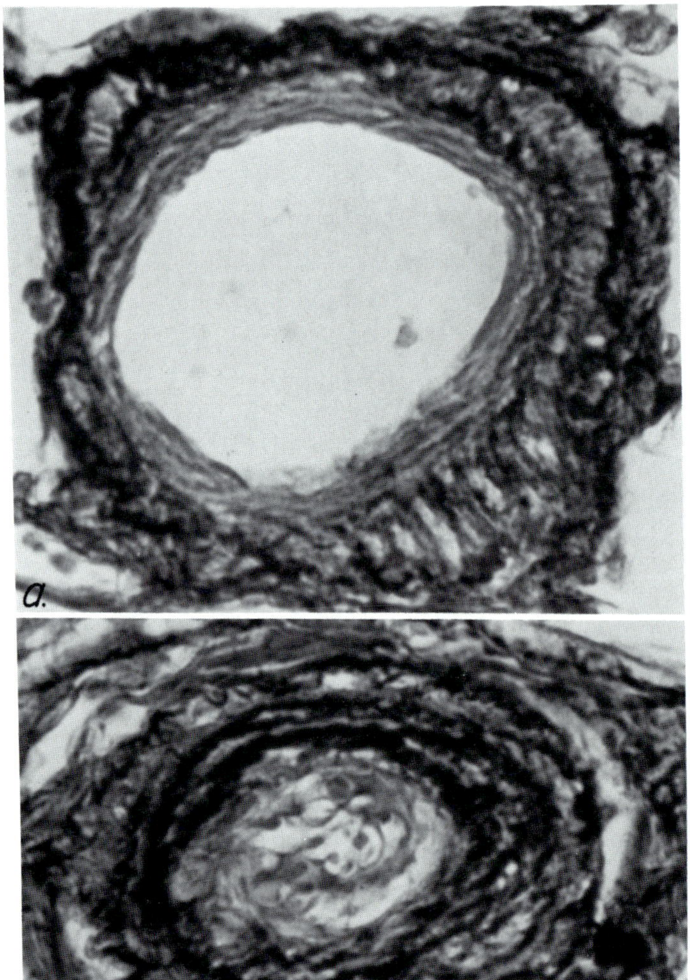

FIG. 14. Changes in small pulmonary arteries in the tetralogy of Fallot eight or more years after institution of Blalock-Taussig anastomosis (from Ref. 53, reproduced by permission, from the American Heart Association). *a*, Focal medial atrophy and mild intimal fibrosis. Elastic-van Gieson, × 400. *b*, Marked intimal fibrosis. Elastic-van Gieson, × 400.

The Blalock-Taussig procedure makes use of a subclavian artery, and the diameter of the anastomosis is determined by the caliber of the artery. With this operation, secondary pulmonary vascular lesions are less common than in operations wherein the aorta is directly anastomosed to a pulmonary artery (ascending aorta in the Waterston procedure and upper descending aorta in the Potts procedure).[28, 53, 55, 63, 78, 85, 100, 104]

COMPLETE TRANSPOSITION OF GREAT ARTERIES

Complete transposition of the great arteries is one of the most serious types of congenital cardiac disease for which corrective surgery is now being applied. Without operation, this condition has a tendency to become complicated at

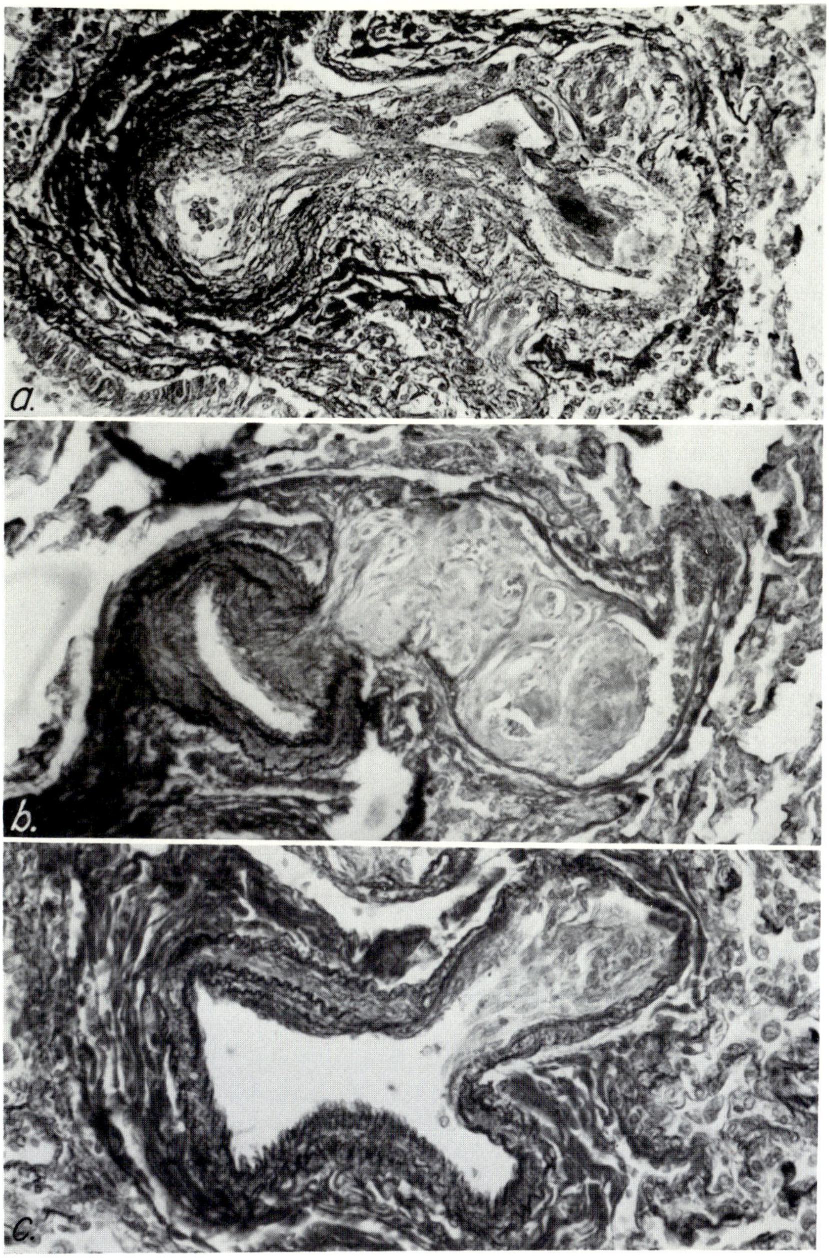

FIG. 15. Plexiform lesions in muscular pulmonary arteries in complete transposition of the great arteries with intact ventricular septum and closed ductus arteriosus. *a*, One-year-old female. *b*, Two and a half-year-old male. *c*, Two and a half-year-old female. Each elastic-van Gieson. *a*, × 180; *b*, × 120; *c*, × 240.

unusually early ages (as young as one year) by severe pulmonary vascular disease of the type that may be seen in the late stages of large ventricular septal defect[20, 29, 30, 60, 76, 97, 106, 121] (Fig. 15, *a–c*).

That these changes may occur in complete transposition even in the presence of an intact ventricular septum and a closed ductus arteriosus is an enigma for which there is as yet no clear explanation. It has been reported that the development of medial hypertrophy of the pulmonary arteries in response to elevated pulmonary arterial pressure is retarded in cases of complete transposition.[121] Although the long-range postoperative functional effects of such pulmonary vascular disease remain to be demonstrated, most investigators suggest performing palliative pulmonary arterial banding or the Mustard operation at as early an age as possible, hopefully before severe pulmonary vascular lesions have developed.

Mitral Stenosis

Either chronic mitral stenosis or mitral insufficiency is associated with hypertension in the entire pulmonary vascular bed. This is manifested by many changes. The pulmonary veins and venules show medial hypertrophy, "arterialization," and intimal fibrosis. There is pulmonary capillary engorgement, lymphatic dilation, alveolar hemorrhages and edema, and pulmonary hemosiderosis. The muscular pulmonary arteries show medial hypertrophy, and focal intimal fibrosis is present. Arterioles develop muscular layers.

Mitral stenosis causes a general increase in pulmonary vascular resistance. Several investigators have demonstrated that precapillary arterial vasoconstriction contributes an additionally significant component of increased pulmonary vascular resistance.[23, 39] After mitral valve replacement, the pulmonary arterial pressure and pulmonary vascular resistance usually fall significantly.[23, 122]

Such responses must mean not only that mitral valvular function is normal but that the precapillary vasoconstrictive response characteristic of mitral stenosis has resolved. In one isolated case studied histologically 11 years postoperatively, Ramirez and associates[80] found that arterial and venous lesions characteristic of mitral stenosis were no longer present. Wagenvoort and Wagenvoort[111] made similar observations in a case studied ten years postoperatively.

REFERENCES

1. Abraham, A. S., Cole, R. B., and Bishop, J. M.: Reversal of pulmonary hypertension by prolonged oxygen administration to patients with chronic bronchitis. *Circ. Res. 23:* 147–157, 1968.
2. Abraham, A. S., Cole, R. B., Green, I. D., Hedworth-Whitty, R. B., Clarke, S. W., and Bishop, J. M.: Factors contributing to the reversible pulmonary hypertension of patients with acute respiratory failure studied by serial observations during recovery. *Circ. Res. 24:* 51–60, 1969.
3. Allen, J. R., and Chesney, C. F.: Effect of age on development of cor pulmonale in nonhuman primates following pyrrolizidine alkaloid intoxication. *Exp. Mol. Pathol. 17:* 220–232, 1972.
4. Annotation: Pulmonary veno-occlusive disease. *Br. Med. J. 3:* 369, 1972.
5. Anderson, R. A., Levy, A. M., Naeye, R. L., and Tabakin, B. S.: Rapidly progressing pulmonary vascular obstructive disease. Association with ventricular septal defects during early childhood. *Am. J. Cardiol. 19:* 854–860, 1967.
6. Arias-Stella, J., and Saldaña, M.: The terminal portion of the pulmonary arterial tree in people native to high altitudes. *Circulation 28:* 915–925, 1963.
7. Berthrong, M., Blount, G. S., and Robinson, J. C.: Pulmonary vascular lesions in "primary" pulmonary hypertension. *Am. J. Pathol. 46:* 31a, 1965(Abstr.).

8. Bessinger, F. B., Jr., Blieden, L. C., and Edwards, J. E.: Hypertensive pulmonary vascular disease associated with patent ductus arteriosus. Primary or secondary? *Circulation 52:* 157–161, 1975.
9. Blank, R. H., Muller, W. H., Jr., and Dammann, J. F., Jr.: Changes in pulmonary vascular lesions after restoring normal pulmonary artery pressure. *Surg. Forum 9:* 356–359, 1959.
10. Blank, R. H., Muller, W. H., Jr., and Dammann, J. F., Jr.: Experimental pulmonary arterial hypertension. *Am. J. Surg. 101:* 143–153, 1961.
11. Blount, S. G., and Vogel, J. H. K.: Pulmonary hypertension. *Modern Conc. Cardiovasc. Dis. 36:* 61–66, 1967.
12. Brantigan, O. C., Kress, M. B., and Goco, R. B.: Pulmonary emboli. A factor in the etiology and pathogenesis of pulmonary emphysema. *Dis. Chest 49:* 491–501, 1966.
13. Bras, G., Berry, D. M., and György, P.: Plants as aetiological factor in veno-occlusive disease of the liver. *Lancet 1:* 960–962, 1957.
14. Braun, A., Greenberg, S. D., Malik, S., and Jenkins, D. E.: Pulmonary veno-occlusive disease associated with pulmonary phlebitis. *Arch. Pathol. 95:* 67–70, 1973.
15. Burwell, C. S., Robin, E. D., Whaley, R. D., and Bickelmann, A. G.: Extreme obesity associated with alveolar hypoventilation—A Pickwickian syndrome. *Am. J. Med. 21:* 811–818, 1956.
16. Byrne-Quinn, E., and Grover, R. F.: Aminorex (Menocil) and amphetamine: Acute and chronic effects on pulmonary and systemic haemodynamics in the calf. *Thorax 27:* 127–131, 1972.
17. Carrington, C. B., and Liebow, A. A.: Pulmonary veno-occlusive disease. *Human Pathol. 1:* 322–324, 1970.
18. Chesney, C. F., and Allen, J. R.: Monocrotaline induced pulmonary vascular lesions in non-human primates. *Cardiovasc. Res. 7:* 508–518, 1973.
19. Clarkson, P. M., Frye, R. L., DuShane, J. W., Burchell, H. B., Wood, E. H., and Weidman, W. H.: Prognosis for patients with ventricular septal defect and severe pulmonary vascular obstructive disease. *Circulation 38:* 129–135, 1968.
20. Clarkson, P. M., Neutze, J. M., Wardill, J. C., and Barratt-Boyes, B. G.: The pulmonary vascular bed in patients with complete transposition of the great arteries. *Circulation 53:* 539–543, 1976.
21. Corrin, B., Spencer, H., Turner-Warwick, M., Beales, S. J., and Hamblin, J. J.: Pulmonary veno-occlusion—An immune complex disease? *Virch. Arch. A Path. Anat. Histol. 364:* 81–91, 1974.
22. Cruz-Jibaja, J., Banchero, N., Sime, F., Peñaloza, D., Gamboa, R., and Marticorena, E.: Correlation between pulmonary artery pressure and level of altitude. *Dis. Chest 46:* 446–451, 1964.
23. Dalen, J. E., Matloff, J. M., Evans, G. L., Hoppin, F. G., Jr., Bhardwaj, P., Harken, D. E., and Dexter, L.: Early reduction of pulmonary vascular resistance after mitral-valve replacement. *N. Eng J. Med. 277:* 387–394, 1967.
24. Dammann, J. F., Jr., McEachen, J. A., Thompson, W. M., Jr., Smith, R., and Muller, W. H., Jr.: The regression of pulmonary vascular disease after the creation of pulmonary stenosis. *J. Thorac. Cardiovasc. Surg. 42:* 722–734, 1961.
25. Edwards, J. E.: The Lewis A. Conner Memorial Lecture. Functional pathology of the pulmonary vascular tree in congenital cardiac disease. *Circulation 15:* 164–196, 1957.
26. Edwards, J. E.: Ventricular septal defect. Unresolved problems. *Am. J. Cardiol. 19:* 832–849, 1967.
27. Evans, T. O., Van Der Reis, L., and Selzer, A.: Circulatory effects of chronic pulmonary emphysema. *Am. Heart J. 66:* 741–747, 1963.
28. Ferencz, C.: The pulmonary vascular bed in tetralogy of Fallot. II. Changes following a systemic-pulmonary arterial anastomosis. *Bull. Johns Hopkins Hosp. 106:* 100–118, 1960.
29. Ferencz, C.: Transposition of the great vessels. Pathophysiologic considerations based upon a study of the lungs. *Circulation 33:* 232–241, 1966.
30. Ferguson, D. J., Adams, P., and Watson, D.: Pulmonary arteriosclerosis in transposition of the great vessels. *Am. J. Dis. Child. 99:* 653–661, 1960.
31. Ferguson, D. J., Berkas, E. M., and Varco, R. L.: Process of healing in experimental pulmonary arteriosclerosis. *Proc. Soc. Exp. Biol. Med. 89:* 492–494, 1955.
32. Fishman, A. P.: Dietary pulmonary hypertension. *Circ. Res. 35:* 657–660, 1974.
33. Fleischner, F. G.: Recurrent pulmonary embolism and cor pulmonale. *N. Engl. J. Med. 276:* 1213–1220, 1967.
34. Fowler, N. O., Black-Schaffer, B., Scott, R. C., and Gueron, M.: Idiopathic and thromboembolic pulmonary hypertension. *Am. J. Med. 40:* 331–345, 1966.
35. Friedli, B., Kidd, B. S. L., Mustard, W. T., and Keith, J. D.: Ventricular septal defect with

increased pulmonary vascular resistance. Late results of surgical closure. *Am. J. Cardiol. 33:* 403–409, 1974.

36. Fritts, H. W., Jr., Harris, P., Chidsey, C. A., III, Clauss, R. H., and Cournand, A.: Estimation of flow through bronchial-pulmonary vascular anastomoses with use of T-1824 dye. *Circulation 23:* 390–398, 1961.
37. Geer, J. C., Glass, B. A., and Albert, H. M.: Pulmonary vascular lesions in the dog produced by autogenous clot embolism. *Exp. Mol. Pathol. 4:* 391–398, 1965.
38. Geer, J. C., Glass, B. A., and Albert, H. M.: The morphogenesis and reversibility of experimental hyperkinetic pulmonary vascular lesions in the dog. *Exp. Mol. Pathol. 4:* 399–415, 1965.
39. Goodale, F., Jr., Sanchez, G., Friedlich, A. L., Scannell, J. G., and Myers, G. S.: Correlation of pulmonary arteriolar resistance with pulmonary vascular changes in patients with mitral stenosis before and after valvulotomy. *N. Engl. J. Med. 252:* 979–983, 1955.
40. Goodwin, J. F., Harrison, C. V., and Wilcken, D. E. L.: Obliterative pulmonary hypertension and thrombo-embolism. *Br. Med. J. 1:* 701–711, 1963.
41. Greiser, E., Jesdinsky, H. J., Backmann, R., Both, A., Dengler, H. J., Gahl, K., and Loogen, F.: Primary pulmonary hypertension and Aminorex. Report on the epidemiological and statistical findings of the cooperative study of the association between ingestion of anorectic drugs and primary pulmonary hypertension, 1975.
42. Grover, R. F., Vogel, J. H. K., Averill, K. H., and Blount, S. G., Jr.: Pulmonary hypertension. Individual and species variability relative to vascular reactivity (editorial). *Am. Heart J. 66:* 1–3, 1963.
43. Harris, P., Segel, N., Green, I., and Housley, E.: The influence of the airways resistance and alveolar pressure on the pulmonary vascular resistance in chronic bronchitis. *Cardiovasc. Res. 2:* 84–92, 1968.
44. Harvey, R. M., Ferrer, M. I., Richards, D. W., Jr., and Cournand, A.: Influence of chronic pulmonary disease on the heart and circulation. *Am. J. Med. 10:* 719–738, 1951.
45. Hasleton, P. S., Heath, D., and Brewer, D. B.: Hypertensive pulmonary vascular disease in states of chronic hypoxia. *J. Pathol. Bacteriol. 95:* 431–440, 1968.
46. Heard, B. E.: *Pathology of Chronic Bronchitis and Emphysema.* Churchill, Ltd., London, 1969.
47. Heath, D.: Longitudinal muscle in pulmonary arteries. *J. Pathol. Bacteriol. 85:* 407–412, 1963.
48. Heath, D., Edwards, C., and Harris, P.: Post-mortem size and structure of the human carotid body. Its relation to pulmonary disease and cardiac hypertrophy. *Thorax 25:* 129–140, 1970.
49. Heath, D., Segel, N., and Bishop, J.: Pulmonary veno-occlusive disease. *Circulation 34:* 242–248, 1966.
50. Heath, D., Swan, H. J. C., DuShane, J. W., and Edwards, J. E.: The relation of medial thickness of small muscular pulmonary arteries to immediate postnatal survival in patients with ventricular septal defect or patent ductus arteriosus. *Thorax 13:* 267–271, 1958.
51. Heinemann, H. O.: Respiration and circulation in patients with portal cirrhosis of the liver. *Circulation 22:* 154–159, 1960.
52. Hicken, P., Heath, D., Brewer, D. B., and Whitaker, W.: The small pulmonary arteries in emphysema. *J. Pathol. Bacteriol. 90:* 107–114, 1965.
53. Hofschire, P. J., Rosenquist, G. C., Ruckerman, R. N., Moller, J. H., and Edwards, J. E.: Pulmonary vascular disease complicating the Blalock-Taussig anastomosis. *Circulation 56:* 124–126, 1977.
54. James, W. R. L., and Thomas, A. J.: Right ventricular hypertrophy and the small pulmonary arteries in chronic lung disease. *Br. Heart J. 25:* 583–588, 1963.
55. Jaques, W., and Singleton, L.: Pulmonary vascular changes in the right lung of a child with a Waterston shunt for 6 years. *Am. J. Path. 70:* 28a, 1973, (abstr.).
56. Kawabori, I., Morgan, B. C., and Guntheroth, W. G.: Reversal of "inoperable" pulmonary hypertension. *Am. Heart J. 89:* 775–778, 1975.
57. Kay, J. M., and Heath, D.: Observations on the pulmonary arteries and heart weight of rats fed on *Crotalaria spectabilis* seeds. *J. Pathol. Bacteriol. 92:* 385–394, 1966.
58. Kay, J. M., Heath, D., Smith, P., Bras, G., and Summerell, J.: Fulvine and the pulmonary circulation. Thorax 26: 249–261, 1971.
59. Khoury, G. H., and Hawes, C. R.: Primary pulmonary hypertension in children living at high altitude. *J. Pediat. 62:* 177–185, 1963.

60. Lakier, J. B., Stanger, P., Heymann, M. A., Hoffman, J. I. E., and Rudolph, A. M.: Early onset of pulmonary vascular obstruction in patients with aortopulmonary transposition and intact ventricular septum. *Circulation 51:* 875–880, 1975.
61. Lalich, J. J., and Merkow, L.: Pulmonary arteritis produced in rats by feeding *Crotalaria spectabilis. Lab. invest. 10:* 744–750, 1961.
62. Leachman, R. D., and Pereyo, J. A.: Decrease in pulmonary vascular resistance following surgical closure of a ventricular septal defect associated with elevated capillary wedge pressure and severe pulmonary arterial hypertension. *Am. Heart J. 76:* 816–819, 1968.
63. Leeds, S. E.: The tetralogy of Fallot in older persons up to the fifth decade. Results of subclavian-pulmonary anastomosis with a five- to ten-year followup. *Am. J. Surg. 96:* 234–245, 1958.
64. Levine, O. R., Harris, R. C., Blanc, W. A., and Mellins, R. B.: Progressive pulmonary hypertension in children with portal hypertension. *J. Pediat. 83:* 964–972, 1973.
65. Liebow, A. A.: The bronchopulmonary venous collateral circulation with special reference to emphysema. *Am. J. Pathol. 29:* 251–289, 1953.
66. Liebow, A. A., Hales, M. R., and Lindskog, G. E.: Enlargement of the bronchial arteries and their anastomoses with the pulmonary arteries in chronic pulmonary disease. *Am. J. Pathol. 24:* 691–692, 1948, (abstr.).
67. Liebow, A. A., Hales, M. R., and Lindskog, G. E.: Enlargement of the bronchial arteries, and their anastomoses with the pulmonary arteries in bronchiectasis. *Am. J. Pathol. 25:* 211–231, 1949.
68. Liebow, A. A., McAdams, A. J., Carrington, C. B., and Viamonte, M.: Intrapulmonary veno-obstructive disease. *Circulation* (Suppl. II) *35, 36:* 172, 1967, (abstr.).
69. Lukas, D. S., and Plum, F.: Pulmonary function in patients convalescing from acute poliomyelitis with respiratory paralysis. *Am. J. Med. 12:* 388–396, 1952.
70. Macartney, F. J., Panday, J., and Scott, O.: Cor pulmonale as a result of chronic nasopharyngeal obstruction due to hypertrophied tonsils and adenoids. *Arch. Dis. Child. 44:* 585–592, 1969.
71. Menashe, V. D., Farrehi, C., and Miller, M.: Hypoventilation and cor pulmonale due to chronic upper airway obstruction. *J. Pediat. 67:* 198–203, 1965.
72. Motley, H. L., Cournand, A., Werko, L., Himmelstein, A., and Dresdale, D.: The influence of short periods of induced acute anoxia upon pulmonary artery pressures in man. *Am. J. Physiol. 150:* 315–320, 1947.
73. Naeye, R. L.: Kyphoscoliosis and cor pulmonale. A study of the pulmonary vascular bed. *Am. J. Pathol. 38:* 561–573, 1961.
74. Naeye, R. L.: Alveolar hypoxia, differential effects on pulmonary arteries of varied size. *Proc. Soc. Exp. Biol. Med. 132:* 558–560, 1969.
75. Naeye, R. L.: Pulmonary hypertension and vascular disease. *In The Heart* (International Academy of Pathology Monograph No. 15), edited by Edwards, J. E., Lev, M., and Abell, M. R. Chapter 15, pp. 297–326. The Williams & Wilkins Co., Baltimore, 1974.
76. Newfeld, E. A., Paul, M. H., Muster, A. J., and Idriss, F. S.: Pulmonary vascular disease in complete transposition of the great arteries: A study of 200 patients. *Am. J. Cardiol. 34:* 75–82, 1974.
77. Olsen, E. G. J.: Repeated pulmonary thromboembolism in rabbits. *Lab. Invest. 32:* 323–329, 1975.
78. Paul, M. H., Miller, R. A., and Potts, W. J.: Long-term results of aortic-pulmonary anastomosis for tetralogy of Fallot. An analysis of the first 100 cases eleven to thirteen years after operation. *Circulation 23:* 525–533, 1961.
79. Peñaloza, D., Sime, F., Banchero, N., and Gamboa, R.: Pulmonary hypertension in healthy man born and living at high altitudes. *Med. Thorac. 19:* 449–460, 1962.
80. Ramirez, A., Grimes, E. T., and Abelmann, W. H.: Regression of pulmonary vascular changes following mitral valvuloplasty. An anatomic and physiologic case study. *Am. J. Med. 45:* 975–982, 1968.
81. Reeve, R., Selzer, A., Popper, R. W., Leeds, R. F., and Gerbode, F.: Reversibility of pulmonary hypertension following cardiac surgery. *Circulation* (Suppl. I) 33, 34: 107–114, 1966.
82. Reeves, J. T., and Noonan, J. A.: Microarteriographic studies of primary pulmonary hypertension. A quantitative approach in two patients. *Arch. Pathol. 95:* 50–55, 1973.
83. Rosenthal, A., Vawter, G., and Wagenvoort, C. A.: Intrapulmonary veno-occlusive disease. *Am. J. Cardiol. 31:* 78–83, 1973.

84. Ross, J., Jr., Morrow, A. G., and Braunwald, E.: Regression of severe pulmonary hypertension after repair of a defect of the ventricular septum in a patient with a bidirectional shunt. *N. Engl. J. Med. 270:* 946–948, 1964.
85. Ross, R. S., Taussig, H. B., and Evans, M. H.: Late hemodynamic complications of anastomotic surgery for treatment of the tetralogy of Fallot. *Circulation 18:* 553–561, 1958.
86. Saldaña, M., and Arias-Stella, J.: Studies on the structure of the pulmonary trunk. II. The evolution of the elastic configuration of the pulmonary trunk in people native to high altitudes. *Circulation 27:* 1094–1100, 1963.
87. Saldaña, M., and Arias-Stella, J.: Studies on the structure of the pulmonary trunk. III. The thickness of the media of the pulmonary trunk and ascending aorta in high altitude natives. *Circulation 27:* 1101–1104, 1963.
88. Sautter, R. D., Fletcher, F. W., Emanuel, D. A., Lawton, B. R., and Olsen, T. G.: Complete resolution of massive pulmonary thromboembolism. *JAMA 189:* 948–949, 1964.
89. Segel, N., Kay, J. M., Bayley, T. J., and Paton, A.: Pulmonary hypertension with hepatic cirrhosis. *Br. Heart J. 30:* 575–578, 1968.
90. Senior, R. M., Britton, R. C., Turino, G. M., Wood, J. A., Langer, G. A., and Fishman, A. P.: Pulmonary hypertension associated with cirrhosis of the liver and with portacaval shunts. *Circulation 37:* 88–96, 1968.
91. Shem-Tov, A., Fine, L. G., Rotem, Y., and Neufeld, H. N.: Occlusive pulmonary vascular disease in a child with a spontaneously closed ventricular septal defect. *Israel J. Med. Sci. 9:* 469–476, 1973.
92. Shepherd, J. T., Edwards, J. E., Burchell, H. B., Swan, H. J. C., and Wood, E. H.: Clinical, physiological, and pathological considerations in patients with idiopathic pulmonary hypertension. *Br. Heart J. 19:* 70–82, 1957.
93. Sieker, H. O., Estes, E. H., Kelser, G. A., and McIntosh, H. D.: A cardiopulmonary syndrome associated with extreme obesity. *J. Clin. Invest. 34:* 916, 1955, (abstr.).
94. Sime, F., Peñaloza, D., and Ruiz, L.: Bradycardia, increased cardiac output, and reversal of pulmonary hypertension in altitude natives living at sea level. *Br. Heart J. 33:* 647–657, 1971.
95. Smith, P., Heath, D., Kay, J. M., Wright, J. S., and McKendrick, C. S.: Pulmonary arterial pressure and structure in the patas monkey after prolonged administration of aminorex fumarate. *Cardiovasc. Res. 7:* 30–38, 1973.
96. Thadani, U., Burrow, C., Whitaker, W., and Heath, D.: Pulmonary veno-occlusive disease. *Quart. J. Med.* (New Series) *44:* 133–159, 1975.
97. Viles, P. H., Ongley, P. A., and Titus, J. L.: The spectrum of pulmonary vascular disease in transposition of the great arteries. *Circulation 40:* 31–41, 1969.
98. Vogel, J. H. K., Grover, R. F., Jamieson, G., and Blount, S. G., Jr.: Long-term physiologic observations in patients with ventricular septal defect and increased pulmonary vascular resistance. *Adv. Cardiol. 11:* 108–122, 1974.
99. Vogel, J. H. K., Weaver, W. F., Rose, R. L., Blount, S. G., and Grover, R. F.: Pulmonary hypertension on exertion in normal man living at 10,150 feet (Leadville, Colorado). *Med. Thorac. 19:* 461–477, 1962.
100. von Bernuth, G., Ritter, D. G., Frye, R. L., Weidman, W. H., Davis, G. D., and McGoon, D. C.: Evaluation of patients with tetralogy of Fallot and Potts anastomosis. *Am. J. Cardiol. 27:* 259–263, 1971.
101. Von Euler, U. S., and Liljestrand, G.: Observations on the pulmonary arterial blood pressure in the cat. *Acta Physiol. Scand. 12:* 301–320, 1946.
102. Wagenvoort, C. A.: Vasoconstrictive primary pulmonary hypertension and pulmonary veno-occlusive disease. *Cardiovasc. Clin. 4:* 97–113, 1972.
103. Wagenvoort, C. A.: Pulmonary veno-occlusive disease. Entity or syndrome? *Chest 69:* 82–86, 1976.
104. Wagenvoort, C. A., DuShane, J. W., and Edwards, J. E.: Cardiac Clinics. 151. Hypertensive pulmonary arterial lesions as a late result of anastomosis of systemic and pulmonary circulations. *Proc. Mayo Clin. 35:* 186–191, 1960.
105. Wagenvoort, C. A., Losekoot, G., and Mulder, E.: Pulmonary veno-occlusive disease of presumably intrauterine origin. *Thorax 26:* 429–434, 1971.
106. Wagenvoort, C. A., Nauta, J., van der Schaar, P. J., Weeda, H. W. H., and Wagenvoort, N.: The pulmonary vasculature in complete transposition of the great vessels, judged from lung biopsies. *Circulation 38:* 746–754, 1968.

107. Wagenvoort, C. A., and Wagenvoort, N.: Primary pulmonary hypertension. A pathologic study of the lung vessels in 156 clinically diagnosed cases. *Circulation 42:* 1163–1184, 1970.

108. Wagenvoort, C. A., and Wagenvoort, N.: Hypoxic pulmonary vascular lesions in man at high altitude and in patients with chronic respiratory disease. *Pathol. Microbiol. 39:* 276–282, 1973.

109. Wagenvoort, C. A., and Wagenvoort, N.: Pathology of the Eisenmenger syndrome and primary pulmonary hypertension. *Adv. Cardiol. 11:* 123–130, 1974.

110. Wagenvoort, C. A., and Wagenvoort, N.: The pathology of pulmonary veno-occlusive disease. *Virch. Arch. A Path. Anat. Histol. 364:* 69–79, 1974.

111. Wagenvoort, C. A., and Wagenvoort, N.: *Pathology of Pulmonary Hypertension.* Wiley Medical, John Wiley and Sons, Inc., New York, 1977.

112. Wagenvoort, C. A., Wagenvoort, N., and Dijk, H. J.: Effect of fulvine on pulmonary arteries and veins of the rat. *Thorax 29:* 522–529, 1974.

113. Walcott, G., Burchell, H. B., and Brown, A. L., Jr.: Primary pulmonary hypertension. *Am. J. Med. 49:* 70–79, 1970.

114. Weidman, W. H., and DuShane, J. W.: Course of pulmonary hypertension following surgical closure of ventricular septal defect. *Adv. Cardiol. 11:* 131–134, 1974.

115. Westcott, R. N., Fowler, N. O., Scott, R. C., Hauenstein, V. D., and McGuire, J.: Anoxia and human pulmonary vascular resistance. *J. Clin. Invest. 30:* 957–970, 1951.

116. World Health Organization. Primary pulmonary hypertension. Report on a WHO meeting. edited by Hatano, S., and Strassner, T. pp. 7–45, Geneva, 1975.

117. Widimský, J., Kasalický, J., Přerovský, I., and Dejdar, R.: Central hemodynamics in recurrent embolism. *Am. Heart J. 71:* 206–215, 1966.

118. Wilhelmsen, L., Bjure, J., Korsgren, M., and Zettergren, L.: Pathophysiology of pulmonary embolism with special reference to recurrent embolism. *Bull. Physio-Path. Resp. 6:* 99–121, 1970.

119. Wilhelmsen, L., Selander, S., Söderholm, B., Paulin, S., Varnauskas, E., and Werko, L.: Recurrent pulmonary embolism. *Medicine 42:* 335–355, 1963.

120. Will, J. A., and Bisgard, G. E.: Haemodynamic effects of oral aminorex and amphetamine in unanaesthetized beagle dogs. *Thorax 27:* 120–126, 1972.

121. Yamaki, S., and Tezuka, F.: Quantitative analysis of pulmonary vascular disease in complete transposition of the great arteries. *Circulation 54:* 805–809, 1976.

122. Zener, J. C., Hancock, E. W., Shumway, N. E., and Harrison, D. C.: Regression of extreme pulmonary hypertension after mitral valve surgery. *Am. J. Cardiol. 30:* 820–826, 1972.

Chapter 14

The Sudden Infant Death Syndrome

RICHARD L. NAEYE

There are an estimated 8,000–10,000 deaths in the United States each year due to the sudden infant death syndrome (SIDS), making it the most frequent cause of death in the first year of life after the neonatal period. It has about one quarter the incidence of congenital heart disease and ten times the frequency of leukemia. Many hypotheses have been generated to explain its etiology. Most of the easily recognized postmortem abnormalities in the victims are in the lungs and they have usually been interpreted as evidence for a sudden, catastrophic event in an otherwise normal infant. Years of speculation about the nature of the catastrophic event have been unfruitful because the easily recognized postmortem abnormalities give few clues to the dynamic events surrounding the deaths.

Short periods of apnea during sleep are normal during infancy while prolonged periods are abnormal. In 1972 Steinschneider[33] reported that several SIDS victims had prolonged periods of apnea during sleep before death. In other disorders such prolonged episodes of apnea are often associated with chronic underventilation of the lungs. This clue led to the finding that more than half of SIDS victims have postmortem evidences of antecedent chronic pulmonary hypoventilation.[21] A plethora of new information has followed, all pointing to chronic abnormalities in the victims. This chapter reviews both the acute and chronic abnormalities in SIDS victims as well as evidence that SIDS has its origins in fetal life.

ACUTE PULMONARY ABNORMALITIES IN SIDS

Until recently, acute pulmonary abnormalities were the focus of attention in SIDS victims. Misinterpretation of these pulmonary abnormalities has misled investigators for many years and has generated emotional problems for parents of the victims. The inflammation and ulcerations found on the vocal cords of some victims have been taken by some as evidence that the deaths were due to acute laryngospasm. A recent study found such vocal cord changes to be as frequent in age-matched cases with known causes of death as in SIDS victims.[6] Pulmonary edema, often hemorrhagic, is common in SIDS victims but it may have no significance since it can develop after death in non-SIDS victims when the interval between death and autopsy is long.[5, 7, 16] Mast cell degranulation, one marker for anaphylaxis, has been found in a few SIDS victims but findings in the thymuses of SIDS victims do not resemble the changes that usually follow anaphylaxis.[1, 8]

Petechiae are found on the surfaces of intrathoracic organs in up to 70% of SIDS victims. They have been taken by some as evidence of antecedent upper airway obstruction and strongly negative intrapleural pressures. Recent experimental studies have shown that upper airway obstruction alone will not produce such petechiae. Hypoxia before cardiac arrest and vigorous respiratory movements are both required to produce them.[14] Finally, acute middle ear and respiratory tract infections are found in up to 45% of SIDS victims but they are almost always too mild to be the direct cause of death.[21, 36] As will be seen later in this chapter, such infections have a likely indirect role in the deaths.

EVIDENCES OF CHRONIC ALVEOLAR HYPOVENTILATION IN SIDS VICTIMS

In 1973 the small pulmonary arteries of more than half of SIDS victims were found to have increased muscle, a characteristic consequence of chronic alveolar hypoventilation and hypoxia[21] (Fig. 1). Alveolar hypoxia increases pulmonary vascular resistance by causing small arteries to contract. When this stimulus is protracted, the medial muscle cells of the arteries undergo both hyperplasia and hypertrophy.[19, 21] The increased pulmonary vascular resistance places an increased pressure load on the cardiac right ventricle. The result is a hyperplasia of myocardial fibers in the right ventricle and chronic cor pulmonale. Those SIDS victims who have increased muscle in their pulmonary arteries also have abnormally heavy cardiac right ventricles[28] (Fig. 2). Unfortunately, neither the increased muscle in the pulmonary arteries nor the cor pulmonale can be recognized by casual observation. A quantitative histologic technique such as point counting is needed to demonstrate the abnormality in the pulmonary arteries.[21] The cardiac ventricles must be separately weighed to demonstrate the cor pulmonale.[28]

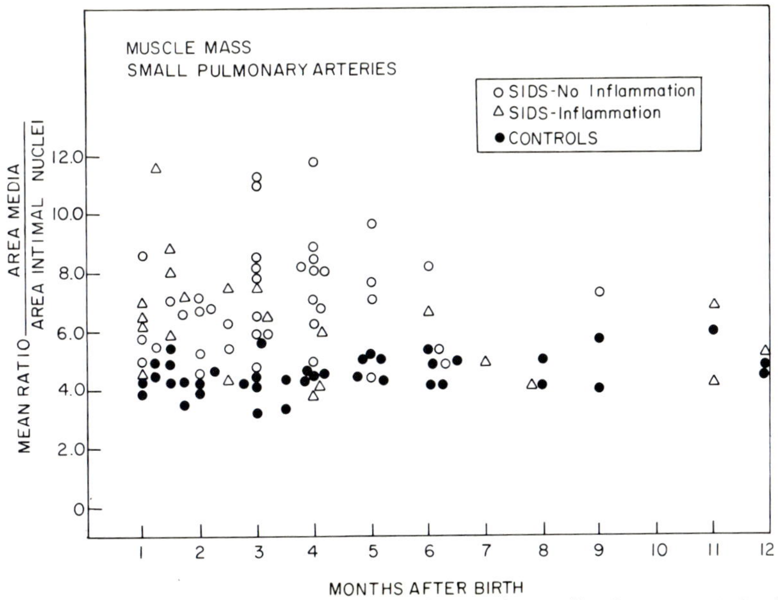

FIG. 1. A ratio reflecting the relative arterial muscle mass for small pulmonary arteries (ordinate) is plotted against age. Mean values for pulmonary arterial muscle mass are greater in SIDS victims than in nonhypoxic controls. (Reprinted by permission, from *N. Engl. J. Med. 289:* 1168, 1973.)

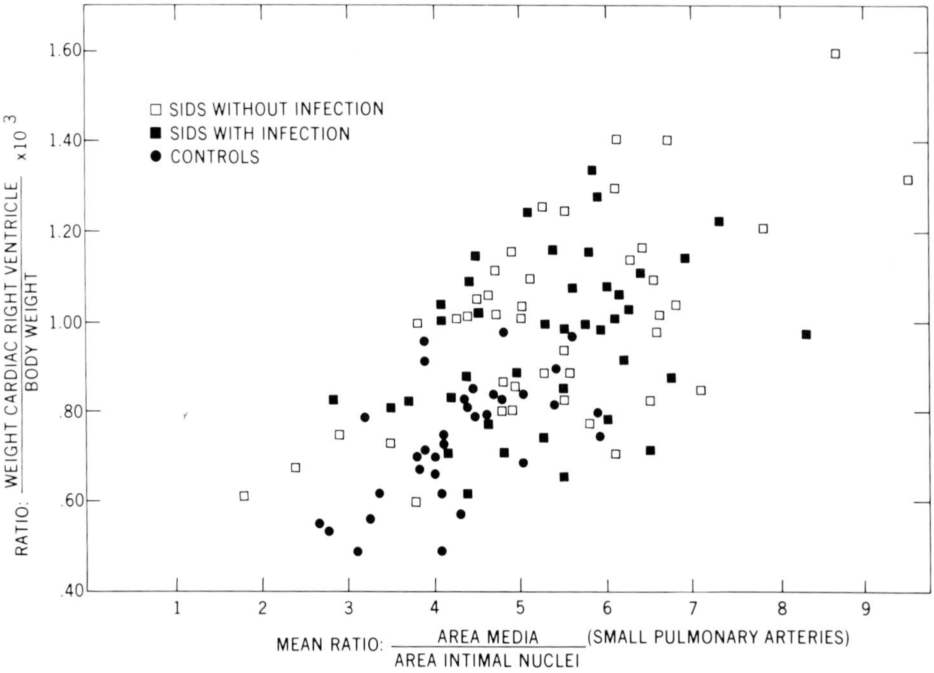

FIG. 2. Relative cardiac right ventricular weights increase with increases of medial muscle in the small pulmonary arteries. Using simple linear regression, the zero order correlation coefficient for these data is 0.60. (Reprinted by permission, from *Am. J. Pathol. 82:* 5, 1976.)

POSSIBLE CAUSES OF CHRONIC ALVEOLAR HYPOVENTILATION IN SIDS VICTIM

Future SIDS victims do not usually have apneic spells or underventilate their lungs when awake so it seems unlikely that the victims have any prime abnormalities in the structures of innervation of the bellows mechanism of the chest. The abnormalities in the victims appear to lie in the central mechanisms of respiratory control or their receptors. Carotid body glomic tissue is hypoplastic in more than half of SIDS victims.[25] All the various glomic cell types are deficient in number. This could constitute the prime defect in some SIDS victims since the organ regulates pulmonary ventilation through its chemoreceptor function. However, the hypoplasia could also reflect a lack of stimulation of the organ through a deficiency of afferent neural impulses from the brainstem respiratory control centers.[25]

A number of structural abnormalities have been found in the brains of SIDS victims. Gadsdon and Emery[11] have reported that fat-laden cells are present in the cerebrospinal fluid of half of SIDS victims. The fat appears to originate in the corpus callosum and the lateral ventricles, where lipid laden macrophages are found among the myelinating tracts. These fat-laden cells are also found in the subependymal zone of the lateral ventricles where they are said to enter the spinal fluid through gaps in the ependyma.

About half of SIDS victims have an abnormal proliferation of astroglial fibers in those areas of the pons and medulla that control respiration[23] (Fig. 3). These

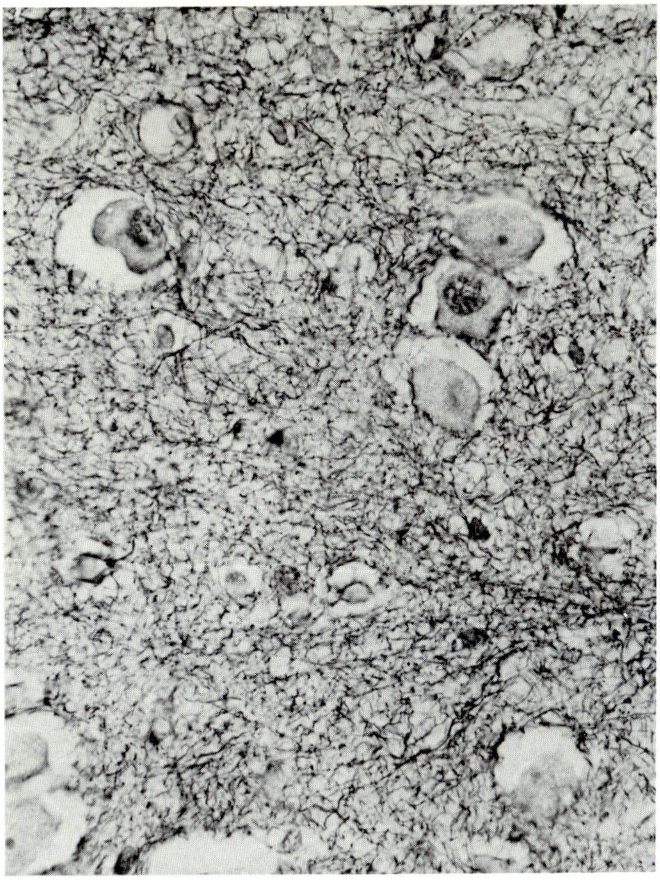

FIG. 3. Marked astroglial proliferation is visible in the medulla of a 3-month-old SIDS victim. Holzer stain, × 600. (Reprinted by permission, from *Am. J. Clin. Pathol. 66:* 528, 1976.)

proliferated fibers may well represent a reaction to chronic hypoxemia which is a consequence of chronic pulmonary hypoventilation. Infants with known chronic hypoxemia before death also have this abnormal proliferation of astroglial fibers in their brainstems.[23] Both the lipid-laden macrophages and proliferated astroglial fibers represent subacute or chronic abnormalities that could not be caused by a single acute, terminal event.

OTHER CEREBRAL ABNORMALITIES IN VICTIMS

If apnea during sleep is a common final pathway of death in SIDS, it would be surprising if it were the only evidence of brain dysfunction because the neural mechanisms that control respiration are not completely isolated from other regulatory mechanisms in the brainstem. Some SIDS victims have recently been reported to have had dysfunction in a number of nonrespiratory control mechanisms before death.[26] These include neonatal abnormalities in temperature regulation, feeding, motor tone, and various neurologic reflexes.[26] These abnormalities did not appear to be related to events in labor or delivery.[26] Some SIDS victims had abnormal cries, were breathless, and were exhausted during feedings long before death.[27] They also had less intense reactions to a variety of environmental stimuli.[27] These behavioral characteristics have been positively correlated with postmortem anatomic markers of chronic hypoventilation and hypoxemia.[27]

CONSEQUENCES OF CHRONIC PULMONARY HYPOVENTILATION

Chronic underventilation of the lungs results in chronic arterial hypoxemia. One half or more of SIDS victims have multiple anatomic markers of such chronic hypoxemia. The first discovered was an abnormal retention of brown fat.[22] The brown fat which surrounds many visceral organs at birth loses most of its mitochondria during the first year of life so that it gradually assumes the appearance of white fat. This transformation is retarded by chronic hypoxemia.[22, 37] Most SIDS victims who have postmortem evidences of antecedent chronic pulmonary hypoventilation have an abnormal retention of brown fat cells about their adrenal glands[22, 39] (Fig. 4). This finding has limited use in the diagnosis of chronic hypoxemia in SIDS victims because the process of fat transformation is not advanced enough during the first three months of life to distinguish hypoxemic from non-hypoxemic cases and just over half of SIDS deaths take place before three months of age.

Most SIDS victims who have an abnormal retention of brown fat have hyperplastic chromaffin tissue in their adrenal medullas.[23] Children with chronic hypoxemia due to cyanotic forms of congenital heart disease also have the adrenal abnormality.[23] An increased release of epinephrine from the hyperplastic chromaffin tissue may be responsible for the brown fat retention because adults with pheochromocytomas that produce catecholamines usually have a reappearance of brown fat at those sites where it was present at birth.[37] This may take place through a stimulation of nerve endings because fat cells at neonatal brown cell

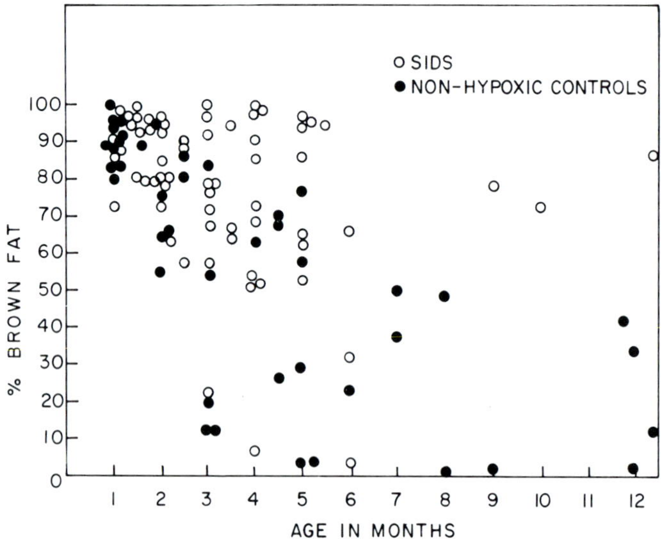

FIG. 4. Percent of periadrenal fat cells which resemble fetal or brown cells decreases with age in nonhypoxic control infants. By contrast, such cells abnormally retain their brown appearance in about half of SIDS victims.

sites do not lose their unique double innervation from the sympathetic nervous system when they lose their mitochondria in the first year of life.

Other markers of chronic hypoxemia in SIDS victims include extramedullary erythropoiesis and an erythroid hyperplasia in the bone marrow. Erythropoiesis in the liver is found in about 17% of SIDS victims.[22, 38] It is found in about the same percent of infants with chronic hypoxemia due to other causes such as cyanotic forms of congenital heart disease.[22] A recent unpublished study from our laboratory found that 23% of the nucleated cells in the bone marrow of 36 SIDS victims were erythroid precursors whereas only 16% of such nucleated cells were erythroid precursors in the bone marrows of 28 age-matched infants who died in fires or in accidents ($P<0.02$).

There are other markers of chronic hypoxemia in SIDS victims. SIDS victims as a group are not significantly growth retarded at birth but often become so after birth.[27, 29, 31] This postnatal growth retardation resembles that seen in experimental animals maintained in a hypoxia environment after birth.[20] It is not due to undernutrition since most SIDS victims have a normal sized thymus gland and a normal amount of subcutaneous fat. A small proportion of SIDS victims have hyperplastic rather than hypoplastic carotid bodies.[25] Such hyperplasia is common in adults with chronic hypoxemia for any known cause.

NONRESPIRATORY MECHANISMS OF DEATH IN SIDS

In the early months of life, bradycardia and sometimes serious arrhythmias have been observed with episodes of sleep apnea.[12, 13] Maron and co-workers[18] have recently found a prolonged Q-T interval on the ECG's of parents and siblings of several SIDS victims. This ECG abnormality is part of a well known inherited syndrome that is sometimes characterized by sudden death in older children and adults.[15] No significant structural abnormalities have been described in the cardiac conduction fibers of SIDS victims to explain arrhythmias in the victims.[17] Sturner and other British investigators have reported increased levels of sodium, chloride, and urea in the vitreous humor of some SIDS victims.[10, 35] These findings which suggest severe dehydration before death have not been found in a study in the United States.[4] Milk formulas are not as well standardized in the United Kingdom as in the U.S. and this has resulted in more cases of dehydration in the U.K. than in the U.S.[32] A few deaths attributed to SIDS are probably homicides. Such cases appear to be very rare.

CORRELATION OF OLDER THEORIES ON SIDS WITH RECENT FINDINGS

It has long been recognized that up to half of SIDS victims have some type of mild infection at the time of death. These infections are usually in the respiratory tract but sometimes involve the middle ear, gastrointestinal tract, or other organs.[3, 21, 25, 27] Viruses and bacteria of many types have been recovered from the infected infants. Many investigators have attributed the deaths to the infections but it has long been clear that most of the infections are too mild to be a simple, direct cause of the deaths. In the past several years a large number of infants who have been continuously monitored have been observed to have more frequent and more protracted apneic spells during sleep following the onset of mild infections.[34] Such infections may exert their effect by interrupting the infant's sleep cycle.[27] Noninfectious interruptions of the sleep cycle also increase the frequency and duration of apneic episodes during sleep in apnea-prone infants.

Before 1974 laryngospasm was the most common explanation for SIDS.[2, 30] This hypothesis has been supported in a few cases by postmortem evidences of struggle and by rare descriptions of stridor just before death. In apnea-prone infants who are continuously monitored, almost all episodes of sleep apnea start with a cessation of chest movement, presumably reflecting a failure of central control mechanisms. In a minority of the infants, occasional apneic periods which start with cessation of chest movements terminate with an apparent sudden closure of the upper airway, perhaps involving the pharynx.[13]

THE ORIGINS OF SIDS

A recent prospective study of pregnancy and infant development provided more than 1000 variables to examine for the causes of SIDS.[24] Interactions were analyzed for those variables that correlated with an increased frequency of SIDS. Seven out of eight factors found to have an independent association with SIDS point to fetal life for the origins of SIDS. These seven factors include: premature birth due to amniotic fluid bacterial infections, maternal cigarette smoking during pregnancy, maternal anemia during pregnancy, few maternal prenatal clinic visits for medical care, membranous insertion of the umbilical cord into the placenta, lymphocytic infiltration of the decidua, and abnormalities in newborns' neurologic tests and muscle tone that persisted through the neonatal period. These abnormalities in neurologic tests and muscle tone presumably originated in fetal life because no increase was detected in the frequency of any noxious event associated with labor or delivery in the SIDS cases.

Infants with blood type B had more than twice the risk of SIDS as infants with other blood types, raising the possibility that some infants may have a genetic susceptibility to SIDS.[24] Finally, SIDS was increased with crowded housing. This association was mainly in victims who had mild respiratory tract infections at the time of death. The crowding may have contributed to the infections by increasing the victims' exposure to infectious agents.

SPECIAL RESPONSIBILITY OF PATHOLOGISTS TO PREVENT LONG-TERM CONSEQUENCES OF SIDS

The impact of SIDS on parents and siblings is often greater than would be expected by the loss of a child. Harsh contacts with police and insensitive interactions with hospital staff, neighbors, and family members often lead to recriminations, intense feelings of guilt, marital discord, and protracted mourning. These problems are often reinforced by physicians who are unable to explain the probable cause of the death or else offer erroneous explanations that generate further feelings of guilt. Pathologists often make the misdiagnosis of interstitial pneumonia in SIDS cases based on the presence of aggregated lymphocytes which are normal in the lungs for the age.[9] This misdiagnosis leads parents to think they missed signs of illness in the infant and were responsible for its death by not seeking medical care. The parents and community are best served by a thorough autopsy that specifically seeks evidences of the chronic abnormalities outlined in this review. When such abnormalities are found and thoroughly explained to the parents, the death will usually be accepted by the parents as unpreventable. Explanations are of course less satisfactory in the approximate one-third of SIDS cases in which no chronic abnormalities can currently be detected postmortem.

REFERENCES

1. Baak, J. P. A., and Humber, J.: Morphology of the thymus in SIDS and the effects of lethal histamine shock on the guinea pig thymus. In *SIDS,* edited by Robinson, R. R. Canadian Foundation for the Study of Infant Deaths, 27–55, 1974.
2. Beckwith, J. B.: Observations on the pathological anatomy of the sudden infant death syndrome. In *Sudden Infant Death Syndrome,* edited by Bergman, A. B., Beckwith, J. B., Ray, C. Seattle, University of Washington Press, 83–102, 1970.
3. Beckwith, J. B.: The sudden infant death syndrome. U.S. Dept. Health, Education and Welfare, Pub. #75-5137, 1975.
4. Blumenfeld, T. A., and Catherman, R. L.: Postmortem vitreous concentration (PVC) of Na, K, Cl, Ca and Mg in sudden infant death syndrome (SIDS). *Pediat. Res. 9:* 347, 1975.
5. Boyd, E. M., and Knight, L. M.: Postmortem shifts in the weight and water levels of body organs. *Toxicol. Appl. Pharmacol. 15:* 119–128, 1963.
6. Cullity, G. J., and Emery, J. L.: Ulceration and necrosis of vocal cords in hospital and unexpected child deaths. *J. Pathol. 115:* 27–31, 1975.
7. Durlacher, S. H., Banfield, W. G., and Bergner, A. D.: Post-mortem pulmonary edema. *Yale J. Biol. Med. 22:* 565–572, 1950.
8. Emery, J. L., and Carpenter, R. G.: Pulmonary mast cells in infants and their relation to unexpected death in infancy. In *SIDS*, edited by Robinson, R. R. Canadian Foundation for the Study of Infant Deaths, 7–19, 1974.
9. Emery, J. L., and Dinsdale, F.: Increased incidence of lymphoreticular aggregates in lungs of children found unexpectedly dead. *Arch. Dis. Child. 49:* 107–111, 1974.
10. Emery, J. L., Swift, P. G., and Worthy, E.: Hypernatraemia and uraemia in unexpected death in infancy. *Arch. Dis. Child. 49:* 686–692, 1974.
11. Gadsdon, D. R., and Emery, J. L.: Fatty change in the brain in perinatal and unexpected death. *Arch. Dis. Child. 51:* 42–48, 1976.
12. Guilleminault, C., Ariagno, R., Souquet, M., and Dement, W. C.: Abnormal polygraphic findings in near-miss sudden infant death. *Lancet 1:* 1326–1327, 1976.
13. Guilleminault, G., Peraita, R., Souquet, M., and Dement, W. C.: Apneas during sleep in infants: Possible relationship with sudden infant death syndrome. *Science 190:* 677–679, 1975.
14. Guntheroth, W. G.: The significance of pulmonary petechiae in crib death. *Pediatrics 52:* 601–603, 1973.
15. James, T. N.: QT prolongation and sudden death. *Mod. Concepts Cardiovasc. Dis. 38:* 35–38, 1969.
16. Lauweryns, J. M., and Bourgeois, N.: Neonatal hyaline membrane disease, light and electron microscopical studies. In *Current Research in Chronic Respiratory Diseases*, pp. 3–30. US-DHEW publ. #1879, 1969.
17. Lie, J. T., Rosenberg, H. S., and Erickson, E. E.: Histopathology of the conduction system in the sudden infant death syndrome. *Circulation 53:* 3–8, 1976.
18. Maron, B. J., Clark, C. E., Goldstein, R. E., Fisher, R. B., and Epstein, S. E.: Sudden infant death syndrome: Potential cardiac mechanisms (in press).
19. Mason, J. M., Mason, L. H., Jackson, M., Bell, J. S., Francisco, J. T., and Jennings, B. R.: Pulmonary vessels in SIDS. *N. Engl. J. Med. 292:* 479, 1975.
20. Naeye, R. L.: Organ and cellular development in mice growing at simulated high altitude. *Lab. Invest. 15:* 700–706, 1966.
21. Naeye, R. L.: Pulmonary arterial abnormalities in the sudden-infant-death syndrome. *N. Engl. J. Med. 289:* 1167–1170, 1973.
22. Naeye, R. L.: Hypoxemia and the sudden infant death syndrome. *Science 186:* 837–838, 1974.
23. Naeye, R. L.: Brain-stem and adrenal abnormalities in the sudden infant death syndrome. *Am. J. Clin. Pathol. 66:* 526–530, 1976.

24. Naeye, R. L. Calculating the risk of the sudden infant death syndrome prospectively (in press).
25. Naeye, R. L., Fisher, R., Ryser, M., and Whalen, P.: Carotid body in the sudden infant death syndrome. *Science 191:* 567–569, 1976.
26. Naeye, R. L., Ladis, B., and Drage, J. S.: Sudden infant death syndrome. A prospective study. *Am. J. Dis. Child. 130:* 1207–1210, 1976.
27. Naeye, R. L., Messmer, J., Specht, T., and Merritt, T. A.: Sudden infant death syndrome, temperament before death. *J. Pediat. 88:* 511–515, 1976.
28. Naeye, R. L., Whalen, P., Ryser, M., and Fisher, R.: Cardiac and other abnormalities in the sudden infant death syndrome. *Am. J. Pathol. 82:* 1–8, 1976.
29. Peterson, D. R., Benson, E. A., Fisher, L. D., Chinn, N. M., and Beckwith, J. B.: Postnatal growth and the sudden infant death syndrome. *Am. J. Epidemiol. 99:* 389–394, 1974.
30. Shaw, E. G.: Sudden unexpected death in infancy syndrome. *Am. J. Dis. Child. 116:* 115–119, 1968.
31. Sinclair-Smith, C., Dinsdale, F., Emery, J.: Evidence of duration and type of illness in children found unexpectedly dead. *Arch. Dis. Child. 51:* 424–429, 1976.
32. Smith, B. A. M.: Feeding overstrength cows' milk to babies. *Br. Med. J. 4:* 741–742, 1974.
33. Steinschneider, A.: Prolonged apnea and the sudden infant death syndrome: Clinical and laboratory observations. *Pediatrics 50:* 646–654, 1972.
34. Stevens, H. L.: Sudden unexplained death in infancy. Observations on a natural mechanism of adoption of the face down position. *Am. J. Dis. Child. 110:* 243–247, 1965.
35. Sturner, W. Q., and Dempsey, J. L.: Sudden infant death: Chemical analysis of vitreous humor. *J. Forensic. Sci. 18:* 12–19, 1973.
36. Tapp, E., Jones, D. M., and Tobin, J. O'H.: Interpretation of respiratory tract histology in cot deaths. *Clin. Pathol. 28:* 899–904, 1975.
37. Teplitz, C., and Chan Lim, Y.: The diagnostic significance of diffuse brown adipose tissue (BAT) transformation of adult human periadrenal fat: A morphologic indicator of severe chronic hypoxemia. *Lab. Invest. 30:* 390, 1974.
38. Valdes-Dapena, M., Gillane, M. M., and Catherman, R.: Abnormal hepatic extramedullary hepatiopoiesis in the sudden infant death syndrome. Dulles *SIDS* Meeting, June, 1975.
39. Valdes-Dapena, M. A., Gillane, M. M., and Catherman, R.: Brown fat retention in sudden infant death syndrome. *Arch. Pathol. Lab. Med. 100:* 547–549, 1976.

Chapter 15

Recent Advances in Neonatal Pulmonary Disease

CLAIRE LANGSTON AND D. G. FAGAN

Pulmonary disease is the most important cause of morbidity and mortality in the neonatal period.[72] Most, but not all pulmonary disease, is seen in the prematurely born, but otherwise normal, infant and is largely related to functional immaturity of the respiratory system. Not only is the lung of the premature infant quite different structurally from that of the adult but it is also different from that of the term infant. There are no doubt corresponding functional differences. However, the pattern of normal lung development must be understood before the contributions of immaturity and/or maldevelopment of the lung to the pathogenesis and sequelae of neonatal pulmonary disease can be assessed adequately.

LUNG GROWTH AND DEVELOPMENT

While there have been several recent review articles on the growth and development of the human infant lung,[40, 61, 67, 71] and its physiology,[6, 7] more is known about lung development in experimental animals than in humans.[4, 16, 24] Although there is considerable interspecies variation in lung development and direct extrapolation from animals to man requires caution, prenatal lung development in the human in general parallels that seen in other mammals. In the earliest or "embryonic period" (up to five weeks gestational age) the lung develops from a vertical laryngotracheal groove in the endodermal tube which evaginates and branches. The bronchial buds continue to divide and subdivide with most bronchial branching occurring between the 10th and 14th weeks. Bronchial development is complete by the 16th week.[15] This stage is called "pseudoglandular" as at this time the lung has a distinctly glandular appearance with airways lined by columnar epithelium separated by abundant undifferentiated mesenchyme. The next, or "canalicular" phase extends to the 24th or 26th week. During this period there is proliferation of the mesenchyme, a rich blood supply develops, and there is irregular flattening of the air space epithelium. Capillaries initially buried deep within the mesenchyme approach and protrude into air spaces producing the thin air-blood barrier of the mature lung in a few places.[49] Type I and Type II epithelial cells become recognizable and rare osmophilic bodies appear in type II cells.[17] The "canalicular" phase is succeeded by the "terminal sac" phase in which the changes become more widespread and the maintenance of respiration becomes possible. Birth occurs during this phase in many species, while in others there is another prenatal phase of alveolar development in which terminal sacs and ducts are transformed into alveolated structures. In the human the time and direction of alveolar development are not completely understood; however, it appears that at least some alveolar development occurs before birth.[29]

The lung of the newborn infant differs from the adult in having a simpler airway structure. Terminal bronchioles are continuous with alveolar ducts which lead into primary saccules. These initially smooth-walled saccules are divided by secondary alveolar crests in late gestation in the human and in the postnatal period in rats, mice and rabbits.[71] These crests are characterized by having an elastic fiber at their free margin.[27, 28] They mark the beginning of alveolar development, although the number of alveoli at birth is markedly less than the adult number. The cells lining air spaces are also different in the newborn from those seen in the adult. Although type I cells increase in proportion near term they still form a relatively low proportion of the airway surface compared to adult lungs. Only type II cells synthesize DNA and incorporate tritiated thymidine. They divide to produce both type I and type II cells,[38] and thus type II cells are the progenitor cells of the alveolar lining. They appear more frequent where growth of lining cells is proceeding more rapidly. Type II cells also are thought to be the site of surfactant synthesis[8, 41] and contain the osmophilic lamellar bodies associated with surfactant. These bodies appear in humans between the 22nd and 26th weeks of gestation.[17] They increase in number with gestational age and become functional at about 34–36 weeks gestation when the appearance of surfactant can be detected in the amniotic fluid. It too increases in amount to term,[21] although there is a marked degree of biologic variability. This functional maturation of the type II cells is most important, for the maintainance of effective respiration in the neonate is dependent, not on the presence of well-developed alveolar structures, but on the presence of sufficient surfactant to stabilize the terminal airways and maintain adequate residual air within the lung on expiration.

ELASTIN DEVELOPMENT

Effective respiration consistent with the stresses imposed by growth and sustained activity, however, must depend upon the structural integrity of the lung. The elastin network in the peripheral pulmonary parenchyma increasingly has been considered to have an important role in alveolar growth and therefore in the ultimate determination of lung structure.[26, 50] A recent study[39] shows that there is an increase in true elastin per gram of dry weight of lung parenchyma related to increasing gestational age and that after full term birth there is a sharp rise in true elastin content to reach adult proportions at about 6 months of postnatal age (Fig. 1). "Polar contaminant" (a protein containing a characteristic proportion of polar amino acids usually mixed with true elastin in the postalkali extraction residue of pulmonary parenchyma in fetal and young animal's lungs) is thought to be microfibrillar material closely associated with developing elastin as well as true elastin as seen by electron microscopy[60, 63] and may have a structural role in the extracellular matrix.[59, 75] The proportion of polar contaminant appears to be related to gestational age with much of the elastin in pre-term lungs actually being polar contaminant (Fig. 2).

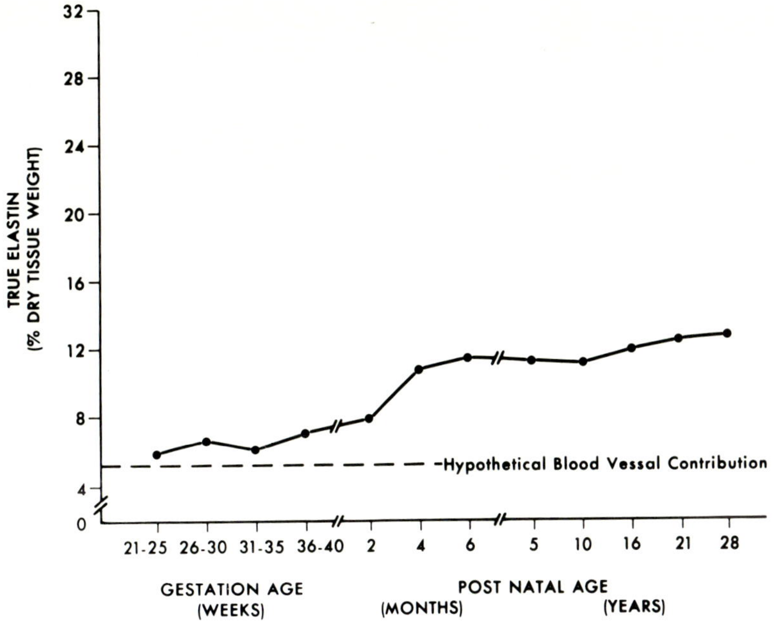

FIG. 1. This graph shows the true elastin content as a percentage of the dry weight of lung parenchyma. The alkali insoluble residue is differentiated into elastin and polar contaminant by amino-acid analysis (see text). The points plotted are grouped mean values.

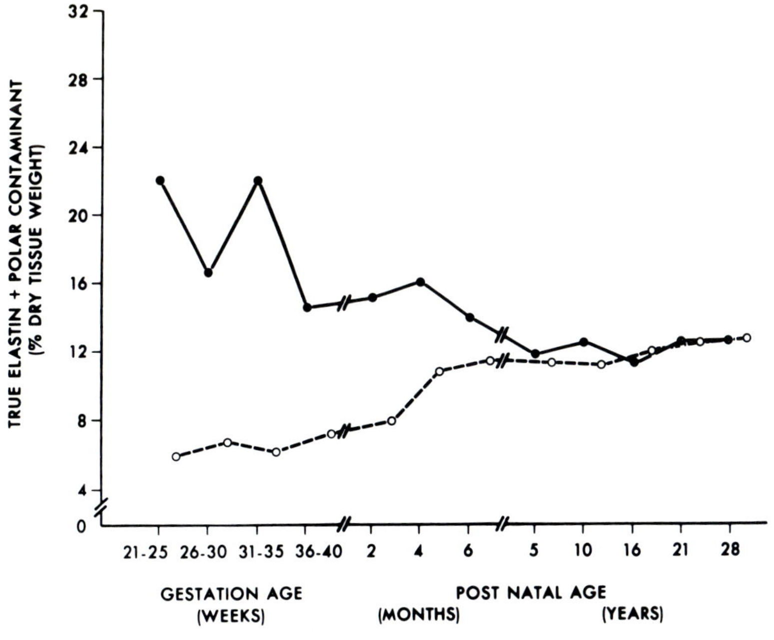

FIG. 2. The *solid line* shows the alkali insoluble polar contaminant as a percentage of dry lung parenchyma weight. The *dashed line* is that of the true elastin shown in Figure 1. The points plotted are grouped mean values.

The biochemical analysis of elastin deposition in developing lungs correlates well with the histologic appearance of elastin in the acinus (Figs. 3–8). At 20 weeks gestation only the proximal bronchioles show elastin deposition (Fig. 3). At 24 weeks the terminal bronchioles show a very thin incomplete elastic lamina with no elastin being present at the saccular parenchymal level except for minimal deposits at the point of bifurcation of the primary saccules (Fig. 4). In the period between 26 and 32 weeks gestation there is a rapid increase in the elastin content of the peripheral parenchyma with the development of secondary alveolar elastin crests (Fig. 5). There is great individual variation in the exact time of the formation of secondary alveolar elastin crests in this period. By 37 weeks gestation (Fig. 6) elastin condensations are complex and intricate in arrangement and differ only in quantity from those seen at term (Fig. 7). By 5 months postnatal age (Fig. 8) an adult proportion of elastin is present. The quantitative biochemical data agree quite well with the subjective impression. There is a slow increase in airway and acinar elastin deposition during intrauterine development, with a rapid acinar increase associated with birth at term, and with adult proportion but not absolute amounts being attained by 4 to 6 months of age.

No abnormality in this sequence of elastin deposition can be shown in preterm infants born after 28 weeks of gestation, that is, after secondary crest alveolar elastin deposition. While it has been suggested that infants with hyaline mem-

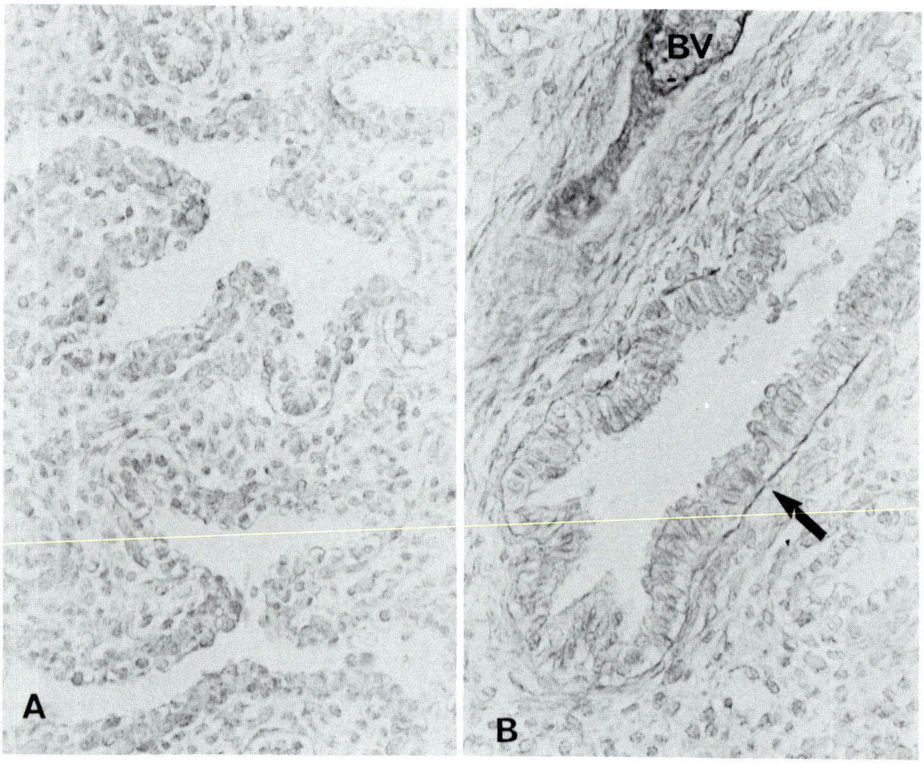

FIG. 3. 19–20 weeks gestation. (*A*) No elastin is seen in the peripheral canaliculi (× 160) but elastin has reached the intermediate bronchioles (*B*), *arrowed* (× 250). Blood vessel elastin is present (*B.V.*).

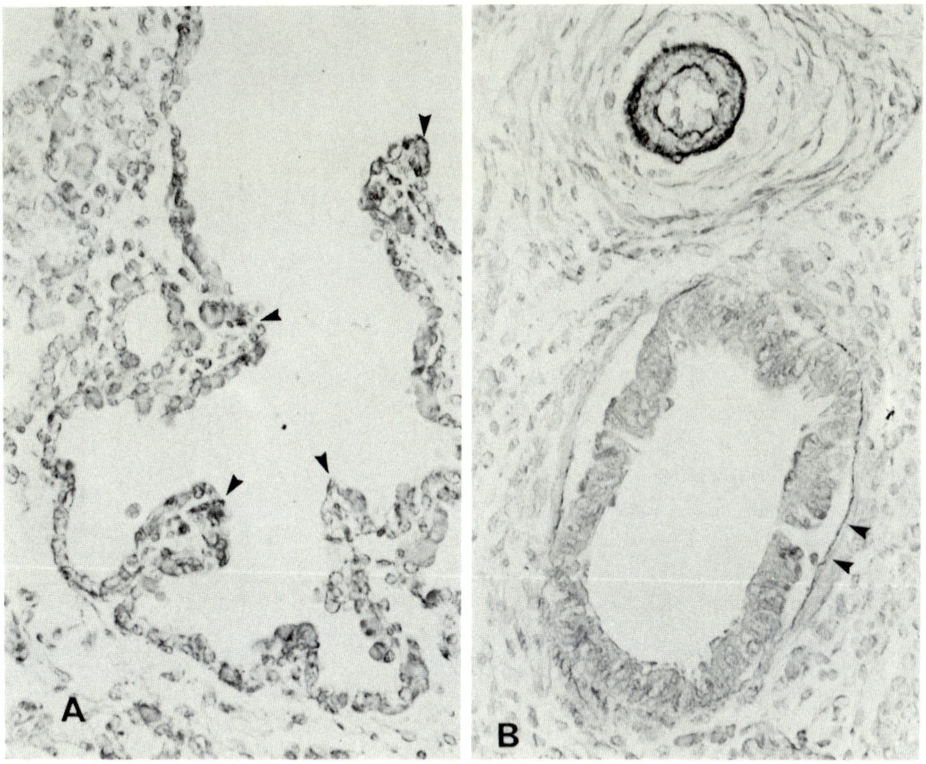

FIG. 4. 24 weeks gestation. (*A*) Elastin is beginning to appear in the terminal bronchioles, and early deposits are seen at the bifurcations of alveolar saccules (× 250). (*B*) Elastin remains constant at the intermediate level (× 250).

brane disease have a deficiency or immaturity of the elastin[30] as well as deficient surfactant production, lungs from cases of hyaline membrane disease showed no difference in elastin composition when compared with age-matched controls.[32] As well, a single case of Wilson-Mikity syndrome and 3 cases of bronchopulmonary dysplasia which were examined showed no abnormality of elastin maturity or proportion.[32] Biochemical assay of elastin in 4 infants born at a gestational age between 26 and 30 weeks and surviving between 2 weeks and 3 months suggests that preterm delivery might be followed by acceleration of elastin development in extra-uterine life.[32] Thus elastin development and concomitant alveolar multiplication may represent in some respects a birth triggered or accelerated phenomenon with the process at the alveolar level being reactive and at least in part dependent on postnatal age.

HYALINE MEMBRANE DISEASE

A variety of factors have been shown to be important in the control of pulmonary growth and maturation.[67] While these have been thought to affect functional maturation within the lung, they are also likely to influence structural development. Indeed, in the case of corticosteroids, which have recently been shown to accelerate functional maturation of the fetal lung,[48] there is, in the rabbit, an accompanying and temporary slowdown in cellular multiplication.[52]

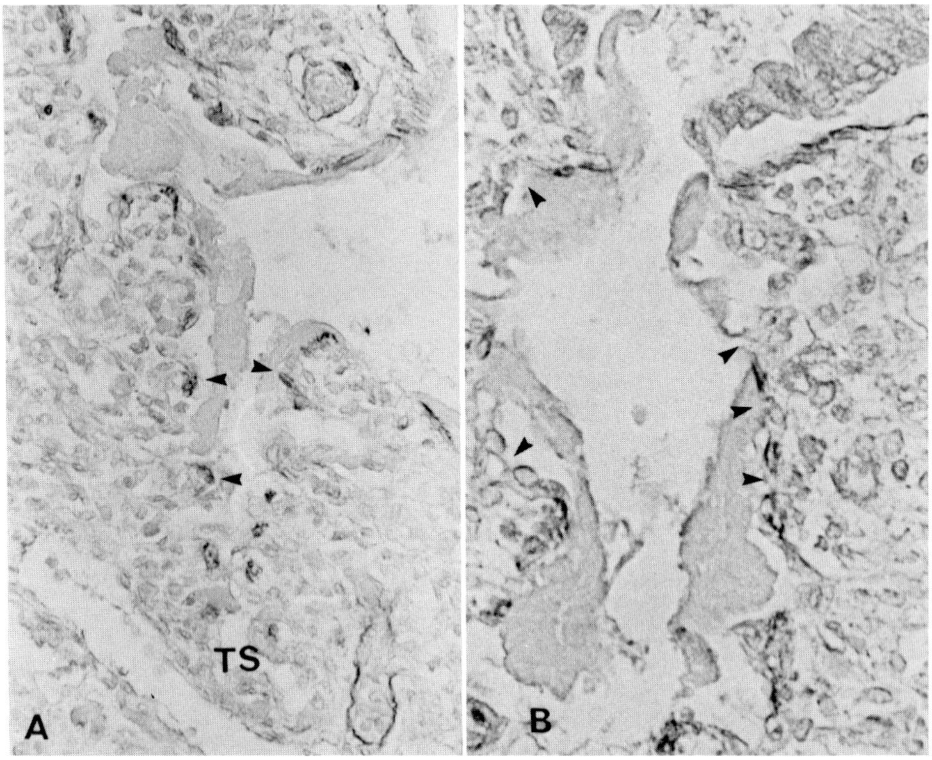

FIG. 5. 28–30 weeks gestation (with hyaline membrane disease). Alveolar elastin "crests" are seen (*A*), but note absence in terminal saccule (*TS*) (× 160). (*B*) Centripetal conversion of terminal bronchiole into a transitional duct appears to be in progress (× 250).

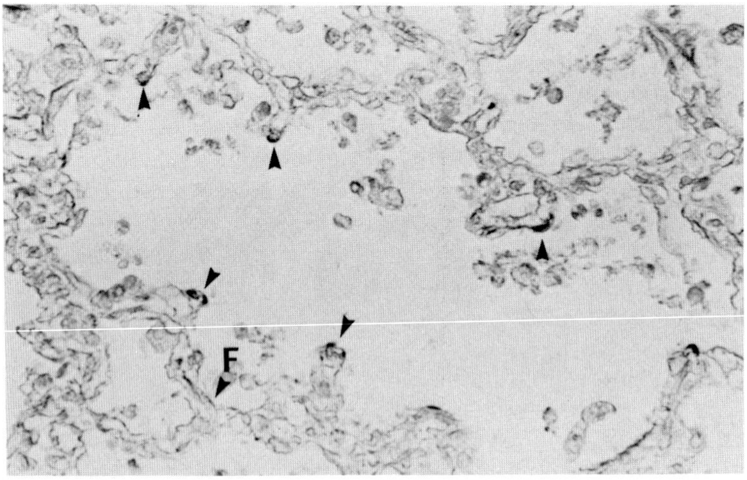

FIG. 6. 36–37 weeks gestational age. Elastin deposition is light, but the arrangement is sophisticated. The "crests", *arrowed*, are at the top of the alveolar septae. Fibrils (*F*) are seen in the walls of the alveolar septae (× 160).

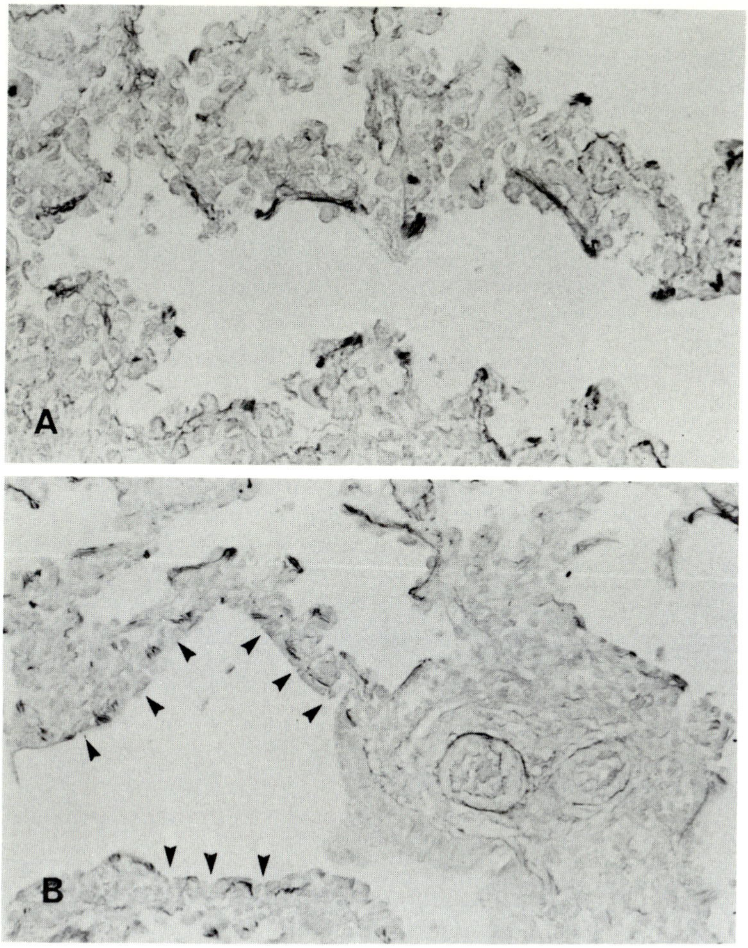

FIG. 7. 40 weeks gestation. (*A*) Elastin deposition is heavier, but the alveolar elastin arrangement is similar to Figure 6 (× 160). (*B*) Centripetal conversion is well marked (× 160).

Much, but not all, of the respiratory distress syndrome of the newborn is seen in the setting of a functionally immature respiratory system, associated with a deficiency in surfactant production. This surfactant deficiency results clinically in the respiratory distress syndrome and produces the pathologic picture of hyaline membrane disease with its typical histology of patchy atelectasis accompanied by hyaline membranes lining terminal air spaces.

While failure of surfactant production is usually the result of interruption of gestational development by premature delivery it may also be seen in the term infant either on a genetic basis or as the result of maternal disease. Primary surfactant deficiency, although the most common, is not the only pathway to the respiratory distress syndrome. Secondary surfactant deficiency may occur in some neonates with marginal or even adequate amounts of surfactant at birth. Initially adequate surfactant may be depleted as a result of inadequate secretion

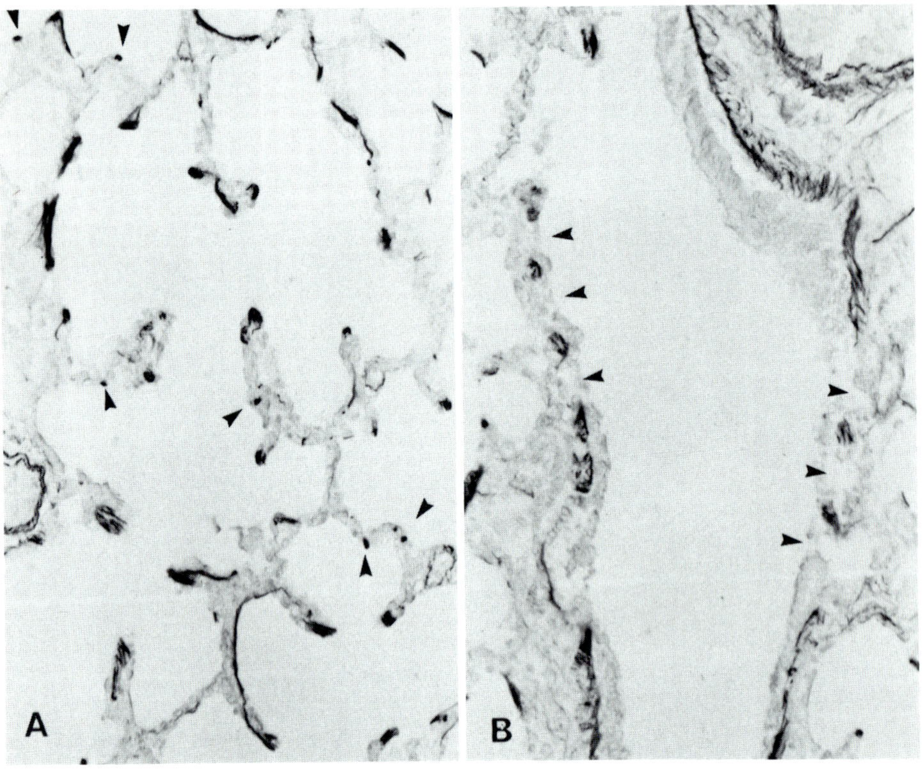

FIG. 8. 40 weeks gestation, 5 months postnatal age. (*A*) shows alveolar elastin "crests" with early subdivision (*arrowed*) into "second generation" alveoli (× 160). (*B*) shows progressing centripetal conversion.

or increased utilization. This may be seen with injury to the surfactant producing cells, usually due to birth-related anoxic injury, but also possibly to chemical injury[33, 47] or infection.[37] Tachypnea or over-ventilation may also deplete marginal surfactant stores.[76] Surfactant deficiency may be short-lived if adequate supportive measures allow survival of the infant over the period necessary for the synthesis and secretion of adequate surfactant. However, without these measures (and occasionally even with them) the infant enters a spiraling course in which the initial surfactant deficiency produces a higher surface tension within the terminal air spaces. This, combined with alveolar retractive forces, produces an increased resistance in pulmonary arteries and arterioles leading to shunting. The consequent hypoperfusion within the lung then further damages the surfactant producing system resulting in still further reductions in pulmonary function, with development of hypoxemia and acidosis, occasionally accompanied by disseminated intravascular coagulation, and the infant's death.[31]

COMPLICATIONS OF THERAPY

AIR-LEAKS

With the recognition of the central role of surfactant deficiency in hyaline membrane disease and a more complete understanding of the pathophysiology of the disease, more effective therapeutic measures became widely employed. These largely consist of attempts to maintain air spaces in expansion during expiration through the use of continuous distending pressure, which may be applied in a variety of ways. The use of continuous distending pressure therapy permits a more rapid decrease in inspired oxygen concentration and the avoidance of respirator assistance in all but the most severe cases. It has resulted in substantially increased survival in hyaline membrane disease.[18] While the mortality from hyaline membrane disease has been markedly reduced with the employment of continuous distending pressures, assisted ventilation, and increased inspired oxygen concentration; these aids are not without attendent complications which may in themselves produce significant morbidity and mortality. The overall trend, however, has been one of reduced mortality.

The rate of lung rupture and a variety of air-leaks have almost doubled with the use of these devices.[11] Rupture of terminal air spaces permits the dissection of air into the interstitial tissues of the lung where it may follow several pathways. It may reach the pleural surface and rupture into the pleural space producing pneumothorax.[69] It may dissect along the pathway of bronchi and vessels into the mediastinum where it may extend into the subcutaneous tissues of the neck, chest and arms producing pneumomediastinum and subcutaneous emphysema[69], it may extend along the pulmonary arteries and rupture into the pericardial sac producing pneumopericardium[14] or it may dissect through the mediastinum into the peritoneum, producing pneumoperitoneum.[46] It is also possible for this air to leak into large blood vessels with the attendent rare complication of air embolism.[20] While many of these air-leaks can and do occur spontaneously, especially with the high intrathoracic pressure generated with the first breaths, their incidence has increased greatly in the period of modern therapy of hyaline membrane disease. There is some suggestion that once these complications occur the improved survival with modern therapy is lost and this group of infants have a less favourable prognosis even when the leaks are aggressively treated.[11]

A new complication due to the long-term presence of air within the interstitial tissues of the lung has recently been described.[66] The continuous presence of air, presumably under pressure, within the interstitial tissues of the lung over a long period of time may induce the formation of cystic spaces accompanied by a granulomatous reaction not unlike that seen with chronic pneumatosis intestinalis. It has been suggested that as many as 10–30% of infants with bronchopulmonary dysplasia may show this additional complication. While conservative medical therapy may close the cysts, in some cases surgery may be necessary. When localized, surgical excision of the affected areas may be effective; but when generalized it may interfere so seriously with pulmonary function that the infant's survival is not possible. Although this condition is not widely recognized, when localized it represents a treatable complication and its wider recognition may lead to earlier surgical intervention and improved survival.

Bronchopulmonary Dysplasia

There have been studies[10, 68] which suggest that mechanical trauma related to ventilator therapy produces the lung injury known as bronchopulmonary dysplasia; however, most investigators feel that the toxic effects of increased inspired oxygen are of primary importance.[5, 13, 62] There is conflicting evidence on the role of artificial ventilation in the pathogenesis of bronchopulmonary dysplasia,[9, 10, 13, 53, 68] and its importance remains to be resolved. The toxic properties of oxygen are now well recognized[23, 33, 53, 64, 74] and there has been a recent suggestion that immature or damaged tissues may be even more susceptible to the toxic effects of oxygen.

Bronchopulmonary dysplasia is seen in infants following several days of intensive respiratory support. It resembles the shock lung state produced in adults in a variety of conditions, and once established probably follows a similar pathway.[36] Immaturity or damage to the infant lung results in clinically evident respiratory distress. Treatment with assisted ventilation and increased inspired oxygen concentration permits survival of the infant over a period of time with a damaged respiratory system. This damage may be further accentuated by the effects of oxygen on pulmonary epithelial cells and blood vessels and by ventilatory pressures which alter the hemodynamics within the lung and result in continued injury to epithelial and interstitial tissues.[9, 54, 57] The pulmonary lesions seen in infants with bronchopulmonary dysplasia are similar to those seen in experimental oxygen toxicity and in a variety of conditions loosely grouped as the "adult respiratory distress syndrome."[9, 36] The lesions are ultrastructurally similar and show a similar progression.[33] The early changes are exudative, with injury to epithelial and endothelial cells leading to pulmonary edema and hyaline membrane formation, while later changes are proliferative involving the epithelial cells of airways and terminal air spaces as well as interstitial cells.[53] These lesions often coexist, as damage is progressive with continuous exposure leading to extensive sloughing of epithelial cells, septal edema, fibrin thrombi, hyperplastic regenerative epithelial changes, and interstitial fibrosis. Ultimately simplification in the pulmonary architecture results perhaps through the obliteration of smaller air spaces.[13, 62] While the precise roles of oxygen and artificial ventilation are not known in this situation, there is compelling evidence in experimental animals for a primary role for oxygen toxicity.[23, 74] Oxygen usually produces change in newborn animals and these changes resemble those seen in adults and are not affected by artificial ventilation.[23] Newborn animals are less susceptible than mature ones to oxygen toxicity; however, when respiratory distress is produced by other means, inspired oxygen tends to increase the severity of that respiratory distress.[64] The evidence, however, is less clear in man and even more complicated in the newborn, most of whom initially have hyaline membrane disease; but the human situation seems analogous to that seen in experimental animals.

The prognosis of infants who survive the respiratory distress syndrome has been a major concern. There have been many studies evaluating the physical, neurologic, and behavioral development of survivors of hyaline membrane disease, and more recently of bronchopulmonary dysplasia.[3, 22, 35, 42, 55, 65] There is evidence that some of these survivors show residual pulmonary abnormalities[22, 42, 65] and that they may also have an increased susceptibility to lower respiratory tract infections in infancy and early childhood.[55] These children in general show no cardiopulmonary disability in early childhood[35] however, the long-term implications of the abnormalities in pulmonary function which have been demonstrated in them[22, 42] remain a concern. A recent study[22] suggests that their functional abnormality is an increase in small airways resistance in childhood. The duration of this abnormality is not known, nor is its implication for the development of pulmonary disease in adulthood.

While it is possible that the gross alterations in pulmonary structure seen in bronchopulmonary dysplasia may produce lasting effects on lung maturation, there has been no demonstration in those who survive that this is so. Whether some of the abnormalities produced in these infants remain as the basis for any of the variety of cystic or fibrotic pulmonary processes is a matter of speculation only. The potential for structural regenerative activity within the infant lung is not known. It is well known in both man and animals, that the residual pulmonary tissue will increase in weight and volume following pneumonectomy[71] and it has recently been demonstrated that this increase in the young rabbit is reflected by the development of new alveoli tending to compensate in numbers for those lost at pneumonectomy.[43] The precise stimuli for alveolar multiplication in this situation are not understood nor is it known what effect age and disease have upon these processes. The potential for the remodeling of injured areas in the infant lung and/or for the development of compensatory alveoli is not known but may exist.

YELLOW MEMBRANES

Yellow hyaline membranes have been the subject of several recent reports[19, 73] and have been discussed as a new variant of hyaline membrane disease. These are not really new observations and were seen by many pediatric pathologists prior to their recent reports in the literature.[73] These yellow membranes are bright canary yellow material which retain this color in both stained and unstained histologic material. They are seen exclusively in infants with the respiratory distress syndrome who survive with continuing disease into the period of diffuse injury and repair (bronchopulmonary dysplasia). While these membranes have not been well analyzed, they resemble ordinary hyaline membranes in many respects. They often appear as a discoloration of the air surface of otherwise typical-appearing hyaline membranes. They stain positively for bile. Ordinary hyaline membranes are formed of necrotic epithelial cells, aspirated amniotic cells and possibly fluid, and a transudate of blood constituents.[44] In addition, yellow membranes contain needle-like structures on electron microscopy, thought to be bilirubin-protein or lipoprotein complexes.[73] With increasing survival, the hyaline membranes appear more sharply delineated and often more deeply stained[44]: this may be associated with water loss from the membrane. A tenuous association with intrahepatic cholestasis has been suggested[19] but has not been supported.[73]

Many of the affected infants have a history of hyperbilirubinemia, but usually only of modest degree. They show no consistent differences in response to therapy from control infants. The only significant difference is that they seem to have survived longer than control subjects.[73] The modern therapy of the respiratory distress syndrome permits greatly prolonged survival in some infants. Prolonged survival with continued disease may present a mechanism for the formation of the yellow membranes. If the period of time of survival with active disease is sufficient, hyaline membranes may become dehydrated enough so that the bilirubin bound to proteins in the transudate may become sufficiently concentrated to become visible as a yellow discoloration. This dehydration would naturally be more pronounced at the air rather than tissue interface of the membrane, thus producing the characteristic appearance. Although many of these infants have only mild hyperbilirubinemia, the process of membrane dehydration would produce sufficient concentration to result in a visible yellow color without a history of serious hyperbilirubinemia.

CONGENITAL PNEUMONIA

In the otherwise normal neonate, incidents surrounding birth may result in impaired respiratory function on an entirely different basis from that seen in the premature. Infection acquired through the aspiration of micro-organisms before or during delivery may result in congenital pneumonia presenting as respiratory distress in the neonate.[12, 45] Pneumonia in these infants remains an important clinical entity.[12] Because the response of the neonate to infection is generally nonspecific, infection remains an important part of the differential diagnosis of respiratory distress in the newborn. It has been generally considered,[45] although without convincing experimental evidence, that pH changes in the amniotic fluid, colloid substances, etc., may produce inflammation in the neonatal lung and that much of what is called congenital pneumonia is produced on this basis. However, it has been shown experimentally that only pathogenic micro-organisms are capable of producing these changes.[45] The response to infection in the neonate, especially in the premature, is much less prominent than in the older child or adult. In newborns the neutrophil infiltrate in the lungs may be scant even when severe pneumonia is present. The best example of this is in the recently recognized syndromes of Group B streptococcal infection in the newborn.[25, 34, 51]

There are two syndromes of Group B streptococcal infection in the newborn.[1, 37] The first is the early onset septicemia type which presents as respiratory distress, resembling the idiopathic respiratory distress syndrome, soon after birth and is characterized by acute pulmonary infection and a high mortality rate. The second is a meningitis of somewhat later onset (days to weeks) and better prognosis. The histologic picture of Group B streptococcal pneumonia in the newborn characteristically shows little in the way of an inflammatory response; instead thick hyaline membranes, often containing numerous bacterial colonies, line terminal air spaces.[1, 37] Mature infants as well as premature may be affected.[1, 37] It has been suggested[37] that the Group B streptococci may play a specific role in the development of a process like hyaline membrane disease in more mature lungs. The suggested mechanism of streptococcal-induced injury to alveolar epithelial cells and capillary endothelial cells by growth within alveoli and tissue invasion could produce exudation of plasma proteins into the alveoli leading to the formation of hyaline membranes. This mechanism is analogous to that proposed for membrane formation in pulmonary oxygen toxicity[33] and other toxic agents in adults.[47]

PULMONARY HYPOPLASIA

While the vast majority of cases of respiratory distress in the newborn period is accounted for by conditions already discussed, occasionally this respiratory distress is the result of an abnormality in pulmonary development. The largest group of these are infants with either unilateral or bilateral pulmonary hypoplasia, often in association with a variety of other conditions. Many of the syndromes have now been grouped together on the hypothesis that a single factor, oligohydramnios, results in the associated pulmonary hypoplasia.[56, 70] The pathogenetic mechanism suggested[70] is compression of the developing lung. The mechanism of compression has been associated with pulmonary hypoplasia seen in association with diaphragmatic hernia, where compression of developing pulmonary structures by the herniated abdominal contents inhibits the later stages of pulmonary development.[70] Compression is also recognized as the mechanism of pulmonary hypoplasia in the syndrome of asphyxiating thoracic dystrophy in which deficient skeletal growth limits pulmonary growth in late gestation.[70] A variety of other syndromes, notably Potter's syndrome, in which pulmonary hypoplasia is seen in association with renal and other anomalies have recently been grouped together with those known to be related to compression.[58, 70] They show no qualitative differences in type of hypoplasia, and changes in histology correlate with severity of growth retardation and not with associated abnormalities.[58] Many syndromes associated with pulmonary hypoplasia have in common a history of oligohydramnios. It is postulated[70] that external compression of the thoracic cage with oligohydramnios may result in retardation of lung growth in late gestation producing pulmonary hypoplasia in much the same fashion as does diaphragmatic hernia or the syndrome of asphyxiating thoracic dystrophy. The mechanism, however, may be somewhat more complex than simple compression. Another possibility[70] is that an accelerated outflow of fetal lung fluid because of altered pressure gradients secondary to oligohydramnios may be a factor in the retarded pulmonary development. The gradient of flow of lung fluid is outward; and this fluid contributes substantially to amniotic fluid.[67] Available space is an important factor in postnatal lung growth[67] and a recent observation[2] with chronic tracheal drainage in fetal lambs suggests that an optimum fluid volume is important in fetal lung growth as well. The distention of the fetal lung by an appropriate volume of fluid may be of paramount importance in normal development.

REFERENCES

1. Ablow, R. C., Driscoll, S. G., Effmann, E. L., Gross, I., Jolles, C. J., Uauy, R., and Warshaw, J. B.: A comparison of early-onset group B streptococcal neonatal infection and the respiratory-distress syndrome of the newborn. *N. Engl. J. Med. 294:* 65–70, 1976.
2. Alcorn, D., Adamson, T. M., Lambert, T. F., Maloney, J. E., Ritchie, B. C., and Robinson, P. M.: Morphologic characteristics of chronic tracheal ligation and drainage in the fetal lamb. *J. Anat. 123:* 649–660, 1977.
3. Ambrus, C. M., Weintraub, D. H., Niswander, K. R., Fischer, L., Fleishman, J., Bross, I. D. J., and Ambrus, J. L.: Evaluation of survivors of respiratory distress syndrome at 4 years of age. *Am. J. Dis. Child 120:* 296–302, 1970.
4. Amy, R., Bowes, D., Burri, P. H., and Thurlbeck, W. M.: Postnatal growth of the mouse lung. *J. Anat.* 1977, (in press).
5. Anderson, W. R., and Strickland, M. B.: Pulmonary complications of oxygen therapy in the neonate. Postmortem study of bronchopulmonary dysplasia with emphasis on fibroproliferative obliterative bronchitis and bronchiolitis. *Arch. Pathol. 91:* 506–514, 1971.
6. Auld, P. A. M.: Pulmonary physiology of the newborn infant. In *Pulmonary Physiology of the Fetus, Newborn and Child,* edited by Scarpelli, E. M., pp. 140–165. Philadelphia, Lea & Febiger, 1975.

7. Auld, P. A. M.: Pulmonary transition from fetal life. In *Reviews in Perinatal Medicine,* edited by Scarpelli, E. M., Cosmi, E. V., pp. 125–148, Baltimore, University Park Press, 1976.
8. Balis, J. U., and Conen, P. E.: The role of alveolar inclusion bodies in the developing lung. *Lab. Invest. 13:* 1215–1229, 1964.
9. Banerjee, C. K., Girling, D. J., and Wigglesworth, J. S.: Pulmonary fibroplasia in newborn babies treated with oxygen and artificial ventilation. *Arch. Dis. Child. 47:* 509–518, 1972.
10. Barnes, N. D., Hull, D., Glover, W. J., and Miller, A. D.: Effects of prolonged positive pressure ventilation in infancy. *Lancet 2:* 1096–1099, 1969.
11. Berg, T. J., Pagtakhan, R. D., Reed, M. H., Langston, C., and Chernick, V.: Bronchopulmonary dysplasia and lung rupture in hyaline membrane disease: Influence of continuous distending pressure. *Pediatrics 55:* 51–54, 1975.
12. Bernstein, J., and Wang, J.: The pathology of neonatal pneumonia. *Am. J. Dis. Child. 101:* 350–363, 1961.
13. Bonikos, D. S., Bensch, K. G., Northway, W. H., Jr., and Edwards, D. K.: Bronchopulmonary dysplasia: The pulmonary pathologic sequel of necrotizing bronchiolitis and pulmonary fibrosis. *Human Pathol. 7:* 643–666, 1976.
14. Brans, Y. W., Pitts, M., and Cassady, G.: Neonatal pneumopericardium, *Am. J. Dis. Child. 130:* 393–396, 1976.
15. Bucher, U., and Reid, L.: Development of the intrasegmental bronchial tree: The pattern of branching and development of cartilage at various stages of intra-uterine life. *Thorax 16:* 207–218, 1961.
16. Burri, P. H., Dbaly, J., and Weibel, E. R.: The postnatal growth of the rat lung. I: Morphometry. *Anat. Rec. 178:* 711–730, 1974.
17. Campiche, M. A., Gautier, A., Hernandez, E. I., and Reymond, A.: An electron microscope study of the fetal development of the human lung. *Pediatrics 32:* 976–994, 1963.
18. Chernick, V.: Hyaline-membrane disease—Therapy with constant lung-distending pressure. *N. Engl. J. Med. 289:* 302–304, 1973.
19. Cho, S. Y., and Sastre, M.: Pulmonary yellow hyaline membrane disease. New variant in premature infants with intrahepatic cholestosis. *Arch. Pathol. Lab. Med. 100:* 145–146, 1976.
20. Chopra, D. R., Baker, P. C., Beam, C. W., and Kassel, S. H.: "Arteriovenous air embolism". A complication of mechanical ventilation in respiratory distress syndrome. *Clin. Pediatr. 15:* 178–180, 1976.
21. Clements, J. A., Platzker, A. C. G., Tierney, D. F., Hobel, C. J., Creasy, R. K., Margolis, A. J., Thibeault, D. W., Tooley, W. H., and Oh, W.: Assessment of the risk of the respiratory-distress syndrome by a rapid test for surfactant in amniotic fluid. *N. Engl. J. Med. 286:* 1077–1081, 1972.
22. Coates, A. L., Bergsteinsson, H., Desmond, K., Outerbridge, E. W., and Beaudry, P. H.: Long-term pulmonary sequelae of premature birth with and without idiopathic respiratory distress syndrome. *J. Pediatr. 90:* 611–616, 1977.
23. de Lemos, R., Wolfsdorf, J., Nachman, R., Block, A. J., Leiby, G., Wilkinson, H. A., Allen, T., Haller, J. A., Morgan, W., and Avery, M. E.: Lung injury from oxygen in lambs: The role of artificial ventilation. *Anesthesiology 30:* 609–618, 1969.
24. de Lorimier, A. A., Magnus, A. G., and Tyler, W. S.: Morphometry of normal and hypoplastic lungs in newborn lambs. *Curr. Top. Surg. Res. 1:* 431–442, 1969.
25. Eickhoff, T. C., Klein, J. O., Daly, A. K., Ingall, D., and Finland, M.: Neonatal sepsis and other infections due to Group B beta-hemolytic streptococci. *N. Engl. J. Med. 271:* 1221–1228, 1964.
26. Emery, J. L.: Connective tissue and lymphatics. In *The Anatomy of the Developing Lung,* edited by Emery, J. L., Chapter IV, pp. 49–73, London, Heinemann Medical Books, 1969.
27. Emery, J. L.: The postnatal development of the human lung and its implications for lung pathology. *Respiration (Suppl.) 27:* 41–50, 1970.
28. Emery, J. L., and Fagan, D. G.: New alveoli—Where and how? *Arch. Dis. Child. 45:* 145, 1970.
29. Emery, J. L., and Mithal, A.: The number of alveoli in the terminal respiratory unit of man during late intrauterine life and childhood. *Arch. Dis. Child. 35:* 544–547, 1960.
30. Evans, H. E., Keller, S., and Mandl, I.: Lung tissue elastin composition in newborn infants with the respiratory distress syndrome and other diseases. *J. Clin. Invest. 54:* 213–217, 1974.
31. Farrell, P. M., and Avery, M. E.: Hyaline membrane disease. *Am. Rev. Resp. Dis. 111:* 657–688, 1975.

32. Fagan, D. G., unpublished observations.

33. Gould, V. E., Tosco, R., Wheelis, R. F., Gould, N. S., and Kapanci, Y.: Oxygen pneumonitis in man: Ultrastructural observations on the development of alveolar lesions. *Lab. Invest. 26:* 499–508, 1972.

34. Hood, M., Janney, A., and Dameron, G.: Beta hemolytic streptococcus group B, associated with problems of the perinatal period. *Am. J. Obstet. Gynecol. 82:* 809–818, 1961.

35. Johnson, J. D., Malachowski, N. C., Grobstein, R., Welsh, D., Daily, W. J. R., and Sunshine, P.: Prognosis of children surviving with the aid of mechanical ventilation in the newborn period. *J. Pediatr. 84:* 272–276, 1974.

36. Katzenstein, A-L. A., Bloor, C. M., Leibow, A. A.: Diffuse alveolar damage—The role of oxygen, shock, and related factors. A review. *Am. J. Pathol. 85:* 210–228, 1976.

37. Katzenstein, A-L., Davis, C., Braude, A.: Pulmonary changes in neonatal sepsis due to group B β-hemolytic streptococcous: Relation to hyaline membrane disease. *J. Infect. Dis. 133:* 430–435, 1976.

38. Kauffman, S. L., Burri, P. H., and Weibel, E. R.: The postnatal growth of the rat lung. II. Autoradiography. *Anat. Rec. 180:* 63–76, 1974.

39. Keeley, F. W., Fagan, D. G., and Webster, S. I.: Quantity and character of elastin in developing human lung parenchymal tissues of normal infants and infants with respiratory distress syndrome. *J. Lab. Clin. Med. 90:* 981–989, 1977.

40. Kikkawa, Y.: Morphology and morphologic development of the lung. In *Pulmonary Physiology of the Fetus, Newborn, and Child,* edited by Scarpelli, E. M., pp. 37–60. Philadelphia, Lea & Febiger, 1975.

41. Klaus, M., Reiss, O. K., Tooley, W. H., Piel, C., Clements, J. A.: Alveolar epithelial cell mitochondria as source of the surface-active lung lining. *Science 137:* 750–751, 1962.

42. Lamarre, A., Linsao, L., Reilly, B. J., Swyer, P. R., and Levison, H.: Residual pulmonary abnormalities in survivors of idiopathic respiratory distress syndrome. *Am. Rev. Respir. Dis. 108:* 56–61, 1973.

43. Langston, C., Sachdeva, P., Cowan, M. J., Haines, J., Crystal, R, G., and Thurlbeck, W. M.: Alveolar multiplication in the contralateral lung after unilateral pneumonectomy in the rabbit. *Am. Rev. Resp. Dis. 115:* 7–13, 1977.

44. Lauweryns, J. M.: "Hyaline membrane disease" in newborn infants. Radiographic, and light and electron microscopic studies. *Human Pathol. 1:* 175–204, 1970.

45. Lauweryns, J., Bernat, R., Lerut, A., and Detournay, G.: Intrauterine pneumonia. An experimental study. *Biol. Neonate 22:* 301–318, 1973.

46. Leonidas, J. C., Hall, R. T., Rhodes, P. G., and Amoury, R. A.: Pneumoperitoneum in ventilated newborns. A medical or a surgical problem? *Am. J. Dis. Child. 128:* 677–680, 1974.

47. Liebow, A. A., and Carrington, C. B.: The interstitial pneumonias. In *Frontiers of Pulmonary Radiology: Pathophysiologic, Roentgenographic and Radioisotopic Considerations.* Proceedings of the Symposium sponsored by Harvard Medical School, April 21–22, 1967, edited by Simon, M., Potchlen, E. J., and Le May, M., pp. 102–141, New York, Grune & Stratton, 1969.

48. Liggins, G. C., and Howie, R. N.: A controlled trial of antepartum glucocorticoid treatment for prevention of the respiratory distress syndrome in premature infants. *Pediatrics 50:* 515–525, 1972.

49. Loosli, C. G., and Baker, R. F.: The human lung: Microscopic structure and diffusion. In *Ciba Foundation Symposium, on Pulmonary Structure and Function,* pp. 194–204, London, Churchill, 1962.

50. Loosli, C. G., and Potter, E. L.: Pre- and post-natal development of the respiratory portion of the human lung with special reference to the elastic fibers. *Am. Rev. Resp. Dis. 80 Part 2: 5–23, 1959.*

51. McCracken, G. H., Jr.: Group B *streptococci:* The new challenge in neonatal infections. *J. Pediatr. 82:* 703–706, 1973.

52. Motoyama, E. K., Orzalesi, M. M., Kikkawa, Y., Kaibara, M., Wu, B., Zigas, C. J., and Cook, C. D.: Effect of cortisol on the maturation of fetal rabbit lungs. *Pediatrics 48:* 547–555, 1971.

53. Nash, G., Blennerhassett, J. B., and Pontoppidan, H.: Pulmonary lesions associated with oxygen therapy and artificial ventilation. *N. Engl. J. Med. 276:* 368–374, 1967.

54. Northway, W. H., Jr., Rosan, R. C., and Porter, D. Y.: Pulmonary disease following respirator therapy of hyaline-membrane disease: Bronchopulmonary dysplasia. *N. Engl. J. Med. 276:*

357-368, 1967.

55. Outerbridge, E. W., Nogrady, B., Beaudry, P. H., and Stern, L.: Idiopathic respiratory distress syndrome. Recurrent respiratory illness in survivors. *Am. J. Dis. Child. 123:* 99-104, 1972.
56. Perlman, M., and Levin, M.: Fetal pulmonary hypoplasia, anuria, and oligohydramnios: Clinicopathologic observations and review of the literature. *Am. J. Obstet. Gynecol. 118:* 1119-1123, 1974.
57. Philip, A. G. S.: Oxygen plus pressure plus time: The etiology of bronchopulmonary dysplasia. *Pediatrics 55:* 44-50, 1975.
58. Reale, F. R., and Esterly, J. R.: Pulmonary hypoplasia: A morphometric study of the lungs of infants with diaphragmatic hernia, anencephaly, and renal malformations. *Pediatrics 51:* 91-96, 1973.
59. Robert, L., and Comte, P.: Aminoacid composition of structural glycoproteins. *Life Sci. Part II. 7:* 493-497, 1968.
60. Robert, B., Szigeti, M., Derouette, J-C., and Robert, L.: Studies on the nature of the "microfibrillar" component of elastic fibers. *Eur. J. Biochem. 21:* 507-516, 1971.
61. Robertson, B.: Pulmonary structure during neonatal adaptation. In *Reviews in Perinatal Medicine,* edited by Scarpelli, E. M., and Cosmi, E. V., pp. 149-164, Baltimore, University Park Press, 1976.
62. Rosan, R. L.: Hyaline membrane disease and a related spectrum of pneumopathies. In *Perspectives in Pediatric Pathology,* Vol. 2, edited by Rosenberg, H. S., and Bolande, R. P., pp. 15-60, Chicago, Year Book Publishers, Inc., 1975.
63. Ross, R., and Bornstein, P.: The elastic fiber. I: The separation and partial characterization of its macromolecular components. *J. Cell. Biol. 40:* 366-381, 1969.
64. Shanklin, D. R.: On the pulmonary toxicity of oxygen. I. The relationship of oxygen content to the effect of oxygen on the lung. *Lab. Invest. 21:* 439-448, 1969.
65. Shephard, F. M., Johnston, R. B., Jr., Klatte, E. C., Burko, H., and Stahlman, M.: Residual pulmonary findings in clinical hyaline-membrane disease. *N. Engl. J. Med. 279:* 1063-1071, 1968.
66. Stocker, J. T.: Persistent interstitial emphysema with giant cell reaction in the neonatal period. *Am. J. Pathol. 82:* 6a-7a, 1976 (abstr.).
67. Strang, L. B.: Growth and development of the lung: Fetal and postnatal. *Annu. Rev. Physiol. 39:* 253-276, 1977.
68. Taghizadeh, A., and Reynolds, E. O. R.: Pathogenesis of bronchopulmonary dysplasia following hyaline membrane disease. *Am. J. Pathol. 82:* 241-264, 1976.
69. Thibeault, D. M., Lachman, R. S., Laul, V. R., and Kwong, M. S.: Pulmonary interstitial emphysema, pneumomediastinum, and pneumothorax. Occurrence in the newborn infant. *Am. J. Dis. Child 126:* 611-614, 1973.
70. Thomas, I. T., and Smith, D. W.: Oligohydramnios, cause of nonrenal features of Potter's syndrome, including pulmonary hypoplasia. *J. Pediatr. 84:* 811-814, 1974.
71. Thurlbeck, W. M.: Postnatal growth and development of the lung. *Am. Rev. Respir. Dis. 111:* 803-844, 1975.
72. Valdés-Dapena, M. A., and Arey, J. B.: The causes of neonatal mortality: An analysis of 501 autopsies on newborn infants. *J. Pediatr. 77:* 366-375, 1970.
73. Valdés-Dapena, M. A., Nissim, J. E., Arey, J. B., Godleski, J., Schaaf, H. D., and Haust, M. D.: Yellow pulmonary hyaline membranes. *J. Pediatr. 89:* 128-130, 1976.
74. Wolfe, W. G., and DeVries, W. C.: Oxygen toxicity. *Annu. Rev. Med. 26:* 203-217, 1975.
75. Wolff, I., Fuchswans, W., Weiser, M., Furthmayr, H., and Timpl, R.: Acidic structural proteins of connective tissue. Characterization of their heterogeneous nature. *Eur. J. Biochem. 20:* 426-431, 1971.
76. Wyszogrodski, I., Kyei-Aboagye, K., Taeusch, H. W., and Avery, M. E.: Surfactant inactivation of hyperventilation: Conservation by end-expiratory pressure. *J. Appl. Physiol. 38:* 461-466, 1975.

Chapter 16

Miscellany*

WILLIAM M. THURLBECK

This chapter is intended to provide recent information that appears relevant and important but which was not covered during the presentations in Toronto or elsewhere in this monograph. It is not intended as an exhaustive review of the recent literature but will stress particular subjects, take points of view, and indicate useful source material. In most sections the heading will contain a reference which reviews the topic.

CELLULAR DIFFERENTIATION AND TRANSFORMATION

In Chapter 1, Kuhn outlined the ultrastructure of type I and type II cells of the lung. The type I cell, being very thin and having a very large surface area, has the primary function of covering the alveolar walls. Also, because it forms tight junctions with type II cells, the alveolar wall is relatively impermeable. Type II cells have the exocrine function of secreting surfactant and, as pointed out in Chapters 1 and 2, are generally less sensitive to toxic agents than type I cells. This is biologically advantageous, since it is now apparent that type II cells are the progenitor cells of type I and type II cells in health as well as disease. Evans[36] et al. and Adamson and Bowden[1] showed that type II cells proliferated following inhalational injury and subsequently gave rise to type I cells. Adamson and Bowden also showed that type II cells, rather than type I cells, were labeled with tritiated thymidine in the latter part of gestation and early postnatal period.[2]

* This work was supported by Grant No. DG-152 from the Medical Research Council.

This occurred despite the fact that rapid lung growth and differentiation were occurring at this time with the resultant formation of many type I cells. If the animals are killed sufficiently long after injection of tritiated thymidine so that cellular division can occur, type I cells will label but will contain half the number of grains found in type II cells of animals killed shortly after injection. Thus, initially, both after injury and in differentiation, type II cells appear and multiply to form further type II cells. At a later stage, and under an unknown stimulus, type II cells then divide to form another type II cell and a type I cell. It is thus fortunate that the type II cell is relatively less susceptible to injury; when type II cells die, regeneration of the alveolar lining epithelium is not possible.

In Chapter 1, Kuhn also discusses the structure and function of Clara cells and indicates that their secretory product may be related to surfactant. Interestingly, this cell appears to be the progenitor cell of the peripheral airways. Evans *et al.*[37] showed that in the early stages following inhalation of NO_2, Clara cells multiplied and at a later stage these cells changed, perhaps by maturation-division, to ciliated and goblet cells in the airways. The situation is complex, however, since Adamson and Bowden[3] have just shown that type II cells may transform to form ciliated cells in the alveolar walls of mice following the administration of a single dose of bleomycin.

ALVEOLAR GROWTH AND MULTIPLICATION[106]

A major area of investigation in the last decade has been the study of the postnatal growth of the lung in humans and in animals. It is now apparent that in dogs, rats, mice, and rabbits the lung is qualitatively very different at birth compared to adult life.[4, 19, 99] In these species, the peripheral lung parenchyma is formed by structures known as primary saccules.[14] These are relatively simple structures with smooth walls and a double capillary layer.[19] They are larger than the smallest adult units, which are multifaceted alveoli with a single capillary layer in their walls. In the postnatal period, primary saccules are subdivided into smaller units by structures termed secondary crests, each of which has an elastic fiber, together with some collagen, at its free margin.[4] Subdivisions produced by the secondary crests are responsible for the formation of alveoli, each of which has elastic fibers around the margin of its mouth. It has thus been suggested that the way in which elastic fibers are laid down may play a key role in alveolar multiplication.[4] Alveoli are also thought to be formed by alveolarization of distal nonrespiratory bronchioles, converting them to respiratory bronchioles.[14]

Investigations initiated in acromegaly[17] and hypopituitarism[53] led to animal investigation. Lung growth has been manipulated experimentally by many investigators recently. Administration of growth hormone[10] or implantation of tumors which secrete growth hormone[15] results in large animals whose lungs are larger than they should be for the age of the animals, but not for the size of the animals. Hypophysectomy produces the reverse result.[16] The pulmonary enlargement that occurs with excess growth hormone is due more to cellular enlargement rather than to cellular multiplication.[15] Although the initial results were controversial, it now appears that animals exposed to hypobaric conditions, and thus hypoxemia, have larger lungs than they should[30] and that high levels of oxygen interfere with lung growth.[106] It is not clear whether alveolar multiplication is altered under these circumstances. The effect of pneumonectomy on the contralateral lung has been studied extensively. It appears that in young animals of most species studied, there is cellular multiplication and lung enlargement so that the contralateral lung has the same weight, volume, and cell number as both lungs of the control animals. The response is more complete in young than in old animals, and is largely complete 7–10 days later.[106] The results concerning alveolar multiplication have been conflicting. We have recently been able to show unequivocal evidence of alveolar multiplication following pneumonectomy in 10-week-old rabbits. We found that 4 weeks later they have the same number of alveoli as in both lungs of control animals.[64] The primary stimulus for lung growth appears to be mechanical stretching since the compensatory response does not occur, or is much diminished, if the pleural cavity on the pneumonectomized side is filled with wax or other material.[28]

Alveolar multiplication similarly occurs postnatally in humans and the data are reviewed in Chapter 15. The factors that affect lung growth and alveolar multiplication in the human are not understood. It may be of great importance. It is now becoming apparent that subjects who have evidence of chronic airflow obstruction in adult life have a history of more frequent and severe respiratory infection in infancy and childhood.[20] It is also apparent that cigarette smoking produces chronic airflow obstruction in some subjects but not in others.[38] It may thus be that childhood infection may impair qualitative and/or quantitative lung growth in infancy and childhood and these infectious may predispose to lung damage and chronic airflow obstruction induced by cigarette smoking in adult life.

THE WAY THE LUNG EXPANDS[108]

The exact way that the lung expands has been controversial. Until recently, there were two schools of thought and now there is a third. The two original ideas were that the lung expanded either as a balloon[33, 35, 44, 59] or as a paper bag.[70, 114] The former way involved isotropic expansion (equal in all dimensions) of all the alveolated part of the lung as well as the peripheral airways in continuity with the elastic framework of the lung. This mode of expansion would apply to the useful range of lung inflation, at least from functional residual capacity to total lung capacity (at low lung volumes alveoli must collapse so that isotropic expansion cannot occur under these circumstances). With isotropic expansion of the lung, surface area must increase to the 2/3 power of the increase in lung volume and linear dimensions will increase to the cube root of the increase in lung volume. Evidence to this effect is available.[35, 59]

Alternatively, the alveoli may open up as paper bags and under these conditions the alveolar surface area would be unchanged as the lung expanded, alveolar shape would alter markedly and the component parts of the lung airways and alveolated tissue might behave differently. Evidence for this method of expansion has been primarily descriptive rather than quantitative.[70, 114]

More recently it has been suggested that the lungs expand by recruitment and deflate by derecruitment of alveoli.[6, 42] That is, as the lung expands, alveoli that were previously closed open up and during expiration alveoli shut. Under these circumstances alveolar surface area would vary directly with lung volume and alveolar size and shape would remain more or less constant. The evidence of this comes from no less a source than Weibel's laboratory[42, 43] but has not yet been confirmed.

NONADRENERGIC (PURINERGIC) INHIBITORY NERVOUS SYSTEM IN AIRWAYS[90]

The thought may be unpalatable to those primarily concerned with the lung but the fact remains that the lung is merely a part of the gut modified for gas exchange. Thus, for example, tracheobronchial mucous glands are analogues of the salivary glands and are therefore heir to those tumors (adenoid cystic carcinoma, mucoepidermoid carcinoma, and pleomorphic adenoma) that occur in the salivary glands, as well as to conditions such as Sjögren's disease. Carcinoids of the lung come from the same cell type as those found in the gut, and perhaps, if the carcinogen of tobacco smoke could be administered internally, one might see oat cell cancer of the intestines as well. The notion of the homology of gut and lung has led to another important discovery in a pathology laboratory.

The nonadrenergic inhibitory nervous system has recently been shown to be the most important nervous inhibitory system in the gastrointestinal tract.[18] It is responsible for relaxation of the internal anal sphincter and the gastroesophageal sphincter and is also responsible for the relaxation phase of peristalsis.[29, 41] The nonadrenergic nervous system and the parasympathetic nervous system develop together in the fetus and both of the systems function well before the development of the adrenergic nervous system. The nonadrenergic nervous system is sometimes referred to as the purinergic nervous system since at one stage it appeared that adenosine triphosphate was the mediator of the system. Very recently, it has been suggested that endorphins (endogenous substances that act on morphine receptors in the brain) may be the mediators.[88]

Dr. John Richardson of McGill University showed that there was a lack of the nonadrenergic inhibitory nervous system in a murine model of Hirschprung's disease.[89] He then reasoned that this system might be the inhibitory nervous system within the lung because of the lung's homology with the gut. Indeed, this is what he found.[90, 91] Using human material, he was able to demonstrate cholinergic excitatory nerves whose effect was blocked by atropine.[90] Electrical field stimulation of airways in the presence of atropine caused relaxation of smooth muscle. This relaxation was not altered by adrenergic blocking agents. Tetrodotoxin blocked the relaxation effect and since this substance blocks axonal transmission, the relaxation effect must have been mediated through nerves and not by a direct effect on muscle. Richardson examined the airways histochemically and could find no evidence of adrenergic nerves. He therefore concluded that the nonadrenergic nervous system was the dominant inhibitory nervous system in human airways. He has also speculated that a defect of this system in the airways would lead to loss of control of smooth muscle in the airways, just as is seen in the gut in Hirschprung's disease. Thus a defect or disturbance of the nonadrenergic nervous system might provide an explanation for the hyperactive airways seen in asthma and some patients with chronic bronchitis. In view of his work, it is difficult to sustain the hypothesis that β-adrenergic blockade is an important cause of asthma. The final twist is related to the possibility that endorphins may be the mediators of the system.[88] Thus there are profound pharmacological and clinical implications to these recent discoveries.

As part of the study, Richardson used human lungs obtained at necropsy and lungs removed at surgery. The patients who provided the latter specimens were treated with a variety of drugs in the immediate preoperative and intraoperative period. Richardson therefore pretreated his lungs with a modified Krebs-Henseleit solution to remove therapeutic agents and to perhaps improve the responsiveness of the necropsy tissue. He found that not only did the Krebs-Henseleit solution improve the pharmacologic responsiveness of lungs removed at necropsy but also greatly improved the appearance of the tissue as seen by transmission electron microscopy.[40] This technique opens up a new area, perhaps even a new era, for exploitation of necropsy tissue.

THE MUCUS BLANKET[110, 113]

It is conventional wisdom that the mucus blanket in the major airways acts as an important protective mechanism. The concept of the mucus blanket is more than 30 years old, and the cilia of the airway lining cells are thought to beat in a sol. On top of the sol phase is the gel phase which is propelled by the beating of the cilia whose tips reach to the gel phase. Inhaled particles of aerodynamic diameter greater than 5 μm are deposited on the mucus blanket and are then transported to the trachea and expelled into the pharynx and swallowed or coughed up. The process is rapid and clearance of particles deposited on the airway takes place in 30 minutes to several hours.

More recently, the details of the mucociliary mechanism have been questioned.[111, 112] The problem is best stated by an oversimplification—the summed circumferences of the terminal bronchioles is of the order of 40–80 meters, whereas that of the trachea is 6 cm.[104] If the thickness of the layer is the same throughout the airways, some mechanism must exist that enables the mucus layer to pass through the ever-narrowing funnel of proximal airways without causing their obstruction. In part, this is accomplished by increasing the velocity of mucus flow in the central airways. However, the increase in flow is only about 4-fold,[113] and apparently some two orders of magnitude too small to accomplish the task by itself. An additional factor may be absorption of fluid from the lining layer and it has been suggested that this may be the function of the "brush" cell of the trachea.[92] However, recent evidence suggests that there is secretion of fluid by the tracheal epithelium rather than absorption.[82] More recently, it has been suggested that the mucus layer increases from 0.1 μ in the peripheral airways to 5 μ in thickness in the central airways.[69] This, together with the increase in mucus velocity would compensate for the decrease in total cross-sectional circumferences of the central airways. To some extent the problem may not be a real one and only apparent because of mistaken assumptions. The peripheral airways are probably mostly lined by surfactant rather than mucus,[42, 71] and mucus probably only becomes a major part of the lining layer at the level of the distal bronchial tree, where mucus glands are first encountered as one proceeds proximally towards the mouth. At this level, the total cross-sectional circumference of all the airways may not be much more than 8–16 times the tracheal circumference.[104] This sort of difference would allow for a ready passage of mucus through the central airways by increased velocity and slight changes in thickness of the mucus blanket, even allowing for the problems of passage around origins of branches and across points of bifurcation. It is also true that one should distinguish between the total thickness (sol plus gel) and the gel or mucus layer. The sol layer may remain fairly constant in position and thickness and need not be taken into account in these calculations.

There is controversy about the appearance of the mucus layer. Direct studies of the rat airway have suggested that mucus existed in plaques rather than as a sheet.[111, 112] More recently, scanning and transmission electron microscopy have, however, suggested that the traditional view of the structure of the mucociliary blanket is correct. Transmission microscopy has shown a layer of mucus which is situated at the tops of the cilia.[118] Material resembling surfactant is encountered in the deeper layers of the blanket (*i.e.,* closest to the cellular lining of the airway) and beneath it (Fig. 1). It seems likely that the electron lucent layer deep to the

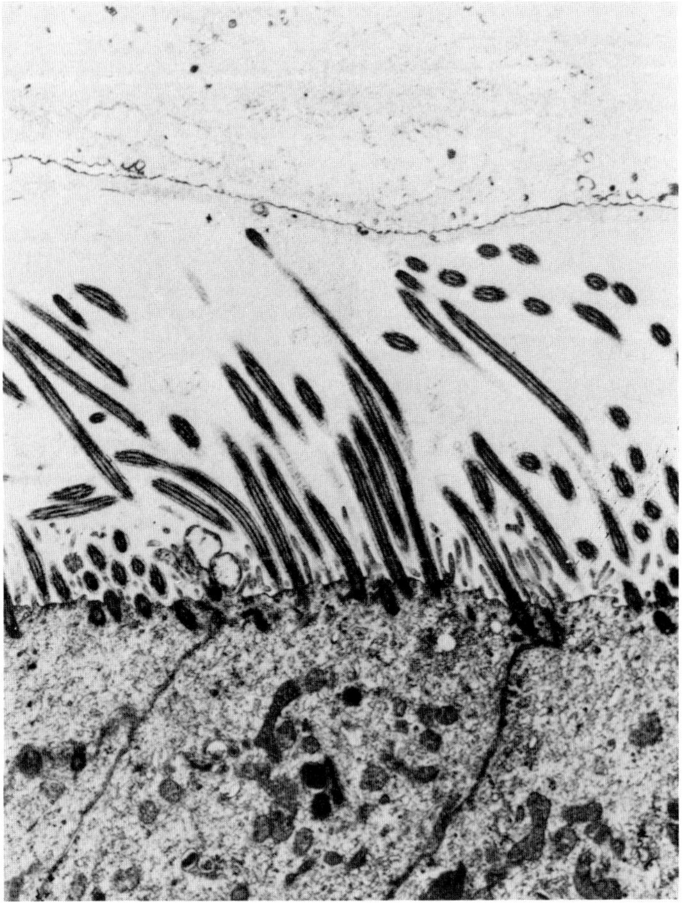

FIG. 1. Transmission electron micrograph of the mucociliary apparatus of the rat. A dense osmiophilic line lies in the depths of a modestly electron dense layer and on an electron lucent layer which lies between the cilia. × 6600. (Reproduced by permission, from Yoneda, K.: *Am. Rev. Resp. Dis. 114:* 837–842, 1976.)

blanket and among the cilia is in the sol phase. Scanning electron microscopy also indicates that the mucus layer overlies the tips of the cilia in the major airways of the rabbit (Fig. 2). More importantly, this study shows that the layer is generally a continuous sheet, consisting of a complex three dimensional arrangement of overlapping layers and fibrous networks.[102] A variety of discontinuities were apparent, especially in the main and lobar bronchi and it is not clear how real these discontinuities were and whether they represented preparation artefacts. Mucus secreted from goblet cells and tracheobronchial glands likely pass as a discrete column through the sol layer to join and merge with the superficial mucus layer.

CHRONIC AIRFLOW OBSTRUCTION[107]

Despite the large volume of material written about it, chronic bronchitis remains a confusing term to the pathologist and it surely must conjure up an image of a chronic inflammatory process of the major airways. However, its usual meaning is chronic mucus hypersecretion, which manifests itself by chronic phlegm production. This specific definition was coined some 20 years ago[26]

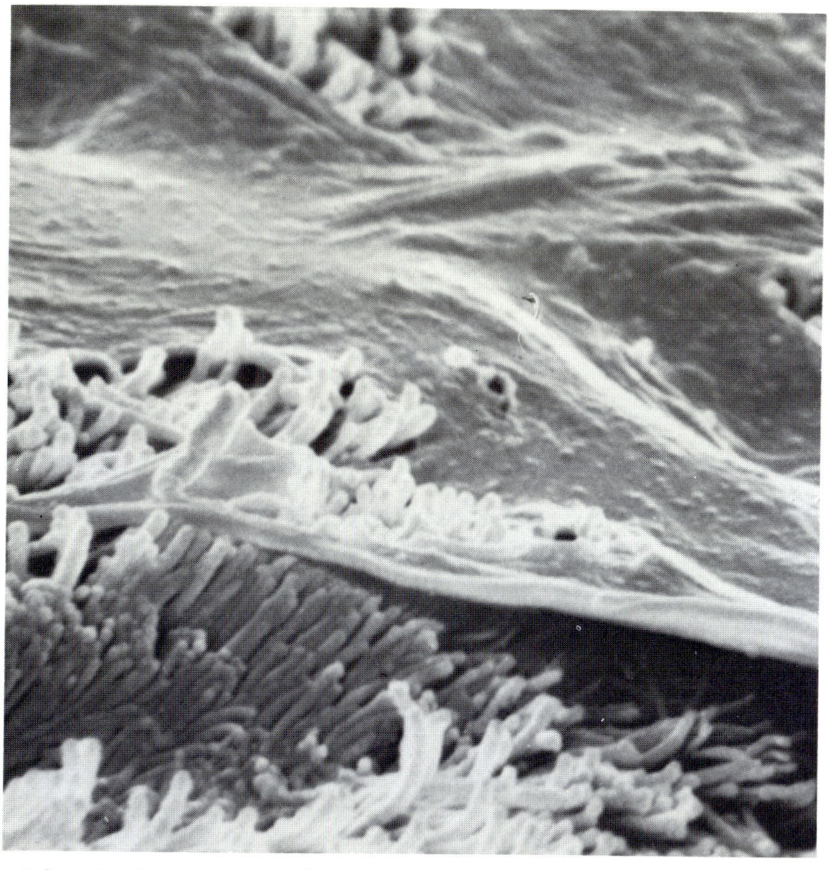

FIG. 2. Scanning electron micrograph of rabbit trachea. The mucus blanket overlies the cilia and the mucus is situated at the tips of the cilia. × 13,270. (Reproduced by permission, from Sturgess, J. M.: *Am. Rev. Resp. Dis. 115:* 819–827, 1977.

because before that, chronic bronchitis was used to mean several different things. Notably, it was used synonymously with chronic airflow obstruction; this was particularly the case in Britain. Chronic bronchitis, defined as mucus hypersecretion, was the subject of extensive epidemiologic investigations and in the intervening period much useful infoımation has been obtained. One of the pioneers has recently published a short monograph that recounts his experience.[38] One of the most notable observations in the monograph is that chronic bronchitis (chronic mucus hypersecretion) *per se* does not seem to be a serious symptom, certainly not in all subjects. It has long been known that patients with mucus hypersecretion have more severe chronic airflow obstruction than those without and also have a worse prognosis. However, when patients are matched by cigarette smoking habit and by degree of airflow obstruction, those with chronic mucus hypersecretion have a prognosis which is no worse than those without mucus hypersecretion. These observations suggest that mucus hypersecretion may be primarily a marker of cigarette smoking and it is likely that associated cigarette-produced disease, either emphysema or peripheral airway lesions, is the major cause of airflow obstruction in these subjects. Fletcher's studies have also indicated that patients whose disease is destined to progress are those who initially have poor levels of function.[38] This has been termed the "horse-race" effect (the horse in the lead is the one that has run the furthest—similarly the patient whose airflow is most obstructed is likely the one whose airway disease has progressed most rapidly), and it may not be too surprising that it has considerable practical implications. Only the minority of smokers will develop severe chronic airflow obstruction: it seems likely that those subjects who have relatively normal flow rates at middle age will have only a very small likelihood of developing crippling chronic airflow obstruction. Conversely, those who will develop severe chronic airflow obstruction will have evidence of significant airflow obstruction in the fifth decade. Since disease in the lungs and airways has to be fairly advanced before conventional tests of chronic airflow obstruction are abnormal, it is important to detect evidence of chronic airflow obstruction earlier in the state of the disease, perhaps when conventional tests of airflow are still normal. This has led to the "cottage industry"[11] of tests of small airway function since it is in these airways that the early lesions are thought to occur in patients with chronic airflow obstruction. This subject is reviewed in Chapter 9. In that chapter, Dr. Niewoehner questions the conventional use of the term chronic bronchitis to mean chronic mucus hypersecretion. Ambiguity results since the same term can be used to describe a patient with chronic mucus hypersecretion who does not have chronic airflow obstruction and who will never develop it, as well as patients who have chronic mucus hypersecretion and die of chronic airflow obstruction. There seems little reason to continue to use an ambiguous term, especially when it really refers to a symptom. The parallel would be to use polyuria instead of chronic pyelonephritis or chronic renal failure. It would be much better to use the term chronic mucus hypersecretion and abandon the term chronic bronchitis altogether, and this idea is gradually receiving wider acceptance.[38, 109]

One of the main thrusts of research in emphysema since the lung was last the topic of the Long Course has been clinicopathologic correlations. The last volume gave support to the then conventional wisdom that there were two distinct clinicopathologic syndromes of chronic airflow obstruction. One was the "blue bloater," who was markedly hypoxemic and developed gross right ventricular failure. This syndrome was thought to occur in patients with severe chronic bronchitis and little or no emphysema. The other syndrome was the "pink puffer" who maintained relatively normal blood gases by dint of markedly increasing minute ventilation. These patients were thought to have severe emphysema which was responsible for their airflow obstruction and little or no bronchitis. It is still true that two separate clinical syndromes exist and that they can be defined fairly precisely. However, even at the clinical level, the majority of patients do not fit either clinical syndrome. What is equally clear, however, is that even in classical examples of both syndromes nearly all patients have both mucus hypersecretion and emphysema. In general, most patients with a type A syndrome (pink puffer) will be found to have moderate or severe emphysema in their lungs at necropsy.[107] In contrast, all degrees of severity of emphysema from none to severe, may be found in patients with the type B syndrome (blue bloaters). In fact, the morphologic differences between the lungs of the two syndromes appears to be becoming smaller and smaller. The most recent information suggests that the amount of emphysema is essentially the same in the two syndromes.[74] These data suggest that it is the patients' response to their disease which may produce the syndromes. The most obvious explanation is altered control of breathing—patients with the type B syndrome do not respond to hypercapnia and hypoxemia by adequately increasing ventilation, and develop pulmonary hypertension, right ventricular hypertrophy and failure, as a consequence of hypoxemia. There is evidence to suggest that this may be the mechanism in at least some patients with type B chronic airflow obstruction. Another suggestion is that patients with type B syndrome have more severe narrowing of the peripheral airways leading to the severe ventilation/diffusion abnormalities so characteristic of this syndrome[12, 34] and this may account for some of the patients. What is true is that the pathologist can never be certain what he will find in the lungs in a patient dying of chronic airflow obstruction. This is what makes chronic airflow obstruction so interesting, but also so confusing.

It has also now become apparent that the severity of emphysema is the major determinant of chronic airflow obstruction and the relationships between the severity of clinical symptoms, alterations in flow rates or lung volumes and the severity of emphysema are moderately close and are much better related than to any other anatomical lesion.[74, 107] The test which relates best to the amount of emphysema in the lungs is the measurement of the diffusing capacity for carbon monoxide. However, even the relationship of this test is not very precise. While emphysema is perhaps the most important association of chronic airflow obstruction, many patients have severe emphysema in their lungs and yet appear, on retrospective analysis of their charts, to have little or no evidence of chronic airflow obstruction.[107] Whether their lungs are functionally normal is less clear; it seems likely, however, that the majority of them would have had evidence of at least mild chronic airflow obstruction during life had they been through the pulmonary function laboratory. At the time of the last Long Course, conventional wisdom suggested that it was possible to recognize radiologically most patients with severe emphysema in their lungs. More recent data suggest that radiology is a rather imprecise instrument for recognizing emphysema.[107]

Alterations in the diaphragm in emphysema have attracted recent interest, but the data are conflicting. Authors have not always distinguished between chronic airflow obstruction and emphysema, and often the quantitation of the lung lesions has been imprecise. Several authors have suggested that the diaphragm is hypertrophied. In one instance, this is an assertion without providing data,[117] and was said to occur in severe emphysema. Ishikawa and Hayes[52] noted significant thickening of the diaphragm muscle in 9 patients with chronic airflow obstruction, compared with 15 patients without chronic airflow obstruction. They also found that the individual muscle fibers had increased diameter in two patients with chronic airflow obstruction. Scott and Hoy[98] contrasted the area of diaphragm muscle fibers as seen on histologic slides in 6 nonemphysematous patients to the area of fibers seen in 18 patients with emphysema varying from mild to severe. They found that the mean muscle fiber diameter was greater in patients with emphysema (1069 μ^2 compared with 851 μ^2) and there was a greater variation in muscle fiber size in patients with emphysema. However, there was no relationship between the extent of emphysema and the increase in area of muscle. All of the patients with emphysema had respiratory symptoms; half died of airflow obstruction. The diaphragm muscle fiber areas were larger in the patients who died of chronic airflow obstruction. Interestingly, there was a positive correlation between weight of the ventricles of the heart and diaphragm muscle size. A correlation between heart weight and diaphragm weight has also been previously recorded.[39]

On the other hand, there is apparently good evidence that the diaphragm decreases in size in emphysema. Diaphragm weight was found diminished in an older study from Germany of 6 emphysematous subjects.[39] Steele and Heard[101] found that the area, volume, and thickness of the muscular part of the diaphragm was decreased in 15 "chronic bronchitics" compared to 23 control subjects. They felt that the amount of emphysema in the lungs was not a significant variable affecting diaphragm weight. These authors found a positive correlation between body weight and diaphragm volume and thickness. The bronchitic patients were underweight but the loss of diaphragm volume was greater than could be accounted for by the loss of body weight. They could see no obvious change in the diaphragmatic muscle histologically. An attempt was made to quantitate muscle fiber size but they found that the great variability of muscle fibers in different parts of the diaphragm made a proper study impossible. The most recent study[21] was also the largest, involving 95 U.S. veterans. This study showed a significant inverse correlation between diaphragm area and the extent of emphysema in the lungs. The reduction involved the muscular portion of the diaphragm particularly. In contrast to the previous study, diaphragm thickness was not reduced.

It is difficult to predict what changes might be expected in emphysema and CAO. The loss of weight characteristically associated with emphysema and diminished diaphragm movement that occurs with emphysema argue for diminished weight. However, the increased work of breathing and the fact that the diaphragm must contract to be low and flat argue for increased diaphragm mass. What is clear, however, is that a study of large numbers of patients will be needed to solve the problem so that the variables of body size, weight, emphysema, and chronic airflow obstruction can be studied independently.

The papain-induced emphysema in animals had been described at the time of the last Long Course[46] but had not received widespread attention. That discovery has led to important advances in the understanding of the pathogenesis of emphysema. We now know that papain produces emphysema by its elastolytic properties and that intratracheal installation of elastase will produce emphysema but intratracheal collagenase will not do so.[54–56] The central role of the lung scleroproteins in maintaining the integrity of the lung is now well established and several laboratories are studying the proteins and proteases of the lung. Of particular interest is the similarity of elastase-induced emphysema to the newborn lung (Figs. 3 and 4). Thus, an emphysematous lung resembles the lung of a newborn animal. From the discussion in the early part of this chapter, this perhaps could be expected. The hypothesis was advanced that the development of the elastic tissue framework of the lung was intimately involved with alveolar multiplication. It is logical therefore to anticipate that destruction of the lung's elastic tissue would result in loss of alveoli and thus mimic the infantile state. A more depressing observation from the elastase model is that the induced emphysema is progressive, even after a single dose.[62] This observation is, of course,

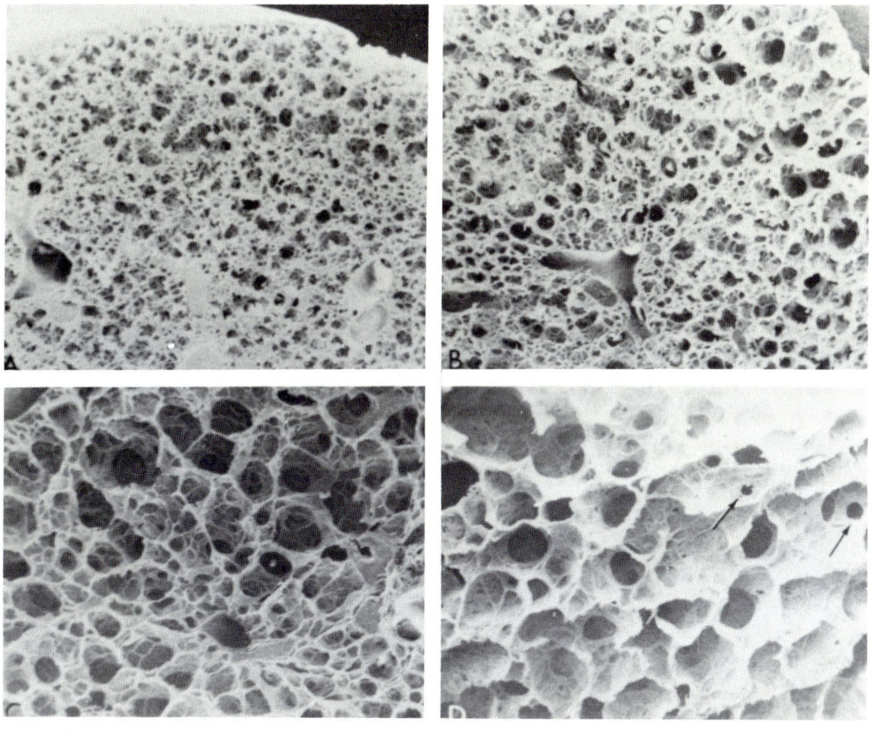

FIG. 3. Scanning electron micrographs of hamster lungs following a single installation of elastase. *A,* 2 days; *B,* 2 weeks; *C,* 2 months; *D,* 1 year after installation. Note progressive enlargement of air spaces. Approximately × 24. Compare to Figure 4. (Reproduced by permission, from Kuhn, C., and Tavassoli, F.: *Lab. Invest. 34:* 2–9, 1976.

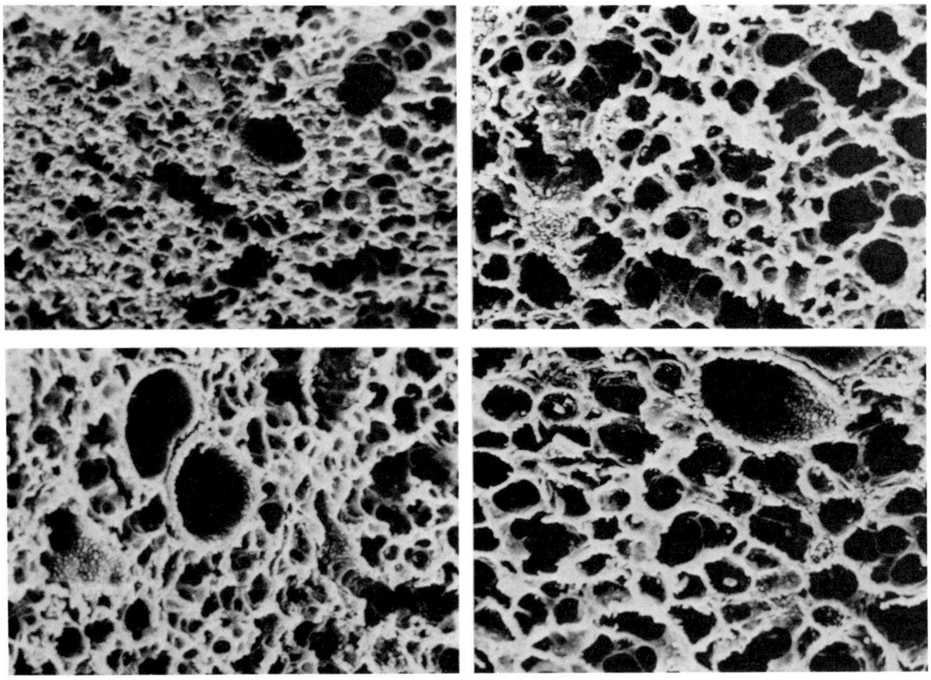

FIG. 4. Scanning electron micrograph of mouse lungs at various ages postnatally. *Top left,* 13 days; *bottom left,* 7 days; *top right,* 5 days; *bottom right,* 36 hours. Note the resemblance between papain emphysema at one year to the newborn mouse lung, approximately × 100. (Reproduced by permission, from Thurlbeck, W. M.: In *Pathology Annual, 1975* (see Ref. 105).

consonant with the progressive nature of the human disease, despite cessation of smoking and adequate therapy.

COAL WORKERS' PNEUMOCONIOSIS (CWP)[75, 76] (See Chapter 6)

The problems of lung disease in coal workers are made more complex by emotion, political overtones and compensation. Despite extensive work over the last 20–30 years, many areas of doubt still exist, although the issues are now much clearer, thanks in large part to the work of Morgan and his colleagues in West Virginia.[75, 76] Regrettably, there is still a notable gap in our knowledge of structure-functional correlations. While the anatomical pathology, the radiology, and the alterations in function are reasonably well known from studies of separate groups of patients, the relationships between radiology, function, and structure are only poorly studied in the same group of patients.

One of the major problems is that coal workers are subject to the usual forms of bronchitis and emphysema as occur in the remainder of the population. Indeed, cigarette smoking plays a dominant role in producing chronic airflow obstruction in miners. The situation is not unlike that in air pollution—it is easy to show the ill effect of cigarette smoking in both the general population and in the miners, but it takes a skilled and careful experiment to show an additional effect due to environment or to dust within the lung.

There are two distinct forms of CWP—simple pneumoconiosis and progressive massive fibrosis (PMF). Simple CWP is also known as focal emphysema and is characterized by the deposition of coal in and around respiratory bronchioles.[49] This results in the formation of a characteristic macule, which appears spidery in shape on cross-section and is associated with enlargement of the respiratory bronchioles. PMF is characterized by the formation of large confluent areas of fibrous tissue within the lung, characteristically in the superior segment of the lower lobe or of the posterior segment of the upper lobe. CWP is thought due to coal alone, and PMF due to complicating tuberculosis or perhaps complicating rheumatoid arthritis.

Despite the controversy of the past, it appears that the following statements are agreed upon:[75]

(1) The amount of dust in the lung correlates with increasing radiologic severity of simple CWP.[96]

(2) The progress of severity of CWP is related to the amount of dust in the mine, although the correlation is not strong.[94]

(3) Increased exposure to dust is associated with reduction in ventilatory capacity.[93]

(4) The degree of disability is closely related to diminution in expiratory flow rates (chronic airflow obstruction).[84]

(5) PMF is closely associated with CAO and disability.[85]

(6) The presence of simple CWP and advancing grades of simple CWP *as assessed radiologically,* produce only subtle changes in pulmonary function. These include an increase in residual volume, minor alterations in gas exchange, and abnormalities in tests of small airway function.[67, 75, 77] Morgan has stated flatly, "The presence of severe shortness of breath in a coal miner with simple CWP is virtually always related to a non-occupationally related disease such as chronic bronchitis or emphysema, rather than to coal mining."[75]

(7) A functional-radiologic-morphologic study of British coal miners has indicated that chronic airflow obstruction is overwhelmingly related to the amount of emphysema in the lungs at necropsy.[97] However, the amount of emphysema in the lungs at necropsy is not related to increasing amounts of simple CWP *as assessed radiologically.*

(8) Exposure to mine dust during a shift produces an acute increase in airflow obstruction in both central and peripheral airways in smoking miners and in the peripheral airways of nonsmoking miners.[66]

(9) The major anomaly exists that while it is possible to show, as mentioned above (a) that there is a relationship between the amount of dust in the lungs and the increasing radiologic severity of CWP, and (b) that there is a relationship between the amount of dust breathed and evidence of airflow obstruction, yet it has not been possible to show a relationship between increasing radiologic severity of simple CWP and severity of CAO. Morgan has suggested that the anomaly can be explained because there is a form of "industrial bronchitis" that affects the function of all miners to some extent and that industrial bronchitis is not associated with evidence of radiologic dust retention.[75] Evidence for this hypothesis includes the high frequency of chronic bronchitis in miners and the fact that central airways appear to be obstructed in them.

An alternative explanation will require detailed clinicopathologic study. It is possible (though unlikely) that emphysema might obscure and alter the chest roentgenogram so that it is no longer possible to discriminate accurately the amount of dust in the lungs. Thus the severity of anatomical CWP might not be directly related to the severity of radiologic CWP. It will be necessary to show that the amount of coal dust in the lungs is directly related to the severity of emphysema but not to the radiologic severity of pneumoconiosis. The major compounding problem, however, as illustrated in the Ryder study[97] is that while emphysema may be the dominant cause of chronic airflow obstruction in miners, in many miners the emphysema may not be the direct result of the dust.

ADULT RESPIRATORY DISTRESS SYNDROME (ARDS)[58, 103]

Although some argue that the term should not be used,[78] ARDS serves the useful purpose of bringing together several conditions that have a common disturbance of function and, more importantly, that require the same skilled management. In general, the syndrome consists of the development of acute respiratory failure in a patient who had apparently normal lung function previously. This concept includes conditions of known etiology such as viral pneumonia, aspiration pneumonia, and fat embolism, as well as causes of ARDS that are less well defined. The common and most important cause of ARDS is nonthoracic trauma with associated circulatory collapse. Characteristically, respiratory failure becomes apparent after circulatory collapse has been treated and stabilized. It is heralded by increasing hypoxemia, increasing lung stiffness and the development of roentgenographic lung opacities. The latter rapidly progress to form a "whited out" lung and hypoxemia becomes so severe that assisted ventilation and oxygen are required for management. With increasing severity, higher concentrations of oxygen are required and patients who die almost invariably have had high levels of oxygen (even 100%) administered for some days before death. Positive end expiratory pressure (PEEP) ventilation has enabled more satisfactory oxygenation with lower levels of inspired oxygen. It is the administration of oxygen that makes the lesions seen at necropsy so difficult to interpret. In Chapter 3, Pratt makes a convincing case that most of what is seen at necropsy in patients with ARDS is due to oxygen. His observations should not obscure the fact that ARDS associated with nonthoracic trauma (shock lung) does exist. It should be noted that the clinical syndrome appears before, and is the reason for, the administration of oxygen. It is also true that the extent of the lesions and the amount of oxygen given are not very closely correlated. The lesions may appear in patients who have had relatively low levels of oxygen for short periods of time and may not appear in patients who had 100% oxygen for long periods of time.[83]

It is questionable whether the lung lesions are directly related to shock and some experts have stated flatly that shock itself is never the cause for ARDS.[23] Factors such as overhydration during resuscitation, aspiration, microemboli of cell aggregates in transfused blood and infection may all play a part in individual patients.[23] Thromboemboli have been found in two-thirds (80%) of patients[50, 83] and diffuse intrapulmonary thrombosis of small vessels has been postulated as playing an important role.[83] Morphologic investigation has generally been disappointing because of the complicating factor of oxygen toxicity and often because there is terminal infection which obscures the lung lesions. Biopsies are now being used more commonly[50, 63, 65] and have provided useful information, as has a fairly recent electron microscopic investigation.[81] Biopsies especially play a significant role in recognizing infection in the lung,[50] which is an important and frequent complicating condition.[5]

The gross findings are characteristic but not specific. The lungs are extremely heavy (usually over 1,800 grams), very congested and airless. Histologically, the findings depend on the stage of the illness, and an exudative phase and a proliferative phase are recognized. The former is characterized by congestion, edema, hemorrhage, and hyaline membrane formation. The latter classically first appear at the tips of alveolar septa in alveolar ducts.[83] Electron microscopically, interstitial edema and necrosis of the type I epithelial cells are seen.[81] It is the last feature that likely leads to massive alveolar edema. Hyaline membranes consist of necrotic cell debris, fibrin, and proteinaceous exudate. Endothelial damage is not a feature. All these changes may be seen in patients who have not been given oxygen at levels generally considered toxic. The proliferative phase consists of proliferation of type II cells to line the airspaces and interstitial and intra-alveolar fibrosis. Interstitial fibrosis is characteristic of oxygen toxicity[57, 80] but it has also been described in patients with ARDS but who have not had high levels of oxygen.[7] Extensive intra-alveolar proliferation of fibrous tissue is a characteristic feature of ARDS (Figs. 5 and 6) associated with trauma,[65, 83] but has generally been described in the setting of high levels of oxygen as noted by Pratt. It should be noted that this lesion is different from that described in experimental oxygen poisoning and thus it may still be a feature of ARDS rather

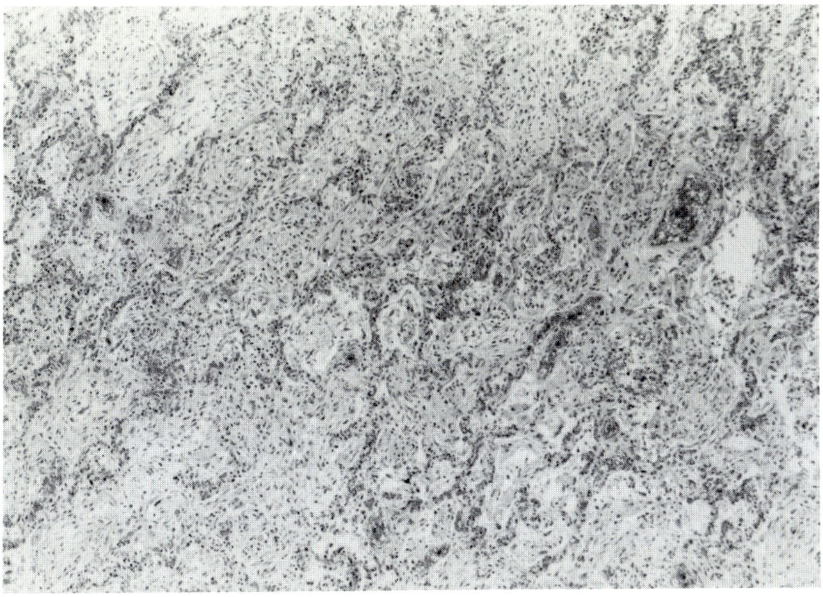

FIG. 5. Patient with adult respiratory distress syndrome. The alveolar framework can be made out because of its capillary network. The air spaces are filled with loose fibrous tissue. Hematoxylin and eosin, × 60.

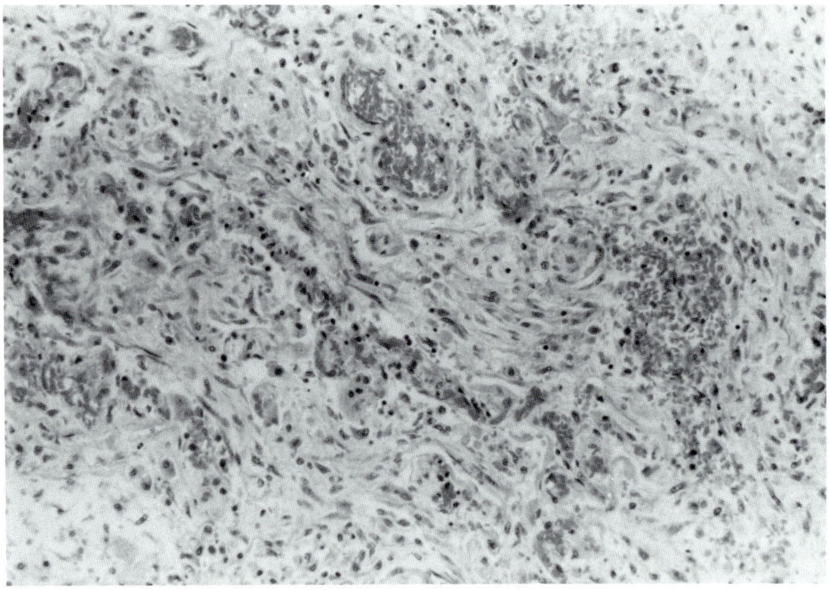

FIG. 6. A higher power view of Figure 5 shows the alveolar walls and the nature of the tissue in the air spaces more clearly. Hematoxylin and eosin, × 150.

than of oxygen toxicity. One of the surprising aspects of ARDS is that those who recover have adequately functioning lungs despite extensive fibrosis, proven by biopsy, occurring during the episode.[63] Residual symptoms are commoner in smokers and in older subjects, suggesting that they may have had pre-existing disease which may (or may not) have been aggravated by the episode. A mild restrictive pattern and some loss of diffusing capacity have been observed.[63] Casts of the pulmonary capillary bed in ARDS have shown extensive obliteration of the microvasculature[23] so that loss of diffusing capacity might be anticipated in survivors. A progressive loss of flow rates suggested increased bronchial reactivity in one patient.[63]

TOPICS OF INTEREST IN SURGICAL PATHOLOGY OF THE LUNG

This monograph started with a tribute to Drs. Liebow and Gough and it seems fitting that it should end with a reference to observations initiated by one of them.

I have been fortunate enough to attend Dr. Liebow's course in pulmonary pathology (now run by Drs. Carrington and Bloor) in La Jolla on several occasions. It is a remarkable experience as one has access to Dr. Liebow's vast collection of fascinating referral material. Some of the wisdom and information imparted by Dr. Liebow and his colleagues is not published and I am taking the liberty of giving my interpretation of both published and unpublished material, the latter often coming by way of informal comment and discussion.

INTRAVASCULAR BRONCHIOLAR ALVEOLAR TUMOR (IVBAT)[32, 45]

These are very characteristic lesions, although their precise origin is still unclear. Originally they were thought to be variants of bronchiolar-alveolar tumors but there is now some question whether they all represent bronchiolar-alveolar tumors with intravascular invasion. The original abstract reported by Drs. Dail and Liebow contained 20 cases seen since 1962.[32] Dr. Dail has seen a further case. Two-thirds of the patients were female and 40% were under the age of 30 years, with an age range of 14–71 years. The condition is slowly progressive with patients dying of pulmonary insufficiency or pleural involvement, and patients have lived up to 12 years from the time of discovery of the lesion.

The lesions are very perplexing when seen for the first time and have often been referred to as examples of chondrosarcoma or chondromyxosarcoma. The lesions are multiple. The center of the lesion classically appears hyaline or amorphous and may be calcified. However, the alveolar framework is relatively preserved as seen with a reticulin stain or even with hematoxin and eosin (Fig. 7). The center still remains modestly cellular due to cells in the alveolar wall as well as scattered cells in the intra-alveolar material (Fig. 7, *B* and *C*). Occasional cells lining the alveolar walls may resemble type II cells with atypical nuclei (Fig. 7*C*). The cells within the matrix are poorly defined and continuous with the amorphous hyaline material which fills the alveoli. The nuclei are often elongated and distorted. In some areas the material in the air spaces takes on a distinctly chrondroid appearance (Fig. 8). At the periphery, the lesion is much more cellular and its margin often resembles a classical bronchiolar-alveolar tumor, although with certain differences. There may be a mild interstitial mononuclear infiltrate and the air spaces are lined by cells with bizarre, hyperchromatic nuclei (Fig. 9). In some areas the air spaces contain only cells. The major difference between these lesions and classical alveolar bronchiolar tumors is the presence of the solid material within the air spaces. A characteristic feature is the invasion and growth within both arteries and veins, and this involvement occurs beyond the tumor masses (Fig. 10). The vascular involvement is often not very conspicuous with hematoxin and eosin stained material but can usually be recognized. In addition, the lesion extends into the bronchioles.

In some instances typical bronchiolar-alveolar tumors were associated with the lesion, hence the use of the term intravascular bronchiolar-alveolar tumor. However, it may be that other tumors may also produce the lesion. Irrespective of its precise histogenesis, the lesion is sufficiently curious and characteristic to warrant its recognition.

Sclerosing Hemangiomas and Plasma Cell Granulomas of the Lung[9, 45]

The terminology of these lesions is unclear. The lung does not appear to have caught up with the popularity of the term fibrous histiocytomas as in other organs and thus the term sclerosing hemangioma is still generally used. There is some confusion in that some authors tend to group sclerosing hemangioma and plasma cell granulomas together, despite the fact that they are clinically and histologically quite different.

Sclerosing hemangiomas characteristically have a papillary appearance (Fig. 11). This may lead to confusion with bronchiolar-alveolar carcinomas. The distinction is important since sclerosing hemangiomas are benign lesions. The distinction is usually easy since sclerosing hemangiomas reveal their true nature by showing areas of dense sclerosis with obliterated capillaries (Fig. 12), have

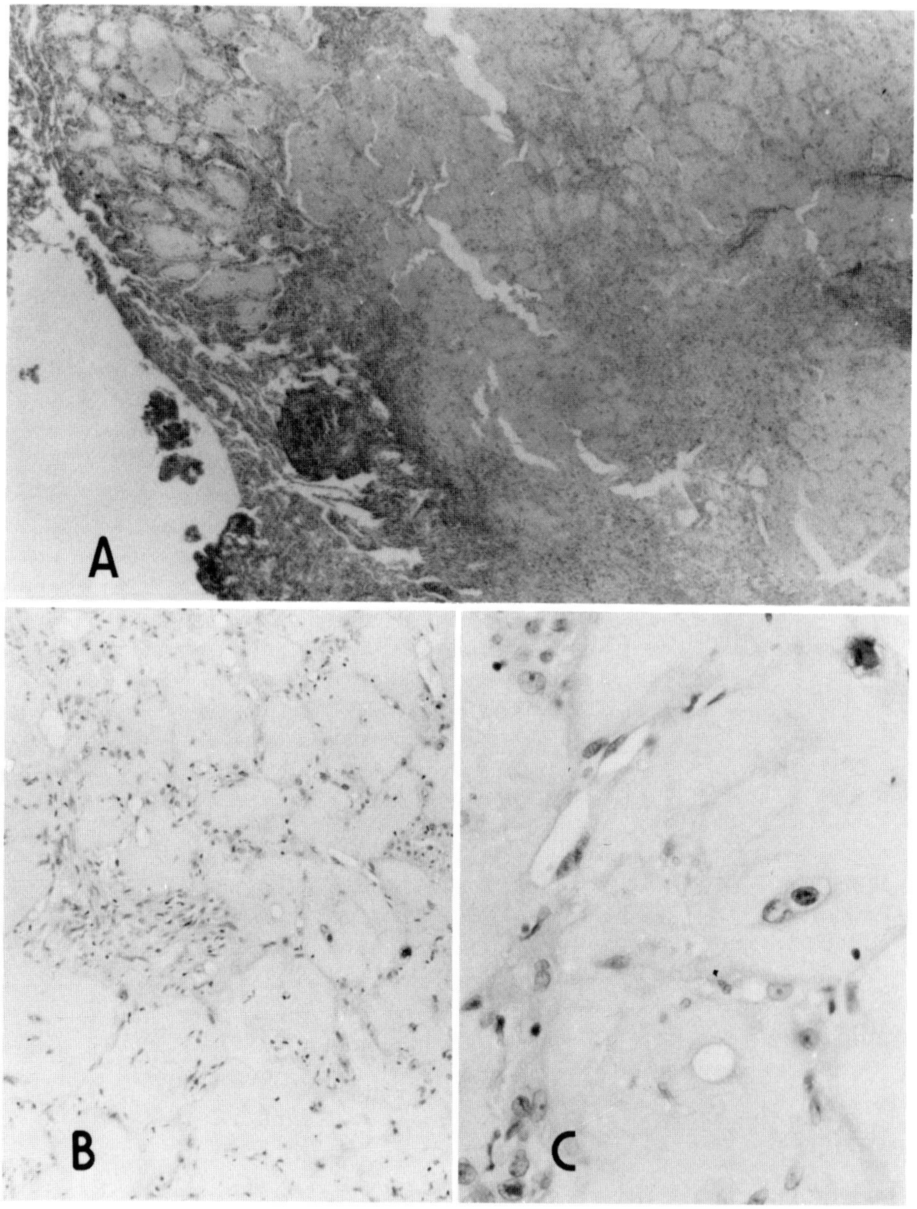

FIG. 7. *A,* A low power view (hematoxylin and eosin, × 40) shows an intravenous bronchiolar alveolar tumor (IVBAT) from its centre (*right*) to its periphery. *B* and *C,* higher power (× 60 and × 150, respectively) views of the center of the lesion show that the alveolar framework is intact and that the spaces are filled with amorphous hyaline material with occasional cells. The alveolar walls are still visible and a lining cell with a hyperchromatic nucleus can be seen. (This case was kindly supplied by Dr. Charles Carrington.)

distinct margins and do not have alveoli as a framework on which to grow. Ossification of the densely sclerotic tissue may occur. In addition, there may be sheets of endothelial cells (Fig. 13). Characteristically, areas of old hemorrhage result in many hemosiderin laden macrophages. Foam cells may be prominent

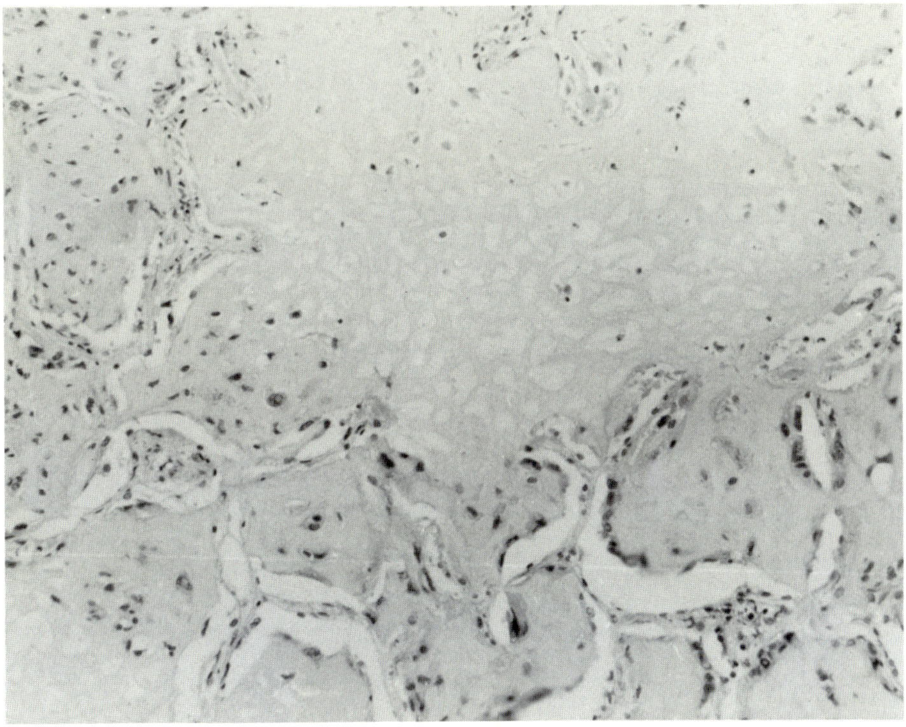

FIG. 8. The airspaces in IVBAT are filled with material that has a distinctly chondroid appearance. Hematoxylin and eosin, × 95.

and give the tumor a yellow color and this feature has also led to the appellation of "histiocytoma". Sclerosing hemangiomas are usually (85%) single and involve all lobes of the lung, although the right middle lobe is involved disproportionately often for its small size. About one-half of the cases occur in the age range of 40–60 years and only about one-sixth of the cases have been found in men.

By contrast, almost 40% of plasma cell granulomas occur in males, and more than one-half of the cases occur under the age of 30 years, and slightly more than one-fourth occur under the age of 10 years. It is thus the common cause of a solitary mass in the lungs of children and adolescents. The lesions are usually single and well encapsulated. Microscopically, these are characteristic and consist of masses of plasma cells with Russell bodies in a stroma of variable nature. It is often whorled and collagenous (Fig. 14), but in some areas may resemble granulation tissue or there may be dense hyalinization with formation of pseudoamyloid. There is an admixture of lymphocytes and mononuclear cells to varying degree. Mononuclear cells may contain fat and hence may be confused with histiocytoma and hence sclerosing hemangioma, but plasma cell granulomas are in reality quite distinct and easily recognizable. These lesions are usually cured by resection and are unconnected with multiple myeloma. Occasional cases extend from the lung to involve the mediastinum.

HEMANGIOPERICYTOMA[8, 72, 73]

With reason, some regard this as a diagnosis of the intellectually destitute. Nonetheless, even when fairly stringent criteria are used, such as have been

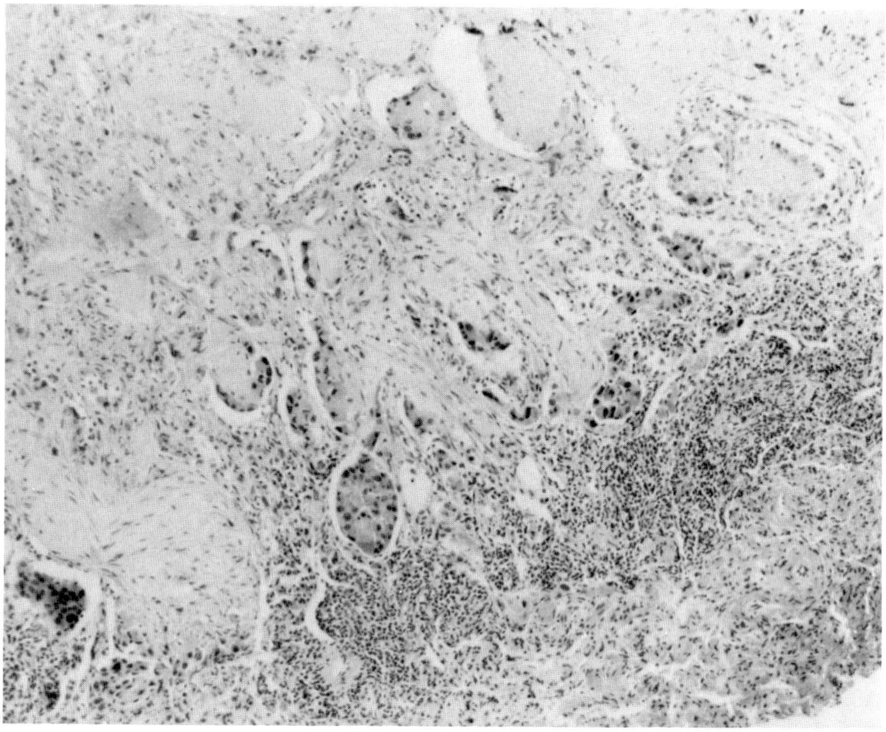

FIG. 9. At the periphery, the lesion is more cellular and cells with atypical nuclei line the air spaces. Mild interstitial inflammation is apparent at the margin of IVBAT and some air spaces are filled with cells whose nuclei are hyperchromatic and atypical. Hematoxylin and eosin, × 95.

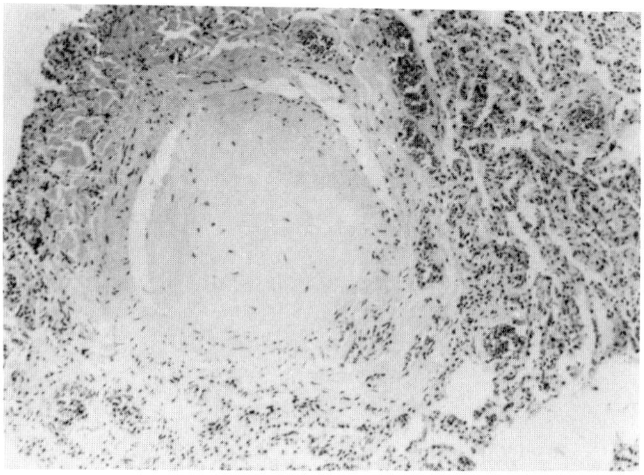

FIG. 10. Intravascular tumor is found separate from the main parenchymal tumor mass in normal lung parenchyma. Hematoxylin and eosin, × 60.

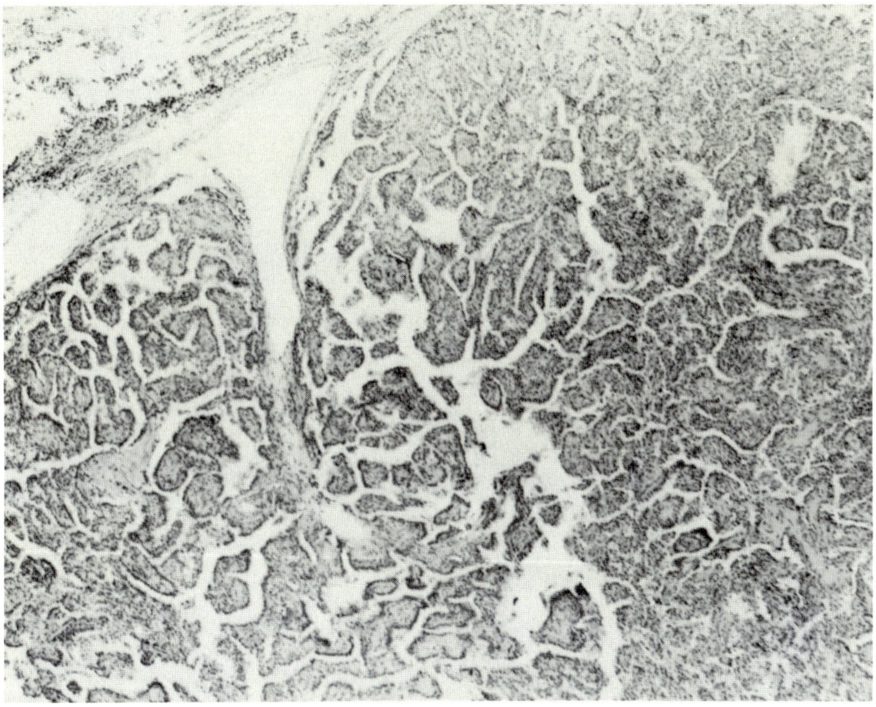

FIG. 11. Papillary appearance of a sclerosing hemangioma of the lung. Hematoxylin and eosin, × 60.

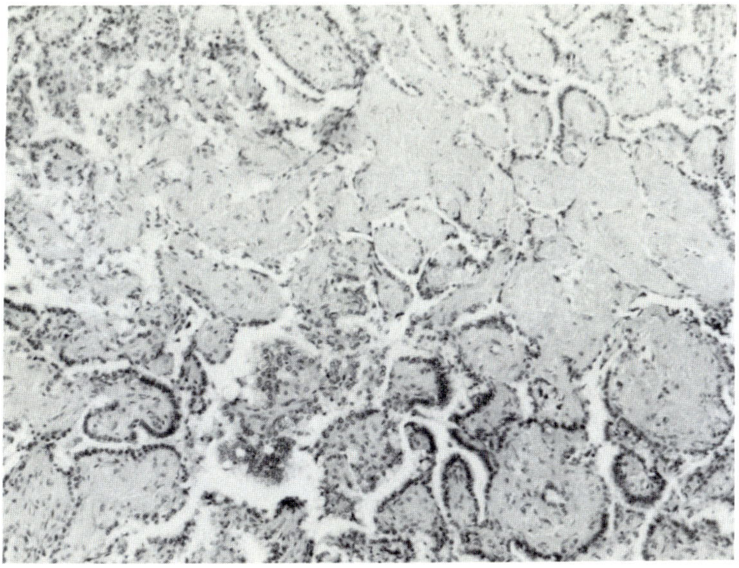

FIG. 12. Sclerosing hemangioma. Dense sclerosis and obliteration of vessels are apparent. Hematoxylin and eosin, × 60.

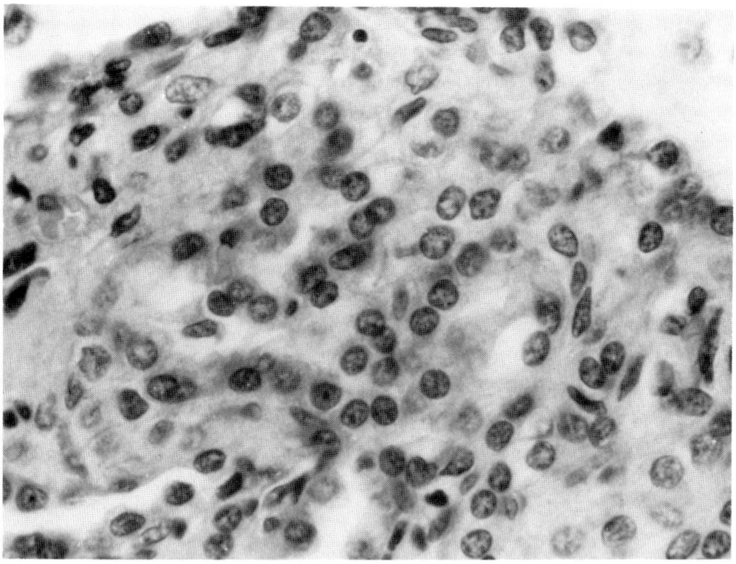

FIG. 13. Sclerosing hemangioma. Sheets of endothelial cells with occasional capillary lumens. Hematoxylin and eosin, × 380.

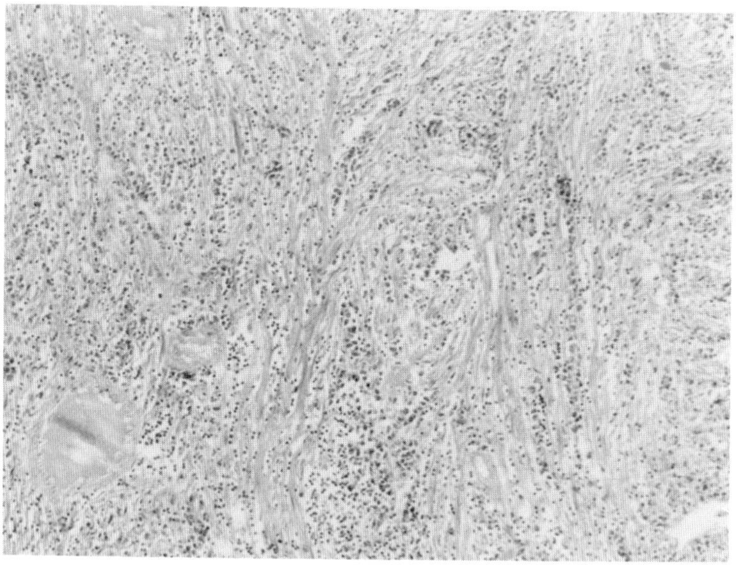

FIG. 14. Plasma cell granuloma shows intertwined bands of collagen with interspersed cells. The inflammatory cells are virtually all plasma cells. Hematoxylin and eosin, × 23.

recently emphasized,[72] hemangiopericytomas occur within and around the lung. Twenty-four cases of hemangiopericytoma of the lung were reported in 1974[73] and these authors found that hemangiopericytoma of the lung occurred predominantly in patients over the age of 40 and were slightly more common in women than men. Mortality from recurrence was higher in men (50%) than women (32%) and large tumors had a worse prognosis than small ones. McMaster *et al.*[72]

emphasized the importance of grading hemangiopericytomas in general into benign, borderline, and malignant and these criteria can be applied usefully to the lung as well. Dr. Liebow has stressed the importance of distinguishing between hemangiopericytoma of the lung and the chest wall. In his experience, hemangiopericytomas of the lung were relatively benign, whereas those of the chest wall occurred at an average age of about 30 years, occurred mostly in women, and behaved in a much more malignant fashion. In their review of the literature, Backwinkel and Diddams[8] grouped hemangiopericytomas of the lung and mediastinum together and noted that their recurrence rate (45.3%) was about that of all hemangiopericytomas (52.2%). However, the recurrence rate of hemangiopericytomas of lung and chest wall in the first year of 36.3% was the highest of any site. The diagram and text in the paper by McMaster *et al.*[72] substantiate Dr. Liebow's view that hemangiopericytomas of the chest wall frequently appear to be malignant on histologic grounds and often lead to the death of the patient.

Chemodectoma-like Lesions of Lung and Bronchial Carcinoids, Tumorlet Type

Familiarly known as Korn-balls (originally described by Korn, Liebow, and others[60]), these lesions have been found in 0.25–0.5% of random autopsies[24, 51, 60] although when careful search is made they have been found in 3–4% of autopsies.[24, 100] Of reported cases 84% have been in females, and they are more commonly found in association with chronic heart or lung disease such as pulmonary thromboembolism, bronchitis and emphysema, mitral stenosis, and chronic heart failure.[24, 100] Usually they are an incidental finding during microscopic examination of the lung, but occasionally they are recognized as 1/2–2 mm yellowish-white nodules scattered through the lung. By light microscopy they resemble chemodectomas very closely. The importance of these lesions and the interest in them arose mainly because the lung *should* have chemoreceptor structures but none has ever been convincingly demonstrated. Thus the occurrence of these tumors was used to support the notion that there is chemoreceptor tissue in the lung, situated somewhere in the pulmonary venous system, since these lesions were characteristically intimately related to small pulmonary veins.[60] Regrettably, recent electron microscopic studies have shown that these lesions bear no resemblance to chemoreceptor tissue.[24, 61] The characteristic secretory granules of chemoreceptor tissue are absent. The tumor cells are large, with long, complex, interwoven cytoplasmic processes as described by Dr. Kuhn in Chapter 1. They have many typical desmosomes, few mitochrondria, and few ribosomes. The associated capillaries are nonfenestrated and basement membrane is lacking. Surprisingly, they resemble meningiomas histologically.[24, 61] The interpretation of these findings is uncertain. Meningiomas occasionally occur outside the cranial cavity.[116] The exact origin of the arachnoidal cell has been ascribed to both mesoderm and neuroectoderm[79] so that these lesions may arise from cells that have aberrantly followed nerves out of the central nervous system.[24, 116] Others have suggested that they may be of mesothelial origin.[27]

These tumors should not be confused with tumorlets of the lung.[115] In common with chemodectoma-like tumors, tumorlets are commonly multiple, occur dominantly in females (78%) and are usually associated with chronic lung disease. The classical association is bronchiectasis[115] where they may be found in up to 20% of cases.[31] On the basis of light microscopy they have long been noted to resemble carcinoids[86, 87] but it is only recently that electron microscopy has disclosed the characteristic neurosecretory granules.[25] These authors also found argyrophilic granules in the cells. Where there is extensive scarring, the origin of these tumors cannot be determined as they tend to exist as multiple discrete foci of tumorlets through the scar. In the absence of extensive scarring, they occur in and near small bronchi and bronchioles. The tumors are unencapsulated and consist of nests and irregular bands of typical carcinoid cells, separated by bands of anastomosing fibrous tissue. Often they appear to invade lymphatic channels although Churg and Warnock suggest that the spaces that they extend into are really distorted air spaces.[25] The question is whether these are neoplasms or a reaction to injury. The benign biological behavior and lack of association with ectopic hormone production suggests that they are really proliferations. However, there are well documented cases with lymph node metastases[25, 47] and peripheral (as opposed to those arising in major bronchi) carcinoids are often associated with tumorlets.[13, 48] Peripheral carcinoids also occur dominantly in females. Churg and Warnock suggest that these lesions should be regarded as small carcinoid neoplasms, differing only in size from peripheral carcinoids. The upper limit of size of tumorlets is undefined; presumably radiographic visualization is an effective operational definition. Churg and Warnock suggest the term "bronchial carcinoid, tumorlet type" for these lesions.[25]

Angiitis in Sarcoidosis and Necrotizing Sarcoid Granulomatosis[68, 95]

Until recently, involvement of the pulmonary vascular system was thought uncommon in sarcoidosis, but has now been found in 42–60% of biopsies from patients with pulmonary sarcoidosis.[95] As a greater proportion of lung tissue is involved by granulomas, vascular involvement becomes progressively more common. The veins are involved in 61% of patients with granulomatous angiitis, both arteries and veins in 31% and arteries alone in only 8%.[95] The granulomas are often in continuity with parenchymal granulomas but may occur separately. Medium to small sized vessels were involved, and all grades of involvement of the wall were noted and focal destruction of elastic tissue of the vascular wall was common. Clinically, these patients had features of sarcoidosis.

Sarcoid-like granulomas occur in about 20% of patients with the limited form of Wegener's granulomatosis[22] but in these cases the lung lesions and the clinical features are usually clearly those of Wegener's granulomatosis. However, a condition may exist which is separate from necrotizing angiitis with sarcoid reaction or sarcoidosis with necrosis or granulomas in vessels. Liebow used the term "necrotizing sarcoid granulomatosis" (NSG) for a group of 11 patients that he studied.[68] None of them had the clinical features of sarcoidosis although two had episodes in the past which could be interpreted as being sarcoid. Clinically, the patients presented with illnesses suggesting infection. Radiologically, there were ill defined pulmonary infiltrates or multiple fine nodules. The disease was unilateral in 2 of the 11 patients. Histologically, there was vascular involvement similar to that described above, but Liebow noted two other forms of vasculitis in addition. One resembled giant cell arteritis except that the outer elastic lamella was involved and lymphocytic and plasma cell infiltrate was seen in the other form. The main distinction morphologically from sarcoid angiitis was the presence of necrosis in the granulomas. As pointed out, the patients were also very distinct clinically. At this point NSG should be regarded as a separate entity and different from sarcoidosis with granulomatous involvement of the vessels.

ACKNOWLEDGEMENT

Drs. David Owen and Ian Robertson read this manuscript and gave much useful advice.

REFERENCES

1. Adamson, I. Y. R., and Bowden, D. H.: The type 2 cell as progenitor of alveolar epithelial regeneration. A cytodynamic study in mice after exposure to oxygen. *Lab. Invest. 30:* 35–42, 1974.
2. Adamson, I. Y. R., and Bowden, D. H.: Derivation of type 1 epithelium from type 2 cells in the developing rat lung. *Lab. Invest. 32:* 736–745, 1975.
3. Adamson, I. Y. R., and Bowden, D. H.: Origin of ciliated alveolar epithelial cells in bleomycin-induced lung injury. *Am. J. Pathol. 87:* 569–580, 1977.
4. Amy, R., Bowes, D., Burri, P. H., and Thurlbeck, W. M.: Postnatal growth of the mouse lung. *J. Anat. 124:* 131–151, 1977.
5. Ashbaugh, D. G., and Petty, T. L.: Sepsis complicating the acute respiratory distress syndrome. *Surg. Gyn. Obstet. 135:* 865–869, 1972.
6. Assimacopoulos, A., Guggenheim, R., and Kapanci, Y.: Changes in alveolar capillary configuration at different levels of lung inflation in the rat. An ultrastructural and morphometric study. *Lab. Invest. 34:* 10–22, 1976.
7. Bachofen, M., and Weibel, E. R.: Basic pattern of tissue repair in human lungs following unspecific injury. *Chest 65:* 14S–19S (suppl. part 1), 1974.
8. Backwinkel, K. D., and Diddams, J. A.: Hemangiopericytoma: Report of a case and comprehensive review of the literature. *Cancer 25:* 896–901, 1970.
9. Bahadori, M., and Liebow, A. A.: Plasma cell granulomas of the lung. *Cancer 31:* 191–208, 1973.
10. Bartlett, D., Jr.: Postnatal growth of the mammalian lung: Influence of excess growth hormone. *Resp. Physiol. 12:* 297–304, 1971.
11. Bates, D. V.: The last link in the chain. *Am. Rev. Resp. Dis. 115:* 139–142, 1977.
12. Bignon, J., Andre-Bougaran, J., and Brouet, G.: Parenchymal, bronchiolar and bronchial measurements in centrilobular emphysema. Relation to weight of right ventricle. *Thorax 25:* 556–567, 1970.
13. Bonikos, D. S., Bensch, K. G., and Jamplis, R. W.: Peripheral pulmonary carcinoid tumors. *Cancer 37:* 1977–1998, 1976.
14. Boyden, E. A. and Tompsett, D. H.: The postnatal growth of the lung in the dog. *Acta. Anat. 47:* 185–215, 1961.
15. Brody, J. S., and Buhain, W. J.: Hormone-induced growth of the adult lung. *Am. J. Physiol. 223:* 1444–1450, 1972.
16. Brody, J. S., and Buhain, W. J.: Hormonal influence on postpneumonectomy lung growth in the rat. *Resp. Physiol. 19:* 344–355, 1973.
17. Brody, J. S., Fisher, A. B., Gocmen, A., DuBois, A. B.: Acromegalic pneumonomegaly: Lung growth in the adult. *J. Clin. Invest. 49:* 1051–1060, 1970.
18. Burnstock, G., and Costa, M.: Inhibitory innervation of the gut. *Gastroenterology 64:* 141–144, 1973.
19. Burri, P. H.: The postnatal growth of the rat lung. III. Morphology. *Anat. Rec. 180:* 77–98, 1974.
20. Burrows, B., Knudson, R. J., and Lebowitz, M. D.: The relationship of childhood respiratory illness to adult obstructive airway disease. *Am. Rev. Resp. Dis. 115:* 751–760, 1977.
21. Butler, C.: Diaphragmatic changes in emphysema. *Am. Rev. Resp. Dis. 114:* 155–159, 1976.
22. Carrington, C. B., and Liebow, A. A.: Limited forms of angiitis and granulomatosis of Wegener's type. *Am. J. Med. 41:* 497–527, 1966.

23. Case records of the Massachusetts General Hospital (Case 22-1977). *N. Engl. J. Med. 296:* 1279–1287, 1977.
24. Churg, A. M., and Warnock, M. L.: So-called "minute pulmonary chemodectoma": A tumor not related to paragangliomas. *Cancer 37:* 1759–1769, 1976.
25. Churg, A. M., and Warnock, M. L.: Pulmonary tumorlet: A form of peripheral carcinoid. *Cancer 37:* 1469–1477, 1976.
26. Ciba Guest Symposium Report: Terminology, definitions, and classification of chronic pulmonary emphysema and related conditions. *Thorax 14:* 286–299, 1959.
27. Costero, I., Barroso-Moguel, R., and Martinez-Palomo, A.: Pleural origin of some of the supposed chemodectoid structures of the lung. *Beitr. Path. Bd. 146:* 351–365, 1972.
28. Cowan, M. J., and Crystal, R. G.: Lung growth after unilateral pneumonectomy: Quantitation of collagen synthesis and content. *Am. Rev. Resp. Dis. 111:* 267–277, 1975.
29. Crema, A., Frigo, G. M., and Lecchini, S.: A pharmacological analysis of the peristaltic reflex in the isolated colon of the guinea-pig or cat. *Br. J. Pharmacol. 39:* 334–345, 1970.
30. Cunningham, E. L., Brody, J. S., and Jain, B. P.: Lung growth induced by hypoxia. *J. Appl. Physiol. 37:* 362–366, 1974.
31. Cunningham, G. J., Nassau, E., and Walter, J. B.: The frequency of tumour-like formations in bronchiectatic lungs. *Thorax 13:* 64–68, 1958.
32. Dail, D., and Liebow, A.: Intravascular bronchioloalveolar tumor. *Am. J. Pathol. 78:* 6a–7a, 1975.
33. D'Angelo, E.: Local alveolar size and transpulmonary pressure *in situ* and in isolated lungs. *Resp. Physiol. 14:* 251–266, 1972.
34. DePierre, A., Bignon, J., Lebeau, A., and Brouet, G.: Quantitative study of parenchyma and small conductive airways in chronic nonspecific lung disease. Use of histologic stereology and bronchial casts. *Chest 62:* 699–708, 1972.
35. Dunnill, M. S.: Effect of lung inflation on alveolar surface area in the dog. *Nature 214:* 1013–1014, 1967.
36. Evans, M. J., Cabral, L. J., Stephens, R. J., and Freeman, G.: Renewal of alveolar epithelium in the rat following exposure to NO_2. *Am. J. Pathol. 70:* 175–198, 1973.
37. Evans, M. J., Johnson, L. V., Stephens, R. J., and Freeman, G.: Renewal of the terminal bronchiolar epithelium in the rat following exposure to NO_2 and O_3. *Lab. Invest. 35:* 246–257, 1976.
38. Fletcher, Charles; Peto, Richard; Tinker, Cecily; and Speizer, Frank E.: *The Natural History of Chronic Bronchitis and Emphysema.* Oxford University Press, New York, Toronto, 1976.
39. Fromme, H.: Systematische untersuchungen iiber die gewichtsverhaltnisse des zwerchfells. *Virchows Archiv. f. pathol. anat. 221:* 117–155, 1916.
40. Ferguson, C. C., and Richardson, J. B.: A simple technique for the utilization of postmortem tracheal and bronchial tissues for ultrastructural studies. *Human Pathol.* (in press).
41. Furness, J. B., and Costa, M.: The nervous release and the action of substances which affect intestinal muscle through neither adrenoreceptors or cholinoreceptors. Recent developments in vertebrate smooth muscle. *Phil. Trans. R. Soc. London, Ser. B. 265:* 123–133, 1973.
42. Gil, J., and Weibel, E. R.: Extracellular lining of bronchioles after perfusion-fixation of rat lungs for electron microscopy. *Anat. Rec. 169:* 185–200, 1971.
43. Gil, J., and Weibel, E. R.: Morphological study of pressure-volume hysteresis in rat lungs fixed by vascular perfusion. *Resp. Physiol. 15:* 190–213, 1972.
44. Glazier, J. B., Hughes, J. M. B., Maloney, J. E., and West, J. B.: Vertical gradient of alveolar size in lungs of dogs frozen intact. *J. Appl. Physiol. 23:* 694–705, 1967.
45. Glenn, William W. L., Liebow, Averill A., Lindskog, Gustaf, E.: *Thoracic and Cardiovascular Surgery with Related Pathology,* 3rd ed. New York, Appleton-Century-Crofts, 1975.
46. Gross, P., Babyak, M. A., Tolker, E., and Kashak, M.: Enzymatically produced pulmonary emphysema: A preliminary report. *J. Occup. Med. 6:* 481–484, 1964.
47. Hausman, D. H., and Weimann, R. B.: Pulmonary tumorlet with hilar lymph node metastasis. Report of a case. *Cancer 20:* 1515–1519, 1967.
48. Heimburger, I. L., Kilman, J. W., and Battersby, J. S.: Peripheral bronchial adenomas. *J. Thorac. Cardiovasc. Surg. 52:* 542–549, 1966.
49. Heppleston, A. G.: The pathogenesis of simple pneumokoniosis in coal workers. *J. Pathol. Bacteriol. 67:* 51–63, 1954.

50. Hill, J. D., Ratliff, J. L., Parrott, J. C. W., Lamy, M., Fallat, R. J., Koeniger, E., Yaeger, E. M., and Whitmer, G.: Pulmonary pathology in acute respiratory insufficiency: Lung biopsy as a diagnostic tool. *J. Thorac. Cardiovasc. Surg. 71:* 64–71, 1976.
51. Ichinose, H., Hewitt, R. L., and Drapanas, T.: Minute pulmonary chemodectoma. *Cancer 28:* 692–700, 1971.
52. Ishikawa, S., and Hayes, J. A.: Functional morphometry of the diaphragm in patients with chronic obstructive lung disease. *Am. Rev. Resp. Dis. 108:* 135–138, 1973.
53. Jain, B. P., Brody, J. S., and Fisher, A. B.: The small lung of hypopituitarism. *Am. Rev. Resp. Dis. 108:* 49–55, 1973.
54. Johanson, W. G. Jr., and Pierce, A. K.: Effects of elastase, collagenase, and papain on structure and function of rat lungs in vitro. *J. Clin. Invest. 51:* 288–293, 1972.
55. Johanson, W. G. Jr., Pierce, A. K., and Reynolds, R. C.: The evolution of papain emphysema in the rat. *J. Lab. Clin. Med. 78:* 599–607, 1971.
56. Johanson, W. G., Pierce, A. K., and Southern, P. M.: Comparison of elastase, collagenase, and papain on lung structure and function. *Amer. Rev. Resp. Dis. 103:* 908, 1971, (abstr.).
57. Kapanci, Y., Weibel, E. R., Kaplan, H. P., and Robinson, F. R.: Pathogenesis and reversibility of the pulmonary lesions of oxygen toxicity in monkeys. II. Ultrastructural and morphometric studies. *Lab. Invest. 20:* 101–118, 1969.
58. Katzenstein, A. L. A., Bloor, C. M., and Liebow, A. A.: Diffuse alveolar damage—The role of oxygen, shock, and related factors. A review. *Am. J. Pathol. 85:* 210–228, 1976.
59. Klingele, T. G., and Staub, N. C.: Alveolar shape changes with volume in isolated, air-filled lobes of cat lung. *J. Appl. Physiol. 28:* 411–414, 1970.
60. Korn, D., Bensch, K., Liebow, A. A., and Castleman, B.: Multiple minute pulmonary tumors resembling chemodectomas. *Am. J. Pathol. 37:* 641–672, 1960.
61. Kuhn, C. III, and Askin, F.: The fine structure of so-called minute pulmonary chemodectomas. *Human Pathol. 6:* 681–691, 1975.
62. Kuhn, C. III, and Tavassoli, F.: The scanning electron microscopy of elastase-induced emphysema: A comparison with emphysema in man. *Lab. Invest. 34:* 2–9, 1976.
63. Lakshminarayan, S., Stanford, R. E., and Petty, T. L.: Prognosis after recovery from adult respiratory distress syndrome. *Am. Rev. Resp. Dis. 113:* 7–16, 1976.
64. Langston, C., Sachdeva, P., Cowan, M. J., Haines, J., Crystal, R. G., and Thurlbeck, W. M.: Alveolar multiplication in the contralateral lung after unilateral pneumonectomy in the rabbit. *Am. Rev. Resp. Dis. 115:* 7–13, 1977.
65. Lamy, M., Fallat, R. J., Koeniger, E., Dietrich, H-P., Ratliff, J. L., Eberhart, R. C., Tucker, H. J., and Hill, J. D.: Pathologic features and mechanisms of hypoxemia in adult respiratory distress syndrome. *Am. Rev. Resp. Dis. 114:* 267–284, 1976.
66. Lapp, N. L., Hankinson, J. L., Burgess, D. B., and O'Brien, R.: Changes in ventilatory function in coal miners after a work shift. *Arch. Environ. Health 24:* 204–208, 1972.
67. Lapp, N. L., and Seaton, A.: Lung mechanics in coal workers' pneumoconiosis. *Ann. N. Y. Acad. Sci. 200:* 433–454, 1972.
68. Liebow, A. A.: The J. Burns Amberson Lecture—Pulmonary Angiitis and Granulomatosis. *Am. Rev. Resp. Dis. 108:* 1–18, 1973.
69. Luchtel, D. L.: Ultrastructural observations on the mucous layer in pulmonary airways. *J. Cell Biol. 70:* 350a, 1976, (abstr.).
70. Macklin, C. C.: The alveoli of the mammalian lung. An anatomical study with clinical correlations. *Proc. Inst. Med. Chic. 18:* 78–95, 1950.
71. Macklem, P. T., Proctor, D. F., and Hogg, J. C.: The stability of peripheral airways. *Resp. Physiol. 8:* 191–203, 1970.
72. McMaster, M. J., Soule, E. H., and Ivins, J. C.: Hemangiopericytoma: A clinicopathologic study and long-term followup of 60 patients. *Cancer 36:* 2232–2244, 1975.
73. Meade, J. B., Whitwell, F., Bickford, B. J., and Waddington, J. K. B.: Primary haemangiopericytoma of lung. *Thorax 29:* 1–15, 1974.
74. Mitchell, R. S., Stanford, R. E., Johnson, J. M., Silvers, G. W., Dart, G., and George, M. S.: The morphologic features of the bronchi, bronchioles and alveoli in chronic airway obstruction: A clinicopathologic study. *Am. Rev. Resp. Dis. 114:* 137–145, 1976.
75. Morgan, W. K. C., and Lapp, N. L.: Respiratory disease in coal miners. In *Lung disease—State*

of the Art, 1975-76, edited by Murray, J. F., pp. 25-53. New York, American Lung Association, 1977.

76. Morgan, W. K. C., and Seaton, A.: *Occupational Lung Diseases.* Philadelphia, W. B. Saunders Co., 1975.
77. Morgan, W. K. C., Seaton, A., Burgess, D. B., Lapp, N. L., and Reger, R.: Lung volumes in working coal miners. *Ann. N. Y. Acad. Sci. 200:* 478–493, 1972.
78. Murray, J. F.: The adult respiratory distress syndrome (May it rest in peace). *Am. Rev. Resp. Dis. 111:* 716–718, 1975.
79. Napolitano, L., Kyle, R., and Fisher, E. R.: Ultrastructure of meningiomas and the derivation and nature of their cellular components. *Cancer 17:* 233–241, 1964.
80. Nash, G., Blennerhassett, J. B., and Pontoppidan, H.: Pulmonary lesions associated with oxygen therapy and artificial ventilation. *N. Engl. J. Med. 276:* 368–374, 1967.
81. Nash, G., Foley, F. D., and Langlinais, P. C.: Pulmonary interstitial edema and hyaline membranes in adult burn patients: Electron microscopic observations. *Human Pathol. 5:* 149–160, 1974.
82. Oliver, R. E., Davis, B., Marin, M. G., and Nadel, J. A.: Active transport of Na^+ and Cl^- across the canine tracheal epithelium in vitro. *Am. Rev. Resp. Dis. 112:* 811–815, 1975.
83. Orrell, S. R.: Lung pathology in respiratory distress following shock in the adult. *Arch. Path. Microbiol. Scand. (Section A) 79:* 65–76, 1971.
84. Ortmeyer, C. E., Baier, E. J., and Crawford, G. M.: Life expectancy of Pennsylvania coal miners compensated for disability as affected by pneumoconiosis and ventilatory impairment. *Arch. Environ. Health 27:* 227-230, 1973.
85. Ortmeyer, C. E., Costello, J., Morgan, W. K. C., Swecker, S., and Peterson, M.: The mortality of Appalachian coal miners, 1963-1971. *Arch. Environ. Health 29:* 67–72, 1974.
86. Prior, J. T.: Minute peripheral pulmonary tumors. Observations on their histogenesis. *Am. J. Pathol. 29:* 703–719, 1953.
87. Prior, J. T., and Jones, D. B.: Minute peripheral pulmonary tumors. A study of eight cases. *J. Thorac. Surg. 23:* 224–236, 1952.
88. Puig, M. M., Gascon, P., Craviso, G. L., Musacchio, J. M.: Endogenous opiate receptor ligand: Electrically induced release in the guinea pig ileum. *Science 195:* 419–420, 1977.
89. Richardson, J.: Pharmacologic studies of Hirschsprung's disease on a murine model. *J. Ped. Surg. 10:* 875–884, 1975.
90. Richardson, J., and Béland, J.: Nonadrenergic inhibitory nervous system in human airways. *J. Appl. Physiol. 41:* 764–771, 1976.
91. Richardson, J. B., and Bouchard, T.: Demonstration of a nonadrenergic inhibitory nervous system in the trachea of the guinea pig. *J. Allergy Clin. Immunol. 56:* 473–480, 1975.
92. Rhodin, J., and Dalhamn, T.: Electron microscopy of the tracheal ciliated mucosa in the rat. *Z. Zellforsch. Mikrosko. Anat. 44:* 345–412, 1956.
93. Rogan, J. M., Attfield, M. D., Jacobsen, M., Rae, S., Walker, D. D., and Walton, W. H.: Role of dust in the working environment in development of chronic bronchitis in British coal miners. *Br. J. Ind. Med. 30:* 217–226, 1973.
94. Rogan, J. M., Rae, S., and Walton, W. H.: *Inhaled Particles and Vapours II,* edited by Davies, C. N., p. 493. Oxford, Pergamon Press, 1967.
95. Rosen, Y., Moon, S., Huang, C., Gourin, A., and Lyons, H. A.: Granulomatous pulmonary angiitis in sarcoidosis. *Arch. Pathol. Lab. Med. 101:* 170–174, 1977.
96. Rossiter, C. E.: Relations of lung dust content to radiological changes in coal workers. *Ann. N.Y. Acad. Sci. 200:* 465–477, 1972.
97. Ryder, R., Lyons, J. P., Campbell, H., and Gough, J.: Emphysema in coal workers' pneumoconiosis. *Br. Med. J. 3:* 481–487, 1970.
98. Scott, K. W. M., and Hoy, J.: The cross sectional area of diaphragmatic muscle fibres in emphysema, measured by an automated image analysis system. *J. Pathol. 120:* 121–128, 1976.
99. Short, R. H. D.: Alveolar epithelium in relation to growth of the lung. *Phil. Trans. R. Soc. 235:* 35–86, 1951.
100. Spain, D. M.: Intrapulmonary chemodectomas in subjects with organizing pulmonary thromboemboli. *Am. Rev. Resp. Dis. 96:* 1158–1164, 1967.
101. Steele, R. H., and Heard, B. E.: The size of the diaphragm in chronic bronchitis. *Thorax 28:* 55–60, 1973.

102. Sturgess, J. M.: The mucous lining of major bronchi in the rabbit lung. *Am. Rev. Resp. Dis. 115:* 819–827, 1977.
103. Teplitz, C.: The core pathobiology and integrated medical science of adult acute respiratory insufficiency. *Surg. Clin. N. Am. 56:* 1091–1133, 1976.
104. Thurlbeck, W. M.: The structure of the lungs. MTP International Review of Science, *Respiratory Physiology,* Physiology Series One, Vol. 2, edited by Widdicombe, J. G., consultant editor, Guyton, A. C., pp. 1–30. Baltimore, University Park Press, 1974.
105. Thurlbeck, W. M.: Lung growth and alveolar multiplication. In *Pathobiology Annual, 1975,* edited by Ioachim, H. L., pp. 1–34. New York, Appleton-Century-Crofts, 1975.
106. Thurlbeck, W. M.: Postnatal growth and development of the lung. *Am. Rev. Resp. Dis. 111:* 803–844, 1975.
107. Thurlbeck, W. M.: *Chronic airflow obstruction in lung disease.* Philadelphia, W. B. Saunders Co., 1976.
108. Thurlbeck, W. M.: Structure of the lungs. In *Respiratory Physiology II, International Review of Physiology,* Vol. 14, edited by Widdicombe, J. G., series editor, Guyton, A. C., pp. 1–36. Baltimore, University Park Press, 1977.
109. Thurlbeck, W. M.: Aspects of chronic airflow obstruction. *Chest 72:* 341–349, 1977.
110. Van As, A.: Pulmonary airway clearance mechanisms: A reappraisal. *Am. Rev. Resp. Dis. 115:* 721–726, 1977.
111. Van As, A., and Webster, I.: The organization of ciliary activity and mucus transport in pulmonary airways. *S. Afr. Med. J. 46:* 347–350, 1972.
112. Van As, A., and Webster, I.: The morphology of mucus in mammalian airways. *Environ. Res. 7:* 1, 1974.
113. Wanner, A.: State of the Art. Clinical aspects of mucociliary transport. *Am. Rev. Resp. Dis. 116:* 73–125, 1977.
114. Whimster, W. F.: The microanatomy of the alveolar duct system. *Thorax 25:* 141–149, 1970.
115. Whitwell, F.: Tumourlets of the lung. *J. Pathol. Bacteriol. 70:* 529–541, 1955.
116. Wolff, M., and Rankow, R. M.: Meningioma of the parotid gland: An insight into the pathogenesis of extracranial meningiomas. *Human Pathol. 2:* 453–459, 1971.
117. Wyatt, J. P., Fischer, V. W., and Sweet, H. C.: The pathomorphology of the emphysema complex. *Am. Rev. Resp. Dis. 89:* 533–560, 1964 (Part I) and *Am. Rev. Resp. Dis. 89:* 721–735, 1964 (Part II).
118. Yoneda, K.: Mucous blanket of rat bronchus. An ultrastructural study. *Am. Rev. Resp. Dis. 114:* 837–842, 1976.

Index

Page references in *italic* type refer to illustrations.